Bioengineering Design Methodology

Carl-Fredrik Mandenius

Bioengineering Design Methodology

A Tutorial Handbook for Training Engineers in Industrial Design Practice

Springer

Carl-Fredrik Mandenius
Department of Physics, Chemistry and Biology
Linköping University
Linköping, Sweden

ISBN 978-3-032-33939-3 ISBN 978-3-032-33940-9 (eBook)
https://doi.org/10.1007/978-3-032-33940-9

This Springer imprint is published by the registered company Springer Nature Switzerland AG
The registered company address is: Gewerbestrasse 11, 6330 Cham, Switzerland

Preface

The content of this book has grown out of many years of practice in teaching and training master's students in bioengineering and engineering biology, with the realistic design of industrial products as the goal. The book is intended as guidance for advanced students as well as for tutors in bioengineering design. However, it is not a traditional textbook for students, although substantial parts of it will help readers better understand the context of engineering design related to biology. Neither are the materials intended as a ready-made curriculum for training; rather, they offer supportive guidance to develop such training. The design cases provided should primarily be used as inspiration to form cases tailored to your own curriculum.

The training methods described have been conceived and carried out in close collaboration with bioindustry professionals who possess vast experience in pharmaceutical companies, startup biotechnology development firms, food and agricultural biotechnology companies, and biotech consultancy organizations. This expertise has been combined with numerous interactions with colleagues who have profound academic and educational backgrounds related to bioengineering.

The outlined training approaches have been successfully applied in master's-level design engineering courses for over 20 years, guiding more than one thousand engineering students.

To maximize the value of this book, the first four chapters should be studied alongside the practical design cases in the final chapter. The following reading cues are suggested to help navigate the content:

- *Chapter* 1 details the purpose of the book and connects it to perspectives on bioengineering within a training context. It defines the vast array of "bioproducts" as goods or services that require engineering principles to be realized.
- *Chapter* 2 outlines the fundamental sciences underpinning bioengineering design. Rather than an exhaustive compilation, it serves as a starting point and a primary threshold for evaluating the scientific realism of new product ideas.
- *Chapter* 3 introduces the most pertinent methodologies for designing novel bioproduct ideas, demonstrating how to refine these concepts into feasible,

sustainable products for industrial production. Two primary avenues guide the design process: applying conceptual thinking and establishing rigorous production-economic evaluation over the formative stages of an idea.

- *Chapter* 4 provides practical advice for tutors and program managers organizing bioengineering design training. Consequently, it is particularly useful for preparing laboratory and design courses.

Ultimately, the content of this book provides a framework for training bioengineers to design industrial products. The chapters should be read with this overarching goal in mind.

I am deeply indebted to Drs. Mats Björkman, Gunnar Hörnsten, and Robert Gustavsson-Lindberg for our countless discussions on the principles of design engineering, industrial applications, and how engineering students perceive project design work and training.

I also highly appreciate the valuable inputs and ideas for design cases provided by my industrially and clinically experienced colleagues and peers. I would especially like to thank Drs. Johan Hyllner, Martin Karlsson, Daniel Aili, Bertil Kågedal, Lasse Jensen, Björn Ekberg, Pierfrancesco Pagella, Jan-Peter Axelsson, Sten Ohlson, and Anders Skoglund.

Special thanks go to Dr. Merry Stuber and her coworkers at Springer Nature Publishing Company.

Needless to say, any shortcomings in this book are entirely my own.

Linköping, Sweden
August 2026

Carl-Fredrik Mandenius

Competing Interests The author has no competing interests to declare that are relevant to the content of this manuscript.

Contents

1 The Purpose of Bioengineering Design Training 1
1.1 Objectives of Bioengineering Design Training 1
1.2 Scope and Diversity of Bioengineered Products 3
1.3 Functionalities of Bioproducts 6
1.4 The Industrial Perspective in the Training 7
1.5 Critical Success Factors in Bioengineering Design 8
References 9

2 Fundamentals in Bioengineering Design 13
2.1 Bridging Fundamental Science and Bioproduct Design 13
2.2 Integrating Fundamental Science with Biological Systems 14
2.3 Adapting General Engineering Design Principles to Bioproduct Design 16
2.4 Managing Kinetic and Operational Constraints in Biodesign 18
2.5 Societal Expectations on Bioengineering Design 22
2.6 Evaluating Economic Conditions for Bioproduct Design 23
2.7 Distinctive Characteristics of Bioengineering Design 27
References 31

3 Methodology for Bioengineering Design 35
3.1 Design Methodologies: Their Purpose and Utility 35
3.2 Implementing Method Frameworks in Bioengineering Design 37
3.3 Design Mission and User Requirements 40
3.4 Translating the Design Mission into Functionality 42
3.5 Conceptualization of the Design 45
3.6 Improving Performance of Biological Systems 48
3.7 Scaling Up Production 50
3.8 Evaluating the Economics of Design Alternatives 53

3.9 Optimizing Design Solutions 55
3.9.1 Optimizing Designs Using Design of Experiments (DoE) 56
3.9.2 Applying Mechanistic Modelling to Bioproduct Design 58
3.9.3 Exploring Other Optimization Frameworks 61
3.10 Validating and Testing Final Designs 62
3.11 Utilizing Digital Design Environments 63
References 67

4 Bioengineering Design Training 71
4.1 Training in Designing Bioproducts and Bioproduction Systems 71
4.2 Objectives of the Design Training 73
4.3 Structure of the Design Training 74
4.3.1 The Training Scenario 74
4.3.2 The Team of Trainees 76
4.3.3 The Design Assignment to the Team 78
4.3.4 The Role of the Academic Tutorial Management 79
4.3.5 The Role of the Industrial Experts 79
4.4 Actions During the Training 80
4.4.1 Conceptualization of the Design Assignment 84
4.4.2 Actions for Detailing Design Alternatives 86
4.4.3 Evaluating Intellectual Property Opportunities of the Design 87
4.4.4 Evaluating the Production Economics of Designs 88
4.4.5 Actions for Optimization of the Design 91
4.4.6 Using SWOT Analysis to Evaluate the Potential of the Design Alternatives 91
4.4.7 Reporting Design Assignments 92
4.5 Other Aspects of the Design Training 92
4.5.1 Managing Project Timescales in Training 92
4.5.2 Adaptation to Vocational Training 94
4.6 Evaluation of the Training Performance 95
4.6.1 Evaluation of the Trainees' General Performance 95
4.6.2 Evaluation of the Trainees' Performance in Applying Biological Aspects 97
4.6.3 Evaluation of the Training Program 97
References 98

5 Design Cases for Training 101
5.1 Applying Design Training in Design Cases 101
5.2 Selection of Cases 102
5.3 The Design Cases and Their Training Purpose 103

6 Case 1: Cost-Efficient Production of a Human Growth Hormone Biosimilar . . . 107
6.1 Assignment: Background, Description, and Objectives . . . 107
6.2 Training Scenario for the Assignment . . . 108
6.3 A Recommended Design Approach for the Assignment . . . 109
6.3.1 Structuring the Assignment and Requirements . . . 109
6.3.2 Conceptualization of the Assignment . . . 111
6.3.3 Detailed Design of the Selected Configurations . . . 114
6.3.4 Production Economics of the Selected Designs . . . 118
6.3.5 Patents or Patent Applications that Could Endanger the Designs . . . 121
6.3.6 Optimization of Growth Hormone Biosimilar Production . . . 123
6.3.7 SWOT Analysis of the Selected Designs . . . 129
6.4 Conclusive Suggestions for *Biopharma* . . . 130
6.5 Tutorial Perspectives on the Assignment . . . 131
References . . . 132

7 Case 2: Design of an Integrated Bioprocess for a Therapeutic Monoclonal Antibody . . . 135
7.1 Assignment: Background, Description, and Objectives . . . 135
7.2 Training Scenario of the Assignment . . . 137
7.3 A Recommended Design Approach . . . 138
7.3.1 Structuring the Assignment and Establishing User Requirements . . . 138
7.3.2 Conceptualization of the Assignment . . . 139
7.3.3 Detailed Design of the Selected Conceptual Configurations . . . 143
7.3.4 Production Economic Evaluation for Three Detailed Designs . . . 146
7.3.5 Optimization of the Selected Recycled Designs . . . 152
7.4 Conclusive Suggestions for *Biotherapeutica* . . . 157
7.5 Tutorial Perspectives on the Assignment . . . 158
References . . . 159

8 Case 3: Using a Xenograft Zebrafish Model for Evaluation of Oncogenic Drug Candidates . . . 163
8.1 Assignment: Background, Description, and Objectives . . . 163
8.2 Training Scenario for the Assignment . . . 165
8.3 A Recommended Design Approach . . . 165
8.3.1 Structuring the Assignment and Establishing User Requirements . . . 165
8.3.2 Conceptualization of the Assignment . . . 168
8.3.3 Detailed Design of Selected Conceptual Configurations . . . 171

8.3.4 Evaluation of Economics of the Testing Service 173
8.3.5 Optimization of the Design of the Testing Service 176
8.3.6 SWOT Analysis for the Scaled-Up Testing Alternatives 180
8.4 Conclusive Suggestions for *Drug Technologies* 181
8.5 Tutorial Perspectives on the Assignment 182
References 182

9 Case 4: Microfluidic Chip for Pharmacological Studies of Organotypic Teeth and Liver Cells 185
9.1 Assignment: Background, Description, and Objectives 185
9.2 Training Scenario for the Assignment 187
9.3 A Recommended Design Approach 188
9.3.1 Structuring the Assignment and User Requirements . . . 188
9.3.2 Conceptualization of the Assignment 191
9.3.3 Detailed Designs of Selected Configurations 195
9.3.4 Production Economics for the Two Selected Design Alternatives 197
9.3.5 Status of Intellectual Property Rights for Microphysiological Systems 200
9.3.6 Optimization of the Microphysiological System Alternatives 203
9.3.7 SWOT Analysis of the In-House and Subcontracted Alternatives 208
9.4 Conclusive Suggestions for *Biochip Engineering* 210
9.5 Tutorial Perspectives on the Assignment 211
References 212

10 Case 5: Production of Ventricular Progenitors from Induced Pluripotent Stem Cells 215
10.1 Assignment: Background, Description, and Objectives 215
10.2 Training Scenario for the Assignment 217
10.3 A Recommended Design Approach 218
10.3.1 Structuring the Assignment and Establishing User Requirements 218
10.3.2 Conceptualization of the Assignment 221
10.3.3 Detailed Designs of Selected Alternatives 223
10.3.4 Production Economic Evaluation of the Detailed Designs 225
10.3.5 Optimization of Manual or Robotized Production 228
10.4 Conclusive Suggestions for *Global Pharma* 233
10.5 Tutorial Perspectives on the Assignment 234
References 235

11 Case 6: Cultured Meat as Novel Food Supply 237
11.1 Assignment: Background, Description, and Objectives 237
11.2 Training Scenario for the Assignment 239
11.3 A Recommended Design Approach 240
11.3.1 Structuring the Assignment and Establishing User Requirements 240
11.3.2 Conceptualization of the Assignment 242
11.3.3 Detailed Design of Selected Conceptual Configurations 246
11.3.4 Economic Evaluation of the Detailed Designs 246
11.3.5 Optimization of the Design Alternatives 250
11.4 Conclusive Suggestions for *Food Bioentrepreneurs* 259
11.5 Tutorial Perspectives on the Assignment 259
References 260

12 Case 7: Design of a Point-of-Care Diagnostic Device for SARS-CoV-2 Infections 263
12.1 Assignment: Background, Description, and Objectives 263
12.2 Training Scenario of the Assignment 264
12.3 A Recommended Design Approach 265
12.4 Conclusive Suggestions for *Diagnostic Incorporated* 282
12.5 Tutorial Perspectives on the Assignment 283
References 284

13 Case 8: A Bedside Sensor for Blood Glucose Testing of Diabetic Patients 287
13.1 Assignment: Background, Description, and Objectives 287
13.2 Training Scenario of the Assignment 288
13.3 A Recommended Design Approach 289
13.4 Conclusive Suggestions for *Medtech Sensorics* 304
13.5 Tutorial Perspectives on the Assignment 305
References 306

14 Case 9: Design of a Novel Hemodialysis System 309
14.1 Assignment: Background, Description, and Objectives 309
14.2 Training Scenario of the Assignment 311
14.3 A Recommended Design Approach 312
14.4 Conclusive Suggestions for *Dialytica* 329
14.5 Tutorial Perspectives on the Assignment 330
References 332

Index 335

Chapter 1
The Purpose of Bioengineering Design Training

The purpose and intent of the book are outlined, providing an overall framework for the subsequent chapters and practical design cases. The scope and definitions applied to bioengineering design are explained in relation to the training of bioengineers. The primary focus is to deliver an industrially relevant training perspective for the design of novel bioproducts, emphasizing engineering methodology and production economy.

1.1 Objectives of Bioengineering Design Training

Design and engineering are tightly connected concepts for engineers across all disciplines (Pahl et al. 2007; Ulrich et al. 2019). However, for biological and life science engineers—or bioengineers, for short—the concept of design can seem broad and ambiguous when viewed from a classical engineering perspective. From an educational viewpoint, bioengineering progresses from basic training to vocational and professional practice. As in other fields of engineering, bioengineering embraces design as a central subject in engineering school curricula.

From the outset, this training must encompass industrial applications, aiming to leverage engineering knowledge and skills to develop products that address societal needs and expectations.

The main purpose of this guidance handbook is to position bioengineering from a perspective of design of bioproducts. Without doubt, much of the fundamental design thinking can be adopted from other engineering fields such as mechanics, electronics, and chemical engineering (Dym et al. 2005; Doran 2013). Established methodologies in teaching and training design can be reused in bioengineering design. This encompasses such general concepts as functionality, transformability, optimization, sustainability, and economy of products and their production (Pahl et al. 2007; Doulougeri et al. 2024).

C.-F. Mandenius, *Bioengineering Design Methodology*,
https://doi.org/10.1007/978-3-032-33940-9_1

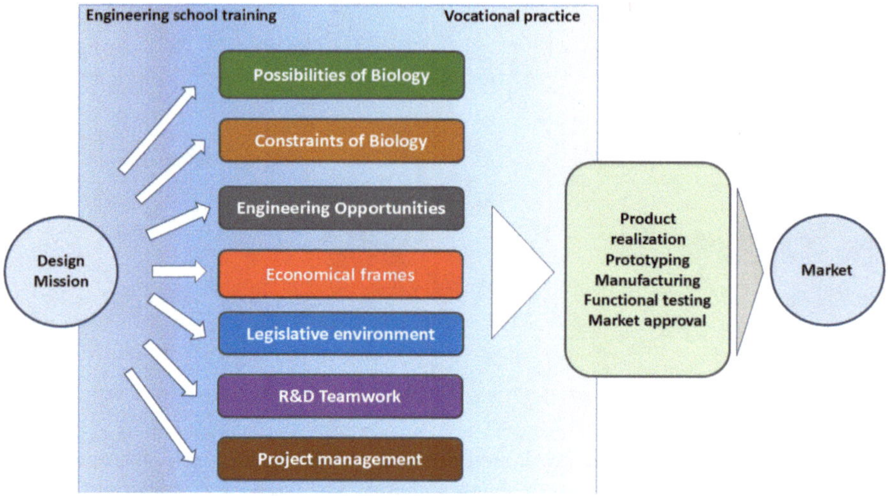

Fig. 1.1 Illustration of the purpose of this guidance: to train engineers in the multifaceted craft of designing products and systems with biology as the driving force, and where many interconnected factors shape the path from the initial design mission to a successful market entry

However, the real challenge in bioengineering design is to creatively explore and exploit the inherent strengths and opportunities of biology and, at the same time, not neglect their weaknesses and limitations.

The bioengineering design training must be able to harness new biological products for the societal demands of economy, market, legislation, and changing conditions and currents. The training must also include project management and team building for running efficient design work. And this know-how must be sustainable over time and a forthcoming vocational life.

The interconnectivity with these matters stems from early well-structured engineering school training, furthered by continuing vocational and professional training and practical experiences. To be successful in bioproduct design, the training needs to cover a variety of skills and insights into the varying demands from the users, industry, and legislative society (Fig. 1.1).

Bioengineering textbooks have thoroughly and clearly explained the fundamentals of biology with technological perspectives (Baily and Ollis 1986; Doran 2013; Ratledge and Kristiansen 2006). The techniques for handling biological systems are, through that, mostly understood in depth. Ingenious molecular and cell engineering approaches for transforming and handling biological systems have successfully been researched and developed in recent decades for a variety of industrial applications and products on a steadily expanding market.

The breadth of this training is extensive, covering a wide range of bioproducts, including pharmaceuticals, food products, diagnostics, and biotechnological devices, each presenting its own inherent biological challenges and technical hurdles. When these products finally reach the market, often after prolonged development cycles, they frequently still suffer from suboptimal performance. This can lead to rejection by regulatory authorities and customers, rapid obsolescence, or failure to compete with superior alternatives. Such shortcomings can be significantly alleviated through robust, proactive training that imparts a deeper understanding of customer needs, product functionality, and production economy (Fig. 1.1).

1.2 Scope and Diversity of Bioengineered Products

To be able to approach the design of bioproducts and their production, it is necessary to have a clear notion of their diversity (Ratledge and Kristiansen 2006).

Bioengineered products are commonly considered those where biology, in some way, is integrated and interacts within the product or its surroundings. Design training must therefore provide a thorough understanding of how the biological components of the product interface with its non-biological components. This profound challenge must be approached wisely by the designer using a structured engineering mindset.

Five different categories of bioengineered products can be distinguished that illustrate these interactions in distinct ways.

First, there is the category of bioproducts that have an intrinsic biology within the product itself and where the products act towards biological surroundings. An example is when human cells derived from pluripotent stem cells are used in regenerative medicine. The bioengineered cells, for example cartilage cells or skin cells, must be able to cope with the biological structure of the receiving body tissue (Tsumaki et al. 2015). Another example is when the product is a delivered service, for example when target cells are used to test the safety of biological drugs in microphysiological systems (Vasanata et al. 2011).

In a second category, bioproducts have an intrinsic biology but act in a non-biological surrounding, where these surroundings influence and interact with the inherent biology of the bioproduct. An example is bioremediation, where a cell culture breaks down non-biological toxic compounds and detoxifies polluted areas (Lea-Smith et al. 2025).

A third category of bioengineered products is those where there is no biology in the product itself, but where it acts in a biological environment. An example is the pacemaker, which must adapt to the physiology of the human heart. The physiological actions of the surrounding cardiac tissues profoundly influence the pacemaker and its performance. Other examples from biotechnology are analytical and preparative instrumentation, such as chromatographic separation materials and bioreactors for microbial cultivations (Jagschies et al. 2017).

A fourth category comprises biomolecular or biological products generated by a biological system. Examples are therapeutic proteins, metabolic compounds, or specific cell cultures produced by cultivation or fermentation techniques.

The fifth and final category is when a non-biological product is generated by a biological production system as in the fourth category, but where that product also

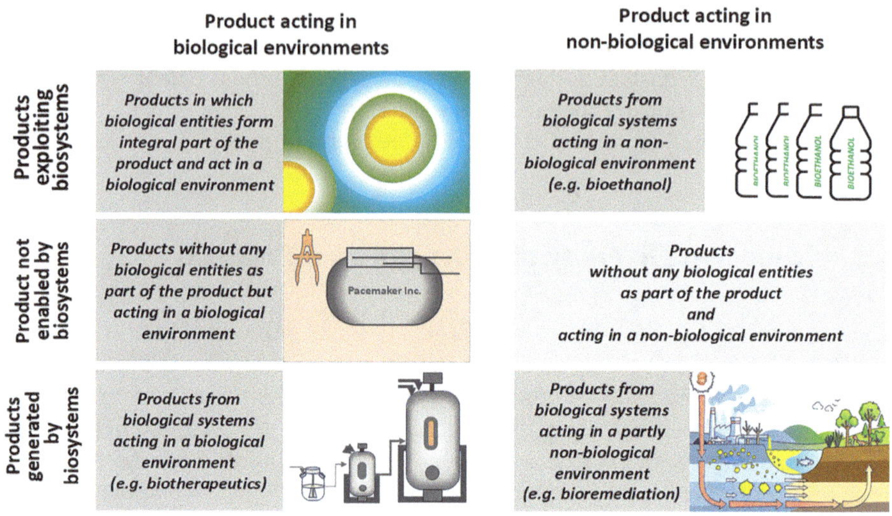

Fig. 1.2 Categories of bioproducts that are subject to bioengineering design. Note especially how biology plays very different roles in relation to the products. (With permission from Matilda and Samuel 2024)

can be produced by non-biological methods. Such products may have a biosynthetic route but, by tradition, have been produced industrially by chemical synthesis. This may include certain organic acids and alcohols, antibiotics, and vitamins.

These five product categories all depend on and interact with biological systems in distinct ways (Fig. 1.2). Present throughout society, these bioproducts result from a wide range of bioengineering design efforts, spanning food, medicine, diagnostics, commodities, and medical devices. While the market conditions for each bioproduct category vary considerably in terms of scale, profitability, quality standards, and regulatory requirements, the underlying engineering design principles, practices, and constraints remain fundamentally similar.

Figure 1.2 also includes a box for a product that contains no inherent biological components and operates strictly in non-biological environments. This explicitly defines the outer limits of the field, highlighting where bioengineering design principles do not apply. Consequently, the primary focus of this text is to teach and train methodologies specifically tailored to the five biologically integrated categories.

For these five bioproduct categories, it is important to realize the difference in how the products undergo development in various branches of industrial biotechnology. Distinct differences may occur if the product is a biopharmaceutical, a diagnostic device, biotech-related equipment or other instrumentation, or a biotech service.

In biopharmaceutical product development, preclinical and clinical trial phases constitute the dominant part of R&D efforts (Jagschies et al. 2017). Prior to initiating clinical trials, regulatory authorities require formal approval, which severely restricts

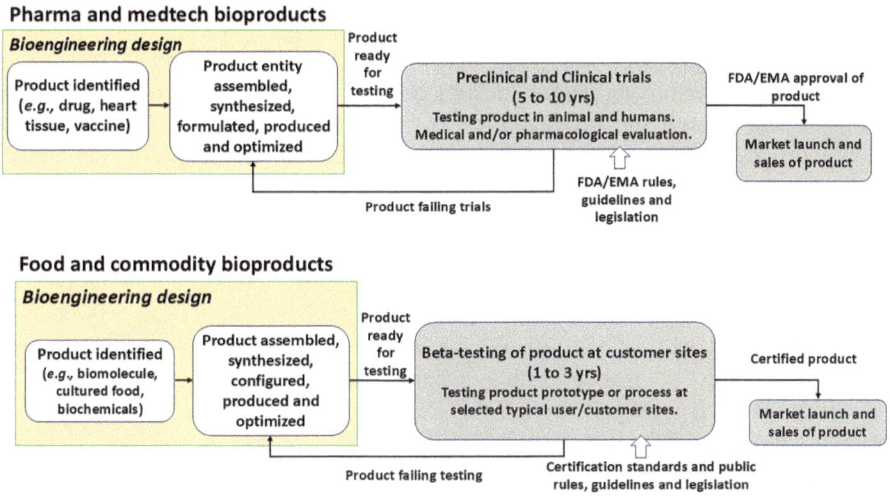

Fig. 1.3 Research and development processes of various biotechnological products. (**a**) Bioproducts regulated by pharmaceutical and medical authorities. (**b**) Bioproducts approved or monitored by other authorities

options for modifying the product or its manufacturing methodology thereafter. Consequently, critical design and manufacturing decisions must be resolved early, typically directly following the drug discovery phase, ensuring that the critical parameters of both the biopharmaceutical product and its process design are locked in before clinical trials begin (United States Food and Drug Administration 2025a) (Fig. 1.3a).

In the R&D process of biotechnical devices, instruments, and equipment, the products are tested at selected testing sites (beta-sites) using prototypes with preliminary protocols (O'Brian 2019). For example, the testing of a device may result in redesigning the device due to observed shortcomings or malfunctions. As for biopharmaceuticals, regulatory approval is necessary but mostly replaced by certification procedures performed by external evaluators (Fig. 1.3b).

If the device is intended for medical usage, such as diagnostic devices, some kind of medical or clinical approval could be necessary (United States' Food and Drug Administration 2025b).

Providing customers with testing results, analytical reports, or other specialized information constitutes what is generally referred to as a service product. In the biotechnology sector, service products, such as subcontracted testing assays or custom synthesis, follow the same design principles as physical products. Consequently, from a development perspective, the design methodologies overlap significantly. Thus, this guidance acknowledges that these service-based products are, from a design perspective, treated by the same design methodologies (Fig. 1.3).

1.3 Functionalities of Bioproducts

A key to successful bioengineering design is mastering the concept of functionality as it applies to both the product and its production system (Pahl et al. 2007; Mandenius and Björkman 2011; Jackson et al. 2024). It is essential to distinguish between (i) product functions from the end-user perspective and (ii) engineering functions required for manufacturing. Establishing the capability to navigate this distinction is a central goal of design training (Fig. 1.4).

Understanding how this duality shapes the learning and training process is particularly critical. In this regard, bioengineering aligns with other engineering disciplines that strive to create functionally outstanding products. Crucially, prioritizing functionality does not exclude managerial, aesthetic, legislative, or other human-centric perspectives. Instead, the elements shown in Fig. 1.4 directly integrate into the broader framework of Fig. 1.1, where all project dimensions converge during the development of a new product.

Thus, Fig. 1.4 underscores a fundamental principle of this guidance: engineering design work must be anchored in and driven by the concept of functionality. Consequently, bioengineering design training should actively cultivate coordinated thinking across these two pillars. This mindset must characterize every stage of design work, from initial concept generation to market-ready products. Conducting a thorough analysis of functionality is a reliable pathway to developing successful biological products.

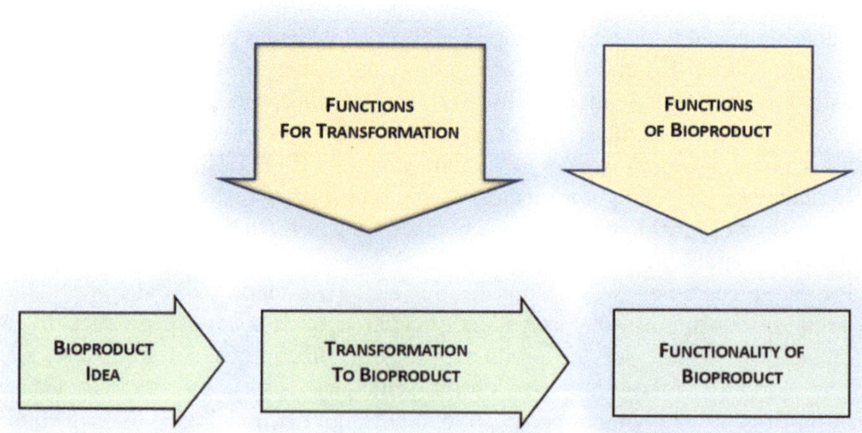

Fig. 1.4 The dual roles of functionality in bioengineering design illustrating the critical intersection between user-oriented functions (the performance, safety, and utility expected by the end-user) and production-oriented functions (the technical mechanisms, scalability, and manufacturing requirements of the bioreactor or processing system)

In essence, while functionality has long been recognized as a pivotal pillar in classical engineering design, it remains a relatively novel focus within bioengineering training (Hubka and Eder 1988).

1.4 The Industrial Perspective in the Training

The industrial perspective must play a central role in advanced engineering curricula. By embedding realistic industry parameters into the training, students become significantly better prepared for professional design environments, allowing them to rapidly adapt and contribute to commercial demands and operational requirements (Fleming et al. 2024; Ulrich et al. 2019).

Furthermore, when the training includes peers or mentors with prior industrial design experience, this practical expertise should be actively leveraged to enrich the learning environment.

Experienced engineers are used to discussing and communicating technical issues. They are also able to "negotiate" in design teams to refine their opinions. Moreover, they have acquired a useful knowledge base from previous experience which they can apply to new design tasks. The training should keep this in mind and take advantage of this when possible.

Consequently, these specific training elements should maintain a broad scope rather than becoming overly specialized. Instead, the curriculum should focus on "game changers" in the application of design methodologies (Heinzle et al. 2006). These include new advanced computer-aided design (CAD) systems, modern technical drawing and visualization tools, applicable artificial intelligence frameworks, and other emerging resources accessible across digital networks.

In bioengineering, the focus should be on biological issues of industrial relevance. That could be access to information about commercial culture collections or repositories; access to systems biology support and how that can be integrated in decision-making; support in statistical experimental investigations (design of experiments, DoE) and examples of how it can be applied in bioengineering; and access to information on the capacity and costs of novel means of bio-analytics, to mention a few aspects that can modernize the way of thinking (Dym et al. 2005).

Training must also address technological shifts in plant equipment, such as the introduction of single-use systems. It is critical to evaluate how their operational performance directly influences facility configurations and cost calculations. While equipment vendors commonly communicate these technical specifications, they seldom analyze the downstream consequences on the entire product lifecycle or the broader production system.

In Chap. 4, a few additional recommendations are given for adapting bioengineering design training to vocational training, based on the above-mentioned ambitions. Importantly, the design training cases described in Chap. 5 can be further extended with goals and tasks that are more qualified and more demanding.

Experienced engineers are accustomed to the tools of designing and will, in a shorter time, be able to judge how to approach a case.

By establishing this framework, this guidance aims to inspire the development of advanced bioengineering curricula dedicated to fostering high professional standards within the bioengineering community. Cultivating these competencies enables the field to deliver superior products to society while optimizing both resource utilization and human capital.

1.5 Critical Success Factors in Bioengineering Design

Figure 1.5 outlines the diverse core capabilities and multidisciplinary skills required to effectively execute novel bioproduct design. This conceptual framework applies universally across all five product categories detailed previously. A specific subset of these capabilities is strictly biological; achieving design excellence depends entirely on a thorough, mechanistic understanding of intricate cellular and metabolic functions. Higher education frameworks must introduce these core competencies early in bioengineering curricula. Programs should systematically reinforce these attributes across university engineering tracks, extending through master's and doctoral-level training. Figure 1.5 highlights these mandatory qualities, indicating that they must be prioritized within educational curricula.

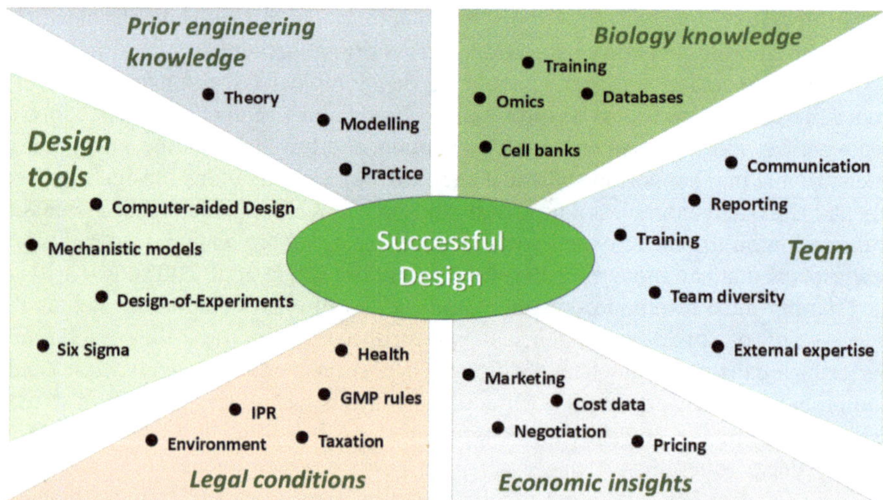

Fig. 1.5 Core factors that must be integrated into bioengineering design to achieve successful bioproduct development, encompassing prior engineering knowledge, biological understanding, regulatory conditions, and insights into production economy. This integration is effectively executed by well-trained design teams utilizing powerful digital design tools

A robust foundation in classical engineering serves as an absolute prerequisite. This baseline must encompass both theoretical principles and mathematical modeling. Students must learn to integrate fundamental engineering disciplines, such as mechanistic modeling, materials science, mathematics, and optimization, with advanced biological systems. Modern training should comprehensively bridge molecular biology, cell line engineering, omics methodologies, bioinformatics database usage, and the practical preservation and deposition of standard cell banks (Pörtner 2021). Furthermore, hands-on competencies must be cultivated through the expert utilization of modern design software. Implementing tools like computer-aided design (CAD), computational fluid dynamics (CFD), and statistical design of experiments (DoE) streamlines product development cycles and accelerates the optimization process (Heinzle et al. 2006; Montgomery 2013).

Parallel to traditional technical metrics, the broader impacts of social, ethical, and legal requirements must be rigorously addressed (Silverman 2004; O'Mathúna 2007; Keswani and Possas 2024). These societal boundaries introduce critical design constraints that engineering teams must address through structured testing and verification protocols. From an industrial standpoint, an innovative idea must prove techno-economically viable to achieve commercial reality (Peters et al. 2003; Towler and Sinnott 2012). Product engineering must be grounded in realistic resource allocations, raw material supply chains, cost structures, and the availability of specialized or proprietary biological systems. Ultimately, production frameworks must align with verifiable market demands where consumers are willing to cover the manufacturing costs.

Ultimately, engineering execution relies on the design team members themselves. Because these individuals are the direct drivers of project execution, they represent the primary target for institutional training efforts (Dym et al. 2005). Professional training curricula must place a heavy emphasis on interpersonal professional skills, specifically focusing on technical communication, precise reporting, inter-team collaboration, and professional negotiation. Curricula must also emphasize managing external expertise, cross-disciplinary consulting, and leveraging the diverse individual strengths within a project team.

The overarching objective of this guidance is to provide a systematic methodology for teaching and training these essential competencies. By guiding the reader from an initial inventive concept to a refined, marketable bioproduct, this text establishes actionable pathways across fundamental scientific principles, structured design methodologies, and realistic economic frameworks.

References

Baily JE, Ollis DF (1986) Biochemical engineering fundamentals. McGraw-Hill, New York

Doran PM (2013) Biochemical engineering principles, 2nd edn. Elsevier, Amsterdam. https://doi.org/10.1016/C2009-0-22348-8

Doulougeri K, Vermunt JD, Bombaerts G et al (2024) Challenge-based learning implementation in engineering education: a systematic literature review. J Eng Educ 113:1076–1106. https://doi.org/10.1002/jee.20588
Dym CL, Agogino AM, Eris O et al (2005) Engineering design thinking, teaching and learning. J Eng Educ 94:103–120. https://doi.org/10.1002/j.2168-9830.2005.tb00832.x
Fleming GC, Klopfer M, Katz A et al (2024) What engineering employers want: an analysis of technical and professional skills in engineering job advertisements. J Eng Educ 113:251–279. https://doi.org/10.1002/jee.20581
Heinzle E, Biwer A, Cooney C (2006) Development of sustainable bioprocesses. In: Modelling and assessment. John Wiley & Sons, Chichester
Hubka V, Eder WE (1988) Theory of technical systems, a total concept theory for engineering design. Springer Verlag, Berlin
Jackson A, Barrella E, Bodnar C (2024) Application of concept maps as an assessment tool in engineering education: systematic literature review. J Eng Educ 113:752–766. https://doi.org/10.1002/jee.20548
Jagschies G, Lindskog E, Lacki K et al (2017) Biopharmaceutical processing development, design, and implementation of manufacturing processes. Elsevier
Keswani C, Possas C (2024) Intellectual property issues in life sciences disputes and controversies. Taylor and Francis Ltd
Lea-Smith DJ, Francis Hassard F, Coulon F et al (2025) Engineering biology applications for environmental solutions: potential and challenges. Nat Commun 16:3538. https://doi.org/10.1038/s41467-025-58492-0
Mandenius CF, Björkman M (2011) Biomechatronic design in biotechnology: a methodology for development of biotechnology products. John Wiley & Sons, New Jersey. https://doi.org/10.1002/9781118067147
Matilda MI, Samuel HS (2024) Bioremediation of oil spill, concepts, methods and applications. Discov Chem 1:24
Montgomery DC (2013) Design and analysis of experiments, 8th edn. John Wiley & Sons, New York
O'Brian D (2019) Engineer 4.0: life science handbook for medical devices and biopharmaceuticals. Independently published. ISBN 9781795753340 (available from www.amazon.com)
O'Mathúna DP (2007) Bioethics and biotechnology. Cytotechnol 53:113–119. https://doi.org/10.1007/s10616-007-9053-8
Pahl G, Beitz W, Feldhusen J et al (2007) Engineering design, a systematic approach, 3rd edn. Springer Verlag, Berlin
Peters MS, Timmerhaus KD, West RE (2003) Plant design and economics for chemical engineers, 5th edn. McGraw-Hill, New York
Pörtner R (ed) (2021) Cell culture engineering and technology. Springer Nature, New York. https://doi.org/10.1007/978-3-030-79871-0
Ratledge C, Kristiansen B (eds) (2006) Basic biotechnology, 3rd edn. Cambridge University Press
Silverman ED (2004) The 5 most pressing ethical issues in biotech medicine. Biotechnol Healthc 1(6):41
Towler G, Sinnott R (2012) Chemical engineering design: principles, practice and economics of plant and process design, 2nd edn. Elsevier, Amsterdam
Tsumaki N, Okada M, Yamashita A (2015) iPS cell technologies and cartilage regeneration. Bone 70:48–54
Ulrich KT, Eppinger SD, Yang MC (2019) Product design and development, 7th edn. McGraw-Hill, New York
United States' Food and Drug Administration (2025a) Innovative designs for clinical trials of cellular and gene therapy products in small populations (draft guidance for industry). U.-S. Department of Health and Human Services, Food and Drug Administration, Center for Drug Evaluation and Research (CDER), Center for Biologics Evaluation and Research (CBER), Center for Veterinary Medicine (CVM), Washington

United States' Food and Drug Administration (2025b) Medical device user fee small business qualification and determination. (guidance for industry). Food and Drug Administration Staff and Foreign Governments. U.S. Department of Health and Human Services, Food and Drug Administration, Center for Drug Evaluation and Research (CDER), Center for Biologics Evaluation and Research (CBER), Center for Veterinary Medicine (CVM), Washington

Vasanata GVA, Roy R, Lelah A et al (2011) A review of product–service systems design methodologies. J Eng Des 23(9):635–659. https://doi.org/10.1080/09544828.2011.639712

Chapter 2
Fundamentals in Bioengineering Design

The fundamental scientific and technological principles that both enable and constrain bioengineering design are outlined in this chapter. It highlights the transition from creative concepts to practical bioproducts through core engineering principles and design methodologies, with a particular focus on bridging fundamental theory and bioproduct execution from a generalized design perspective. Crucially, the text presents only those aspects directly relevant to bioengineered products and systems, including production economics, societal expectations, and risk assessments. By focusing on the biological system parameters that influence overall design quality, this chapter establishes the operational framework for the nine subsequent case studies presented in Chap. 5.

2.1 Bridging Fundamental Science and Bioproduct Design

Successful bioengineered product design must be anchored in fundamental scientific principles (Moorthy 2017; Saterbek et al. 2018; Swamy 2015). Once these scientific prerequisites are secure, established bioengineering methodologies can shape the product concept to achieve the intended functional outcomes. Developing a deep awareness of this relationship is a primary objective of bioengineering design education.

Inventive concepts for bioproducts must strictly adhere to basic scientific and technological principles. These ideas are sequentially refined through structured design methodologies prior to physical implementation and realization (Fig. 2.1). In this guidance book, this core philosophy underpins the overarching approach to design thinking (Dym et al. 2005; Mandenius and Björkman 2011; Ulrich et al. 2019). Fundamental science and technology act as critical filters for every innovative idea before it is structured and refined into a sustainable new bioproduct.

For bioproducts, this filtering process applies specifically to the principles of bioscience and biotechnology (Saterbek et al. 2018; Swamy 2015; Doran 2013;

C.-F. Mandenius, *Bioengineering Design Methodology*,
https://doi.org/10.1007/978-3-032-33940-9_2

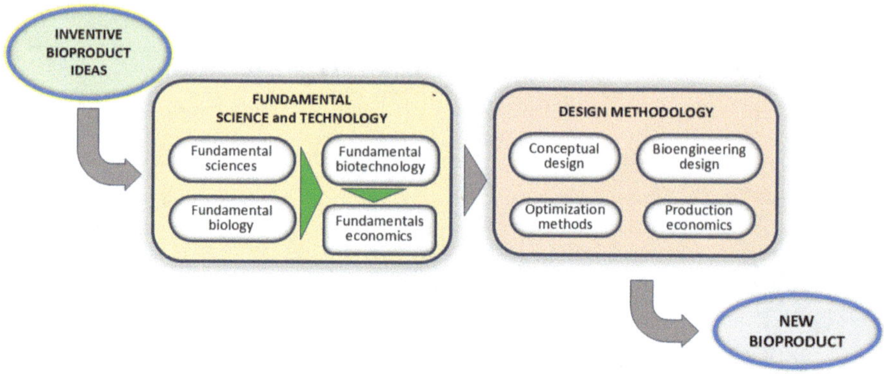

Fig. 2.1 Inventive ideas must first adhere to bioscience and biotechnology tenets before undergoing sequential refinement through design methodologies. This filtering process ensures that final bioproducts are technically viable, production processes are optimized, and the resulting systems satisfy both market demands and economic constraints

Sneppen 2014; O'Brian 2019). If a novel idea violates these biological tenets, it must almost certainly be rejected.

Realizing new bioproducts also demands rigorous focus on manufacturing design, which requires highly optimized production processes. Consequently, process design and product design are inextricably intertwined.

To maintain market competitiveness, bioproducts must be continuously improved and adapted to evolving consumer needs. Managing this recurrent challenge in bioengineering design requires careful proactive planning when initial concepts are being structured (Pahl et al. 2007).

Finally, this framework must incorporate an understanding of economic factors and their direct influence on product and production system design. Because these economic realities dictate global marketing and commercialization strategies, modern bioengineering design must be tightly integrated with economic and business thinking (Ray et al. 2022).

2.2 Integrating Fundamental Science with Biological Systems

As emphasized above, transforming an inventive concept into a viable bioproduct requires a realistic refinement process firmly anchored in scientific principles. For design purposes, the boundaries between biological science, biotechnology, and bioengineering need to be precisely defined.

With *biological science,* we refer to the knowledge and understanding of biological systems, and how they are governed, diversified, and structured in nature (Alberts et al. 2019). The methods to study the natural systems, either at a

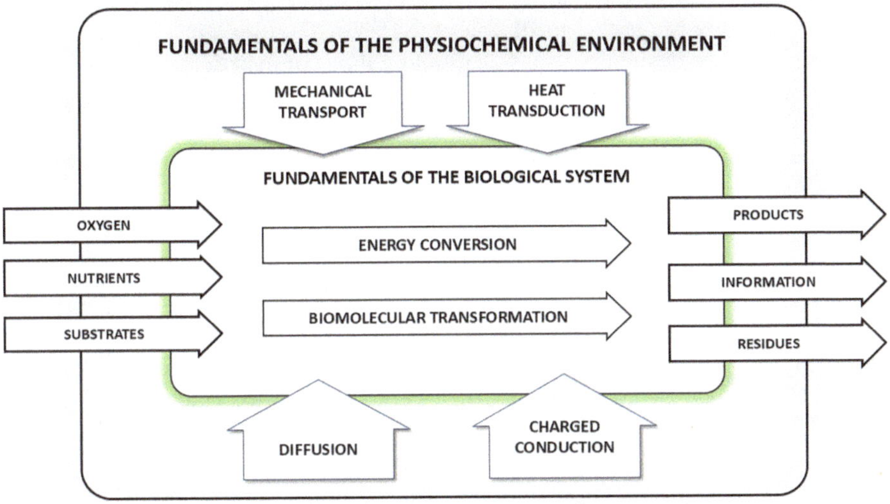

Fig. 2.2 The interplay between physical and chemical components, conditions, and flows in the physicochemical environment is vital for driving the functions of the biological system

microscopic or macroscopic scale, provide the prerequisites for being able to use and exploit the systems technologically. This includes a variety of techniques to observe, analyze, collect, and prepare the biological systems.

Building upon this, *biotechnology* applies these natural systems within a technological framework, introducing methods to modify and adapt biological environments at the biomolecular, metabolic, and physiological levels (Goldman 2022). With *bioengineering,* we extend these biotechnological methods into rigorous engineering workflows (Ratledge and Kristiansen 2006). By directly engineering the biological system itself, bioengineering encompasses a broader operational scope than biotechnology. It couples biological transformation with the technical, industrial scale-up methods necessary to cultivate, select, recover, separate, and purify complex biological systems.

The concepts of biotechnology and bioengineering may overlap. The precise borderline is, at least from a design perspective, of minor importance.

Of importance, however, is to understand and use basic science and engineering in physics, chemistry, and other sciences for developing and exploiting biotechnology and bioengineering for a design purpose.

The physicochemical environment drives and controls the biological systems in the generation of bioproducts or biological information (Fig. 2.2). Several critical features of the physicochemical environment must be carefully considered due to their direct impact on the design process:

- Energy generates heat; sensitive biological systems can be harmed. Thus, heat must be avoided or reduced. In design, heat transduction may be utilized. Key

denominators for this are surface area versus volume, heat capacity of culture media, and flux of cooling media.
- Gradients in the designed systems caused by flows of materials or by energy and heat gradients are well described by general physical laws.
- Mechanical stress exerted on biomolecules, cells, and tissues may harmfully act on the performance of the biological systems. Alleviating such stress is an important design issue and sometimes a great challenge.
- Physical pressure because of expanding gases is likely to negatively influence biological systems. Especially cells are vulnerable to such pressure. The design of the biotechnical systems can decisively reduce such effects.

Many bioengineering textbooks deal with the interface between physics, chemistry, and biology and provide the theory and advice of relevance for these designs (Atkins et al. 2023; Beard and Qian 2010; Parke 2020; Price et al. 2001; Williams 2014).

2.3 Adapting General Engineering Design Principles to Bioproduct Design

When designing bioproducts, established design engineering principles should be applied. General engineering design is based on three fundamental steps relevant to all kinds of products (Dym et al. 2005; Hubka and Eder 1988):

- Conceptualize the design idea and identify options with the users in focus. Interpret the purpose and objectives for finding a wide range of alternatives and converge these into the favorable alternatives.
- Analyze the alternatives by applying fundamental perspectives. Decide what the best alternatives are for realizing the original design concept to become a sustainable product and prototype these alternatives.
- Test and validate the prototypes to assess their performance and sustainability.

These three steps are applicable in all design work, from the construction of buildings, vehicles, and chemical molecules as well as to biological products. Figure 2.3 illustrates the flow of the design work and its relations with key activities and design tools.

In bioengineering design, the steps are strongly interconnected with biological challenges. These interconnections balance between:

- Intrinsic fundamentals of biology, biologically derived actions and reactions of cells, proteins, and other biomolecules.
- Intrinsic fundamental issues of non-biological systems, such as chemical and physical laws and rules of non-biological materials or objects.
- Production economics, market, and socio-economic issues involved in a bioproduct.

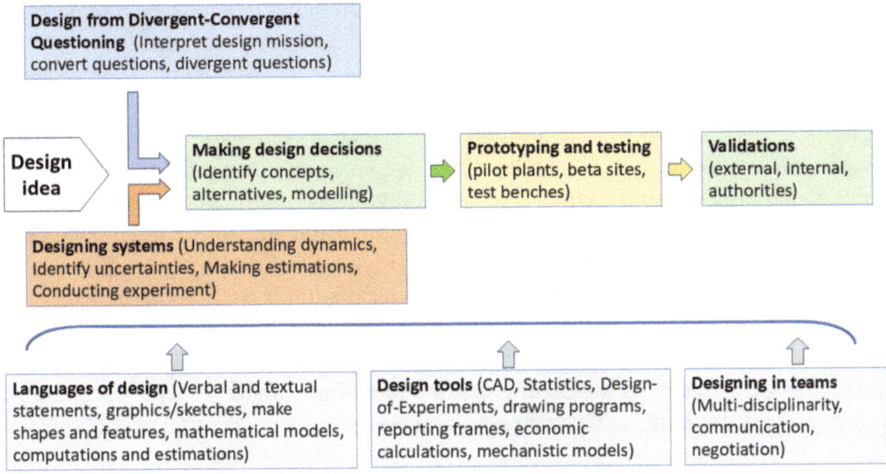

Fig. 2.3 Activities in design projects, from ideas to validated products. Decision-making, prototyping, and validation are based on design skills, tools, and a competent team. The sequential processing of a design idea passes through design decisions, prototypes, and validations (middle part), while a variety of design expressions, tools, and teamwork (lower part) enable the implementation of the design idea

Figure 2.3 highlights another central principle: divergence and convergence in engineering design (Pahl et al. 2007). This methodology requires initially generating a broad spectrum of alternative design solutions (divergence) before systematically filtering and selecting the options that best satisfy the project's objectives and constraints (convergence). This selection process must be guided by a comprehensive understanding of end-user needs. In this context, "users" comprise a diverse group of stakeholders who utilize, interact with, or depend on the final design.

To guide these activities, several fundamental questions must be addressed regarding user requirements:

- What are the users' most critical requirements?
- Are the users able to tell what their critical target values are for these requirements? (Note, these can be qualitative targets defined by yes/no, color, or else.)
- Are there requirements the users have neglected that will be decisive at a later stage? The designer should try to figure out if so and which these are.

These users are seldom a homogeneous group. For pharmaceuticals, it involves users of the healthcare system, with medical doctors and other healthcare professionals and administrators as well as providers of healthcare capital. In the food sector, the distribution chain of food is involved. The regulators of drugs and foods are, by legislation, obliged to ensure that product quality is secured. The manufacturers of the product have demands at a variety of stages: the conditions at the plant for the operators and responsibility for the plant management; the marketing organization of the selling company has its priorities; the business economic management of the company and the financiers have defined expectations.

Figure 2.3 also illustrates the critical process of *decision-making*. At a systemic level, design thinking relies on executing decisions within a structured conceptual framework (Mandenius and Björkman 2011). These frameworks are specifically designed to evaluate product functionalities, user requirements, and specified needs, while balancing available technical resources against economic constraints.

The convergence phase of the design process culminates in the development of prototypes. Built upon rigorous decision-making and validated user requirements, these prototypes are evaluated primarily to verify that their operational performance aligns with the original design intent. Furthermore, Fig. 2.3 underscores the essential role of design tools, including graphics, technical drawings, and predictive modeling, alongside specialized digital engineering tools for calculation and computation, collaborative teamwork, and communication skills.

2.4 Managing Kinetic and Operational Constraints in Biodesign

In bioengineering, successful design requires integrating the general design principles described in Sect. 2.3 with the unique biological characteristics of the bioproduct (Mandenius and Björkman 2011; Saterbek et al. 2018; Swamy 2015). This section outlines the fundamental constraints and operational challenges inherent to this integration.

When applying engineering design to biological products, several technical methodologies must be evaluated. These approaches must be tailored to satisfy user requirements across a variety of criteria, such as the following: Which properties of the biological system are most critical to the expected design outcome?

- Which *properties of a biological system* are most critical to the expected design outcome? These properties are associated with the capacity of the biological system. But what should be included in the term capacity, and what kind of biological capacity has an impact on the product performance? The answer to this will direct the biological part of the design work. The designer must manage to find or shape the biological systems into becoming a better *enabler of performance and quality* of a new product.
- What would be the *most efficient means* or techniques to do this? This should focus on the technological possibilities of *changing a biological system's capacity* or trying to identify other biological systems that can do this.
- The cell factory with its inherent metabolic or transformative capacity constitutes the platform of the bioproduct (Fig. 2.4a). Cell biology and molecular biology provide a wide range of opportunities and methods that are applicable to the designing efforts of shaping a new product. Part of the cell factory, for example, individual proteins or sequences of enzymes, may solve this satisfactorily

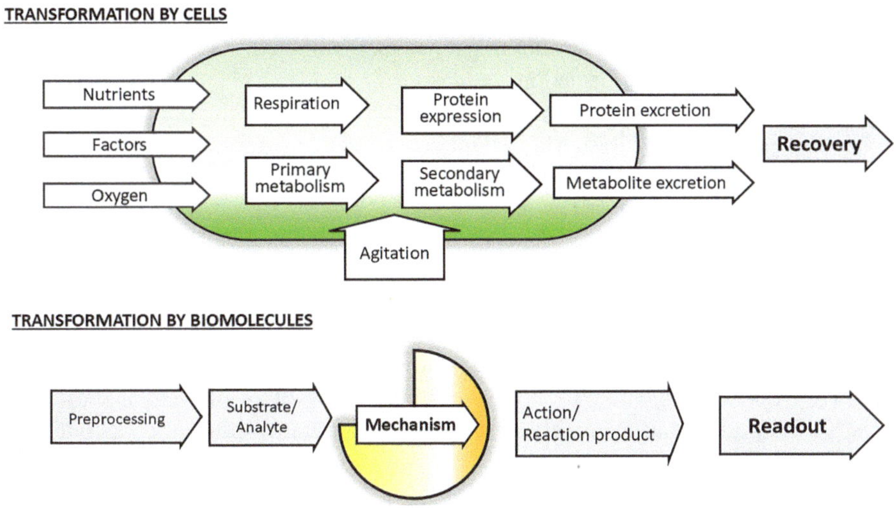

Fig. 2.4 Flows transformed by or within biological systems. The cell factory (top) illustrates metabolic conversions typically in bioproduct manufacturing, such as the production of biotherapeutics and therapeutic cells. The biocatalytic transformation of components by biomolecules (bottom), including enzymes, antibodies, and nucleotides, as applied in diagnostic devices and biosensors

(Fig. 2.4b). Knowledge and methodology should be systematically approached, evaluated, and judged.

From an engineering perspective, these issues can be combined in a resourceful and powerful way to enhance biological rates and activities (Nielsen et al. 2011). It should then be appropriate to funnel these opportunities into such qualities that progressively improve the design, for example through:

- *Conversion rate* in the biological system: This is directly related to the time factor for how long it takes to produce a defined quantity of a target product molecule or bioanalytical information.
- *The host cell factory*, with its inherent metabolic or transformative capacity, serves as the core bioproduct platform (Fig. 2.4a). Cell and molecular biology offer a diverse array of methodologies to guide design efforts when engineering a new product. Subcellular components, such as isolated proteins or specific enzyme cascades, can also fulfill these design requirements effectively (Fig. 2.4b). Consequently, biological knowledge and methodologies must be approached, evaluated, and applied systematically.

From an engineering perspective, these biological features can be integrated synergistically to maximize metabolic rates and productivity (Nielsen et al. 2011). Designers must channel these biological capabilities into specific, quantifiable performance metrics that progressively refine the system design, such as:

- *Biological conversion rate:* This metric directly determines the time required to generate a specified quantity of a target product molecule or to produce a defined unit of bioanalytical information.
- *Expansion* of the biological system: This is related to two important parameters: (i) the capacity of the biological system to expand and (ii) the capacity of the same system to express the target product, whether it is to express a protein, a metabolite, or the cell itself.
- *Saturation effects* of the biological system: Any biological system has limits which we can refer to as a state of saturation. For example, there is a maximum capacity of the cell to grow or express a product, usually due to the cell's nutrient uptake capacity or respiration. These limits should be known and understood in a way that negates any unrealistic design solution to the product's biological part.
- *Purity* of the biological system: Preparations of the biological systems must have sufficient purity to allow an efficient and unbiased transformation to its outcome (biologicals or information).
- *Stability* of biological system: A biological system is more vulnerable to its environment than most physical or chemical systems. The loss of stability then becomes a critical design parameter that one must investigate and, if necessary, counteract. The alternatives for this are many.
- *Reproducibility* of biological transformations: This is directly related to stability. Either it is a transformation of a biological production system with a target product, or a biological system used for analytical purposes, for example, transforming a sample to an analytical readout. Reproducibility becomes the decisive performance. Without high reproducibility, the quality is compromised.

Table 2.1 overviews the quality properties of the biosystems that must be considered in any design mission. All are linked to the products' performance.

Note that these biological properties can be expressed as quantitative metrics, frequently defined by mathematical relationships. The two most widely applied biological transformations in bioengineering are as follows: (i) a cell lineage generating a target product and (ii) a single-step biocatalytic reaction producing an analytical readout (Fig. 2.4). The key process parameters in these systems are consistently coupled with reaction rates, fluid volumes, and biological material quantities.

To design an effective bioproduct, one must understand the distinct and unique characteristics of biological design. To nonbiologists, it may seem unusual that biology maintains a distinct status compared to other sciences and technologies in engineering design. One might wonder if a biological framework could simply be viewed as any other technical system governed by standard functions, or treated merely as a collection of variables, constants, and responses within mechanistic and statistical models. From an engineering standpoint, evaluating these unique characteristics reveals the distinct nature of biological systems and highlights the specific factors that must be integrated into the design (Ratledge and Kristiansen 2006).

Living cells possess immense complexity due to a myriad of interconnected metabolic reactions and continuous interactions with their microenvironment. This

Table 2.1 Critical quality measures for bioengineering design

Quality measure	Relevance for design
Productivity of bioproduct and cells	The higher the productivity of the biosystem, the better the economy can be expected of the bioproduct, both concerning plant size and consumption of consumables and energy
Stability of bioproduct	The better the stability of the bioproduct, the longer the lifespan can be expected after production by customers, during production, of plant operation and size. The impact of product economy is substantial
Cellular transformation fidelity	Transformation of cells, either by growth and expansion or by differentiation and maturation, increases yield of the cellular product, its quality, and usefulness for customers. The impact on the economy can be considerable
Stability of producing biosystem	Cells used for generating the bioproduct exhibit better performance the longer they maintain their stability
Utilization of stabilizers and factors for promotion of productivity	In cellular processes, expenditures for growth-promoting factors tend to be high and increase with scale. All efforts to reduce this favor economy.
Yield of product on raw materials	Due to costs of raw materials and other utilities, their minimization enhances production economy
Cell density	Density of producing cells per plant volume favors economy if productivity per cell remains unchanged
Bioproduct rate	Bioproduct formation rate is a result of the cells' productivity and closely related to the above metrics
Biomolecular affinity	The ability to capture target molecules is a decisive parameter in bioanalytical methods
Analytical sensitivity	Analytical sensitivity can be enhanced by sensitive detectors or by sensitive and amplifying biosystems
Analytical selectivity	Biomolecular discrimination of target versus nontarget molecules is a measure of analytical performance

complexity directly governs how bioengineered products and devices must be designed to ensure their operational utility; without a deep understanding of these cellular dynamics, successful design is unachievable. Therefore, the impact of design choices on these biological systems must be evaluated across several key properties:

- Variations in biological reaction rates are driven by fluctuations in environmental conditions, such as temperature, pressure, and moisture content. Most of these variables are intensive parameters, meaning they are independent of the system's total mass or volume. While some of these parameters are straightforward to monitor online, others present significant measurement challenges.
- Variations in biological reaction rates are driven by fluctuations in environmental conditions, such as temperature, pressure, and moisture content. Most of these variables are intensive parameters, meaning they are independent of the system's total mass or volume. While some of these parameters are straightforward to monitor online, others present significant measurement challenges.

- Different microorganisms and cell lines exhibit distinct variability governed by their genetic profiles. This characteristic can be strategically exploited by selecting specific strains from culture collections. Selection and optimization can be performed at both the molecular and protein levels to match the desired design outcomes.
- The manufacturing and fabrication consequences of these biological traits must be evaluated with high precision. Understanding these effects allows engineers to accurately adjust physical and operational properties during process scale-up.

To systematically manage these biological variables, four core methodologies are widely utilized (and are discussed in further detail in Chap. 3). First, strain screening from natural sources involves isolating microorganisms or cells from natural environments, plants, animals, or human tissues, allowing critical performance parameters to be measured and compared for selection purposes. This is frequently complemented by recombinant and cell line engineering, which modifies these screened or established host strains obtained from official repositories by leveraging state-of-the-art techniques for transfection, gene insertion, and metabolic pathway amplification. At a molecular level, protein engineering can then be applied to alter the primary, secondary, or tertiary structure of a target protein, optimizing specific operational parameters to improve functional performance. Finally, stabilization methodologies employ chemical or biochemical formulations to extend the operational lifespan of these biological systems within the manufacturing process or to preserve the stability of the final product itself.

2.5 Societal Expectations on Bioengineering Design

Bioproducts and their production must comply with the public legal, ethical, and safety requirements (O'Mathúna 2007; Kuszler 2006). Society's expectations and legislation must be considered in the design of a bioproduct and its production. Especially when the scale of production grows, the impact of these demands increases.

Most bioengineered products and their production are surrounded by a variety of national and international legal rules, recurrently surveilled by regulatory authorities. It is the producer that has the responsibility to ensure that legislative and ethical considerations comply with current standards.

Regulatory frameworks governing ethics, consumer protection, occupational health and safety, public environmental impact, and other legal domains constrain the design process, yet they also provide essential guidance for systematically implementing these critical requirements (Ahmad et al. 2015).

These design considerations benefit from being integrated early into the design work.

Of special concern in recent years has been the use of embryonic stem cells. As a result of active stem cell research, this has now been surpassed by induced pluripotent stem cells, solving the ethical question around the use of human embryos (Silvermann 2004; Santoro 2012).

The spread of genetically modified cells to humans or the environment has been intensively discussed and resulted in legislative procedures that industrial users must obey together with other ethical rules or conventions of relevance to bioengineering. Close to these concerns are (i) ethical acceptance of using human individual materials of genetic or other origin (embryos, human samples), and (ii) ethical acceptance of using individual data (sample data, individual information).

An important role in upholding the societal legislation and expectations is played by regulatory organizations, such as the United States' Food and Drug Administration (FDA) and the European Medicines Agency (EMA) for food and pharmaceuticals. Adjacent to these are organizations such as the International Council of Harmonization (ICH) that cooperate with similar objectives and ambitions. The activities are focused on:

- Production methods and production sites (US Food and Drug Administration 2011; European Medicines Agency 2016).
- Products used in healthcare.
- Toxicity and quality of consumer products (International Council of Harmonization 1995; European Medicines Agency 2016).
- Approval of release of products by rules for validation (US Food and Drug Administration 2011).

Their surveillance of private and public commercial activities and distribution of biotechnology products is widely and globally recognized. The design cases in Chap. 5 highlight these issues.

2.6 Evaluating Economic Conditions for Bioproduct Design

Economics is one of the most decisive constraints in designing. But economics must be balanced. Economics represents one of the most critical constraints in engineering design, yet it must be continuously balanced against other vital project constraints. Consequently, bioengineering design must successfully reconcile the following economically driven aims:

- High quality of the product from the user's perspective.
- An acceptable market price for the users.
- To creatively exploit the inherent power of biological systems.

These three aims are intertwined and either supportive or contradictory from an economic perspective. They are intimately associated with product development and production. In product design, these relations must be thoroughly analyzed and, when relevant, carefully compared between design solutions (Peters et al. 2003; Kristiansen 2006; Towler and Sinnott 2012; Ray et al. 2022).

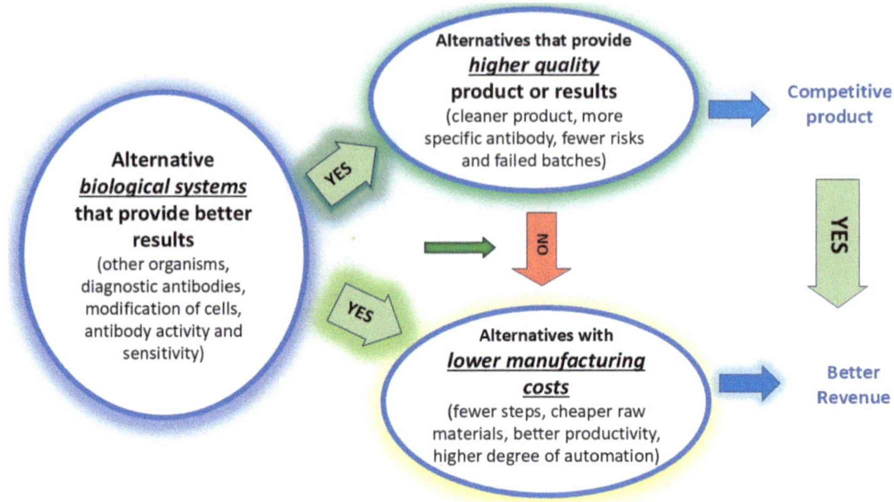

Fig. 2.5 The interplay between quality, costs, and biological power in product development should result in more competitive products and better revenues

For most bioproducts, quality is extremely critical. It involves demanding quality assurance and quality control, with a significant impact on the final cost of the product. However, a higher cost for better quality is often paid back by promoting successful sales and higher confidence in a product. Consequently, it is necessary, especially for a completely new bioproduct, to consider the quality-economy relationship.

Moreover, precise control of biological power supports high product quality and can, if wisely applied, reduce costs. However, biological power may also increase costs for a novel product. Design engineering must seriously leverage and balance these aims (Fig. 2.5).

Several economy-related questions must be asked:

- *What price is the customer ready to pay for the desired functionality*? The customers are not always able to verbalize this but will most probably have an idea of its value in their own context or application.
- *What are the market and production costs for alternative products*? It will require market studies on the product to answer this. It will take investment in time, but this will be paid back.
- *Are critical/indispensable raw materials available within the cost frame*? Thus, the designer needs to study this issue and find out how raw material cost can be reduced.
- *Is the manufacturing scale economically realistic*? It must be possible to see the chance of a continuing future net income, at least as a payback of the capital invested.

Table 2.2 Economic definitions of relevance to bioengineering design

Concept/term	Definition and rationale for new bioproducts and designs
Investments	Capital spent on acquiring equipment, facilities, and commodities used permanently over an extended period (typically exceeding the payback period). This includes installation, project engineering, and the acquisition of patent or intellectual property rights
Upfront costs	Initial expenditures required for process and product development (PR&D). This includes early-stage research, technology transfers, and the initial acquisition or licensing of intellectual property rights (IPR)
Revenue	The total income generated from bioproduct sales, calculated net of sales, taxes, and duties. This gross inflow must cover production costs, overheads, and all commercialization expenses
Payback	In this guidance, this refers to the payback of investments in product development and production facilities from the sale of the product. The payback is usually distributed over a period of 5–10 years, resulting in an annual cost. Sometimes this is referred to as "depreciation," originally an accounting term for the decreasing value of assets
Net income	The final profit remaining after deducting all operational costs, taxes, depreciation, and interest from revenue. This surplus is distributed as dividends to shareholders or reinvested into the company
Sales price	The market price paid per unit by the customer. This value fluctuates based on market competition, volume discounts, and applicable regional tax structures
Brutto income	Total revenue minus the direct cost of goods sold, before accounting for administrative overhead, interest, and corporate taxes. This metric must be clearly defined based on local accounting standards and jurisdictions
Production costs	The direct expenses required to manufacture a product. This strictly includes raw materials, consumables, manufacturing utilities, direct labor, quality control, analytics, and facility maintenance
Operational cost	The total ongoing expenses to run the business. This encompasses all production costs plus indirect expenses such as annual IPR/license fees, logistics, shipping, marketing, and sales administration

- *Will there be risk takers for developing a production to an assumed but uncertain market*? Considerable capital investments are required to set up a new product. In that context, the design of the new product must convince the risk takers. Thus, investors become a kind of user with requirements regarding the quality of the design. They must be convinced that the market likes the product because it is well designed and lives up to the appropriate functionality.
- *Are there design tools that allow proper and reliable investigations of alternative designs*? Conceptual design methodology is such a tool. Its inherent systematics can, if properly applied, reach this.

It is important to be well-oriented about those economic concepts or terms that could influence the design work (Table 2.2). Here, these economic concepts and definitions are mainly used due to their relevance in designing.

In a wider economic scope, companies with many products may sometimes influence the design approach.

Larger companies have a long-term perspective on their product development. For example, pharmaceutical companies often use their revenues from one generation of products to develop the next generation of the product.

The opportunities to economize the design of bioproducts and their production are partly overlapping with previous challenges. Using established cell lines or strains in culture collections, from public or proprietary collections, experimental work can be sped up at modest costs.

Several questions can be asked about the opportunities and potential risks in relation to the economy:

- Can systematic development of culture media, e.g. by using DoE techniques as will be further described in Chap. 3, improve economy rates and yields (Brereton 2003)?
- Can optimization of culture conditions and procedures improve production economics?
- Can the downstream recovery and purification stages, stabilization methods, with similar approaches, be optimized with substantial effect on the economy?
- Due to the sensitive stability of bioproducts, can *stabilizing* the biological entity with, e.g., a film, the formulation in a tablet, a filling material, a sensor, or other analytical machine, or a microfluidic system have an impact on the economy?
- *Can development costs for the biological system be kept at acceptable levels, resulting in an affordable product price for customers*? The higher the development costs, the smaller the margin for return on investment or margin to present a competitive market price. On the other hand, poor quality of development and output design results in a less competitive product on the market.
- *Can biological raw materials be acquired at a reasonable price, not making the final sales price unrealistic*? Production design could certainly encompass looking at alternative raw materials where availability and price for such may vary considerably. This may concern culture media, which for some cell systems, such as mammalian cells and stem cells, require very costly media components. The cost of raw materials will most often influence the price of the final product (Towler and Sinnott 2012).
- *Can the product with its biological system be produced in such a number as the market requests*? The size of the market, the success of the product on the market, the competitive situation, and the correctness of estimating the need for the product are surely difficult to predict and are also interplaying considerably. Usually, the issue from the designer's perspective becomes a matter of the scalability of the production. Most biological systems can be scaled up linearly. The limit is the size of equipment and plant. Often, maximal utilization is desirable. To run a production plant on suboptimal capacity (over time or use of full size) may seem uneconomic but does not leave space for upscaling. It then becomes a matter of decision-making and risk-taking.

Process scale-up represents a critical stage where economics, design, and manufacturing meet (Harmsen 2013; Harnish and Ross 2022). Scaling up production demands capital-intensive, larger-capacity unit operations for biological processing, alongside expanded equipment for non-biological operations. This transition fundamentally poses a core engineering question:

- *Can the production scale easily be adapted to a changing market*? The question ends up in a multiplicity factor. Is it realistic to plan for a tripling of the market or of any other factor? Also, what happens with the production economy if the market is decreasing? It is not necessary to only consider reengineering the same plant. Other alternatives are using parallel or subcontractor manufacture. It will require transfer of production method and regulatory costs for approval but could still be a realistic alternative.

Finally, a few strategic economic issues must be raised that could affect future business with the bio product:

- *Does any other alternative to producing the product exist that could endanger the survival of the suggested design*? This must be a permanent concern after the launch of any product. Competitors will constantly work to achieve this. Biosimilar pharmaceuticals are examples of this.
- *For how long will the technology remain state-of-the-art and not become surpassed by other technologies with better performance, and will that time suffice to quantify the development costs of the product*? If the payback time is around 5 years, it seems reasonable that the plant should remain in operation at least another 5 years, before being replaced or upgraded.
- *Is there a convincing good continuation for newer versions of the product?* Not only may the production process need to be replaced, but also the product itself may be superseded by better products. Can the own company be responsible for these, or even the inventor? Can they be produced in the same or a modified plant?

2.7 Distinctive Characteristics of Bioengineering Design

The uniqueness of bioengineering design is that it is grounded on the condition that there is a factory in microformat embedded in the macro-factory. It is This microfactory, often referred to as the "cell factory," is able, within a single volume of the cell, to carry out reactions that in other technical systems are performed in significantly larger volumes and across an array of stages in separate reaction vessels (Gong et al. 2017). The cell factory encloses this in a single micro-compartment and even smaller sub-compartmental units. This microsystem comprises miniaturized functional surfaces endowing the cell factory with astonishing precision and yields. Each cell factory unit can be multiplied in billions in a short time by efficient culturing. This fundamental uniqueness has remarkable and unprecedented industrial potential. It may, if skillfully exploited, supersede the power of non-biological alternatives, such as industrial production of chemical compounds with chemical

Table 2.3 Ambitions, objectives, and challenges characterizing the design of bioproducts

Ambitions	Objectives	Challenges
Identifying the cell factory with powerful biological systems	Employing the existing repository of biological systems in nature	Managing observability by bioanalytical means
Refining the identified biosystem	Recover and transform the powerful properties of the biosystem for operability of the bioproduct	Applying cell engineering
Optimizing the performance of the biosystem	Ascertain conditions in the bioproduct that favor its operation	Applying genetic engineering Optimization
Enhance the interplay between the biosystem and the environment	Ensure that the biosystem can utilize its environment	Observability
Enclose and demarcate the active biosystems	Contain the bioproduct safely with remaining biological activity	Mechanical engineering and entrapment
Ensure competitive economic conditions in the design	Use raw materials and energy transformed into the bioproduct with high yield factors	Understand mass and energy balance in production and operation
Secure affordable bioproduct quality	Make the decisive quality of the bioproduct possible to generate and maintain at a realistic cost	Procurement and optimal use of means
Make the biosystem within the bioproduct stable and reproducible	Ensure that vulnerable biological action is protected in the lifespan of the bioproduct	Immobilizing or optimally enclosing the biosystem
Scale up the biological functions for a growing market	Allow the bioproduct to grow unchanged in size for an increasing market request	Make conditions scalable without endangering quality and production costs

reactions. The design of the biomolecular-based products depends on the proficiency of exploiting the micro-factory.

It also means that a range of decisive and influential design issues should be brought up, and that connects to the ambitions, objectives, and challenges of the cell factory (Table 2.3).

However, within the five product categories established in Chap. 1, bioproducts that act on or within a biological system but are non-biological themselves (Category II, in Fig. 1.2) do not contain an embedded cell factory.

Basically, five aspects of design with relevance to the Cell Factory should be appraised:

1. How to *find*, refine, and prepare a biological system for the functionality of the bioproduct.
2. How to *optimize* the performance of the biosystem by its interplay with the environment within and around the bioproduct.
3. How to ensure a *high quality* of its functions and performance in its environment.
4. How to *stabilize* the performance over the operative timespan.

5. How to *economize* the production, assembling, and operation of the bioproduct and allow scaling to the market volume in terms of production methods or else.

To *identify and find the biological systems* capable of solving the challenges and, if possible, modify and prepare these for the intended product is the ultimate key for successful bioengineering design. This can be diversified into the following three aspects:

- *Which are the feasible biological systems for new or refined products*? There are always many plausible alternatives. A ranking of these is necessary, but this must be according to several relevant criteria. Those criteria are set by both the users of the product and its manufacturers.
- *How can biological systems, such as cellular micro-factories, be best exploited to fulfil the users/customers' needs*? What alternative solutions can be considered? Of course, a cellular micro-factory approach can always be compared with a chemical or biosynthetic sequence of reactions where critical parameters may be more controllable and reproducible.
- *Are such desired biological systems available in Nature or must they be engineered by using state-of-the-art genetic and cell engineering techniques*? This is a matter of judgement on what will be the most demanding and laborious approach. Maybe it is better to engineer a new biosystem, provided the skills are at hand in the developer's own lab, or possibly to be acquired from collaborating partners.

Usually, this is to provide the optimal design or to configure the design. When exploiting the "cell factory"—concept *optimization* is a valuable approach to leverage the performance.

- The optimization can be accomplished by increased reaction density of a biosystem (Fig. 2.3). More cells per volume or higher reactivity within the cells could ensure optimal reaction density (Pörtner 2021).
- This could be the availability of metabolic paths, either existing in an original biosystem or by creating new pathways. These possibilities are unique for biosystems (Nielsen et al. 2011).
- The result of changing conditions, through optimizations or genetic manipulation, must be possible to observe. This could be by utilizing various omics techniques (Mann 2018).

Ensuring high product quality is a multifaceted challenge. Paramount to this effort is the ability to maximize biological activity per product unit, which is typically quantified through specific reaction rates (as outlined in Table 2.2). Access to precise analytical methods is therefore indispensable for monitoring quality. Key to these measurements is the ability to compare the reactivity or conversion rates of alternative systems both before and after genetic modification. This verification process requires micro-scale biological experiments to validate expected performance improvements.

The fact that products not involving biological systems usually have better *long-term stability* than biological products makes it pivotal to enhance and maintain the stability of the biological system. Understanding stabilization and causes of instabilities is therefore very important.

- The stability of the produced bioproduct, especially when this is a metabolite, a protein, or other vulnerable biopolymer, restricts the design of the product as well as the production process, although the critical issue is the finally formulated product.
- Methods are either formulation with additives that stabilize the structure, or immobilization methods for stabilizing the 3D structure by binding to supports of an otherwise vulnerable protein. If the protein is an active analytical protein in an assay, a biosensor, or else, binding to membranes or other solid supports could be an efficient methodology to apply.
- Storage stability should necessarily be maintained over extended periods of time until the expiry date. This will be a critical quality criterion for a bioproduct, whatever use is concerned (drugs, food, test materials, etc.).

Does the biological system favor the stability and repeatability of performance that makes the product reliable? Frequently, these operational boundaries are strictly defined by regulatory agency requirements.

Can biological systems survive in a new product under the anticipated user conditions and timespan? This information is typically obtained directly from users or regulatory bodies. Thus, the conditions at the site of the user, such as temperature and isolation, become critical design factors.

A plethora of possibilities exist that can be employed to approach the challenges mentioned (Fig. 2.6). These possibilities are all well established in modern bioengineering. As illustrated, diverse metabolic and genetic engineering strategies can be deployed to enhance the performance capacity of the host cell factory. Additionally, multi-omics techniques enable engineers to precisely identify rate-limiting pathways and quantify metabolic fluxes, providing actionable targets for system optimization.

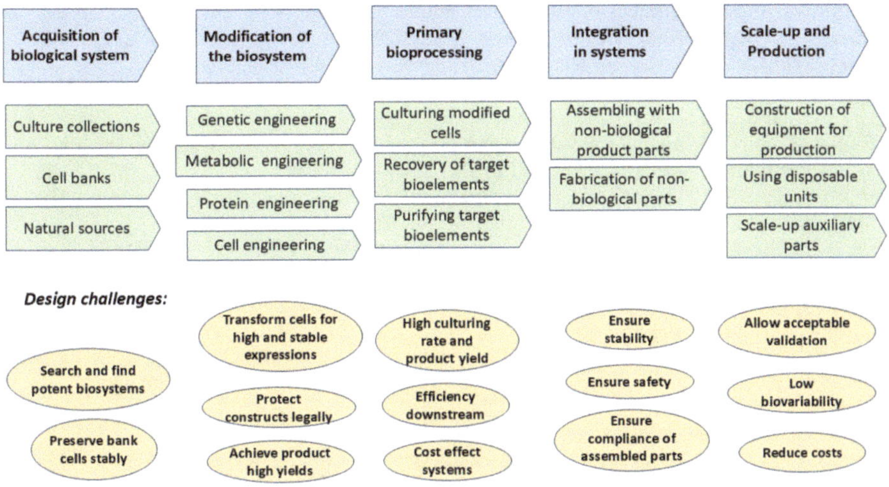

Fig. 2.6 Bioengineering design requires a deep understanding of biological system operations. Irrespective of the specific bioproduct under development, the elements requiring the greatest design attention are fundamentally driven by their underlying biological properties. The targeted biological system must be identified, refined, produced, and rigorously verified and validated. Resolving the associated challenges (indicated by yellow circles) directly relies on the multidisciplinary skills of the design team

References

Ahmad HM, Rashid M, Rahman MU et al (2015) Ethical issues of biotechnology, possible risks and their management. J Biol Agricult Healthcare 5(11):49–54. ISSN 2225-093X

Alberts B, Hopkin K, Johnson A et al (2019) Essential cell biology, 5th edn. Norton & Co, New york

Arivaradarajan P, Misra G (2018) Omics approaches, technologies and applications: integrative approaches for understanding omics data. Springer

Atkins P, Ratcliffe G, Wormald M et al (2023) Physical chemistry for the life sciences. Oxford University Press, Oxford

Beard DA, Qian H (2010) Chemical biophysics, Quantitative analysis of cellular systems. Cambridge University Press, Cambridge

Brereton RG (2003) Chemometrics, data analysis for laboratory and chemical plants. Wiley, Chichester, UK

Doran PM (2013) Biochemical engineering principles, 2nd edn. Elsevier, Amsterdam. https://doi.org/10.1016/C2009-0-22348-8

Dym CL, Agogino AM, Eris O et al (2005) Engineering design thinking, teaching and learning. J Eng Educ 94:103–120. https://doi.org/10.1002/j.2168-9830.2005.tb00832.x

European Medicines Agency (2016) European medicines Agency's guideline on process validation for the manufacture of biotechnology-derived active substances and data to be provided in the regulatory submission. European Medicines Agency, London

European Medicines Agency (2025) European Medicines Agency's scientific quality guidelines. https://www.ema.europa.eu/en/human-regulatory-overview/research-development/scientific-guidelines/quality-guidelines. Retrieved October 2025

United States' Food and Drug Administration (2011) Current Good Manufacturing Practices (CGMP): guidance for industry process validation: general principles and

practices. U.S. Department of Health and Human Services, Food and Drug Administration, Center for Drug Evaluation and Research (CDER), Center for Biologics Evaluation and Research (CBER), Center for Veterinary Medicine (CVM), Washington
Goldman J (2022) Textbook on biotechnology. Larsen and Leller Education, New York. ISBN 978 164 172 261 22
Harmsen J (2013) Industrial process scale-up. A practical Innovation guide from idea to commercial implementation, Elsevier, Amsterdam. ISBN 9780444627261
Harnish V, Ross S (2022) Scaling up compensation: five design principles for turning your largest expense into a strategic advantage. Forbes Books, Charleston
Heinzle E, Biwer A, Cooney C (2006) Development of sustainable bioprocesses. Modelling and assessment. Wiley, Chichester
Hubka V, Eder WE (1988) Theory of technical systems, a total concept theory for engineering design. Springer Verlag, Berlin
International Council of Harmonization (1995) International Council of Harmonization's (ICH) quality guideline Q5C. Quality of biotechnology products Stability testing, 5th edn.
Jagschies G, Lindskog E, Lacki K et al (2017) Biopharmaceutical processing development, design, and implementation of manufacturing processes. Elsevier, Amsterdam
Kristiansen B (2006) Process economics. In: Ratledge C, Kristiansen B (eds) Basic biotechnology, 3rd edn. Cambridge University Press, Cambridge, pp 239–252
Kuszler PC (2006) Biotechnology entrepreneurship and ethics: principles, paradigms, and products. Med Law 25:491–502. https://digitalcommons.law.uw.edu/faculty-articles/419
O'Mathúna DP (2007) Bioethics and biotechnology. Cytotechnol 53:113–119. https://doi.org/10.1007/s10616-007-9053-8
Mandenius CF, Björkman M (2011) Biomechatronic design in biotechnology: a methodology for development of biotechnology products. Wiley, Hoboken. https://doi.org/10.1002/9781118067147
Mandenius CF (ed) (2016) Bioreactors: design, operation and novel applications. Wiley VCH, Weinheim
Mann R (2018) Genetic engineering and biotechnology. Callisto Reference ISBN 9781632399205.
Moorthy K (2017) Fundamentals of biochemical calculations, 2nd edn. CRC Press, Boca Raton
Nielsen J, Villadsen J, Lidén G (2011) Bioreaction engineering principles, 3rd edn. Springer-Nature, New York
O'Brian D (2019) Engineer 4.0: life science handbook for medical devices and biopharmaceuticals. Kindle Edition ISBN-13: 978-1795753340
Pahl G, Beitz W, Feldhusen J et al (2007) Engineering design, a systematic approach, 3rd edn. Springer Verlag, Berlin
Parke VC (2020) Biophysics, a student guide to physics of the life sciences and medicine. Springer, New York
Pörtner R (ed) (2021) Cell culture engineering and technology. Springer Nature, New York, USA. https://doi.org/10.1007/978-3-030-79871-0
Peters MS, Timmerhaus KD, West RE (2003) Plant design and economics for chemical engineers, 5th edn. McGraw-Hill, New York
Price NC, Dwek RA, Ratcliffe RG et al (2001) Principles and problems in physical chemistry for biochemists. Oxford University Press, Oxford
Ray SC, Chambers RG, Kumbhakar SC (2022) Handbook of production economics. Springer Nature, New York
Ratledge C, Kristiansen B (eds) (2006) Basic biotechnology, 3rd edn. Cambridge University Press, Cambridge
Santoro FA (2012) Ethical considerations when prescribing biologics in dermatology. Clin Dermatol 30:492–495. https://doi.org/10.1016/j.clindermatol.2011.06.018
Sneppen K (2014) Models of life. Dynamics and regulation in biological systems. Cambridge University Press, Cambridge

Saterbek A, San KY, McIntire LV (2018) Bioengineering fundamentals, 2nd edn. Pearson Education, New York

Swamy AVN (2015) Fundamentals of biochemical engineering. Student edn. BS Publications

Silvermann E (2004) The five most pressing ethical issues in biotech medicine. Biotechnol Healthcare 1(6):41–46. (December 2004)

Towler G, Sinnott R (2012) Chemical engineering design: principles, practice and economics of plant and process design, 2nd edn. Elsevier, Amsterdam

Ulrich KT, Eppinger SD, Yang MC (2019) Product design and development, 7th edn. McGraw-Hill, New York

United States' National Institute for Medical Research (2023) The human genetic mutant cell repository: list of genetic variants, chromosomal aberrations and normal cell cultures submitted to the repository, 4th edn. United States National Institute for Medical Research, Legare Street Press, Camden. ISBN: 10-102149335X, ISBN-13: 978-1021493354

Williams D (2014) Essential biomaterials science. Cambridge University Press, Cambridge

Gong Z, Nielsen J, Zhou YJ (2017) Engineering robustness of microbial cell factories. Biotechnol J 12(10):1700014. https://doi.org/10.1002/biot.201700014

Chapter 3
Methodology for Bioengineering Design

The methodological frameworks pivotal to successful bioengineering design are described. Once initial bioproduct ideas have been appraised through fundamental scientific principles, they must be refined using structured and versatile design methodologies. When applied wisely, these methods transform inventive ideas into sustainable, commercially viable bioproducts.

The methodological approaches encompass conceptual design—focusing on functional architectures and user requirements—alongside specialized biotechnological methods for improving biological systems. Production conditions are especially highlighted from upscaling to market demands, validation and testing of products, and production economic perspectives. The utility of digital tools is also critically appraised, providing specific implementation recommendations for design work.

The methodologies will subsequently be integrated into the training procedures and applied in the design cases described in the two forthcoming chapters.

3.1 Design Methodologies: Their Purpose and Utility

Bioengineering design work relies on applying powerful methodologies once a new inventive idea has been analyzed by fundamental principles. The methodologies must be distinctly defined and their utility for bioproduct design explained before they are used in training (Doran 2013; Pahl et al. 2007; Nielsen et al. 2011; O'Brian 2019; Ulrich et al. 2019).

Once a new inventive bioproduct idea is found to comply with fundamental scientific and engineering principles as described in the previous chapter, established design methodologies should be applied for the idea's realization into a functional bioproduct. These methodologies are all well-established and widely demonstrated and can thus be exploited for bioengineering design purposes. At the stage of implementation and construction of the design, they also become enabling development tools to evaluate and test the products, prototypes, or pilot processes.

C.-F. Mandenius, *Bioengineering Design Methodology*,
https://doi.org/10.1007/978-3-032-33940-9_3

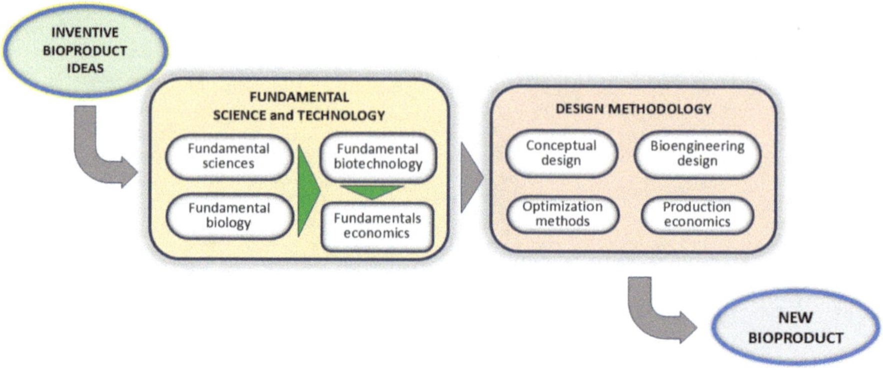

Fig. 3.1 Flow of design work from ideas to new bioproducts where design methodologies such as conceptual design, optimization, and production economy analysis shape the ideas into a new viable bioproduct

The design methodologies include methods for conceptual design, functional design, mathematical modelling, optimization, product testing and validation, scale-up of production, and digital techniques for drawing, construction, and production economics (Ulrich et al. 2019; Mandenius 2016; Heinzle et al. 2006; Peters et al. 2003).

As already emphasized in Chap. 2, it is the fundamental scientific principles that should be the first filter to test the solidity of the inventive product idea. That should be followed by implementing and refining the design using appropriate design methodologies with the aim of leveraging the functionality of the idea (Fig. 3.1).

The methodologies should ensure that the design reaches several critical criteria:

- *To satisfy* the users' demand for functionality of the product
- *To ensure* that all potentially viable design options are reviewed and evaluated at a conceptual level
- *To pave the way* for a technical realization of the concepts
- *To assess* the economic feasibility for manufacturing the product
- *To ensure* that the production can be scaled up to volumes requested by the market
- *To plan* for optimizing the properties, shape, and performance of the final product

These six criteria are all dependent on the ability to apply design methodologies for reaching the intended outcome (Table 3.1). The ensuing part of this chapter provides the methodological approach for this. The design cases in Chap. 5 will further demonstrate how the methodologies are applied for a variety of bioproduct examples.

Table 3.1 Design purposes of a new product by applicable methodologies and intended outcomes

Purposes	Methodologies	Intended outcome
Align with user needs and market requirements	Market research, stakeholder interviews, functional requirement identification, benchmarking, and demand prioritization/specification	Act as an initial filter to eliminate unfeasible design concepts with low market viability
Critically evaluate potential design solutions	Systematically map functional architectures to identify configuration options and evaluate feasibility using existing technologies	Develop a refined set of viable design configurations optimized against user criteria
Evaluate economic feasibility	Perform techno-economic assessments of manufacturing costs relative to projected sales volumes	Act as an economic filter to eliminate cost-prohibitive design variants
Assess process and product scalability	Model production volumes against bioreactor/process sizing metrics and capital/operating expenses	Define production cost margins across realistic and projected market scales
Optimize products and production processes	Investigate parametric optimization strategies to maximize product yields and manufacturing efficiencies	Forecast the long-term potential for cost reduction across the product life cycle
Predict and mitigate technical risks	Conduct strengths, weaknesses, opportunities, and threats (SWOT) analyses to assess design sensitivities	Identify systemic vulnerabilities and establish proactive mitigation strategies
Validate end-user performance	Execute user-acceptance testing and real-world performance validation protocols	Establish an empirical validation filter to finalize the design solution

3.2 Implementing Method Frameworks in Bioengineering Design

The methodologies most vital to bioengineering design encompass systematic techniques and digital tools for conceptual refinement, parameter optimization, process scale-up, and techno-economic assessment (Petrides 2015; Martins and Ning 2021; Harnish and Ross 2022; Towler and Sinnott 2012). To maximize efficacy, these analytical frameworks must be deployed in a disciplined, sequential order that remains consistent across all bioengineering design missions (Fig. 3.2):

- Best practice dictates that designers initially evaluate a novel, innovative bioproduct concept entirely from the end-user's perspective. Trained and insightful engineers must analyze the inventive idea conceptually, leveraging this overview to converge the design into superior, more functional alternatives that respect the boundaries of specific consumer and market constraints (Fig. 3.2a).
- Once these overarching design objectives are framed and the underlying user requirements are thoroughly defined and clarified, the core biological and engineering functionalities required for system execution can be systematically identified. This is done primarily with respect to the required biology and technology. Aspects of biological systems are considered first and are followed by aspects of technical systems.

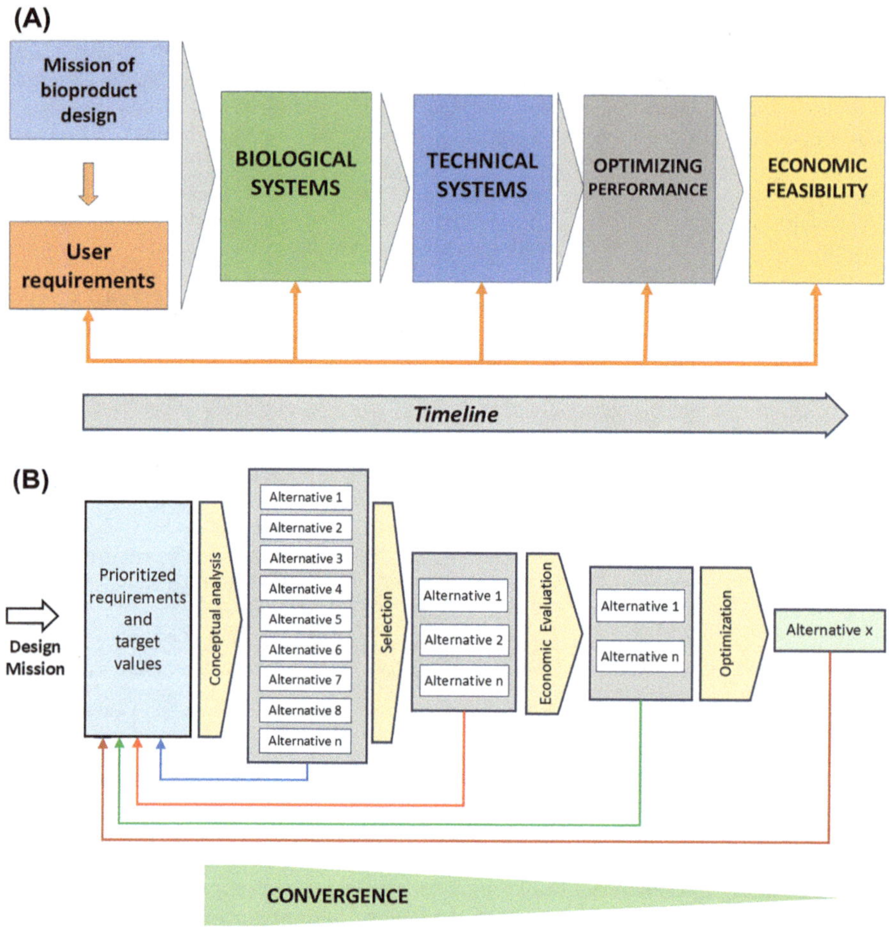

Fig. 3.2 (**a**) The typical order of work in a bioengineering design mission where powerful methodologies are used to develop, refine, and optimize the design from biological, technical, and economic aspects. (**b**) The convergence of emerging alternative design solutions into a prioritized alternative

- This should be followed by studying critical aspects of how the number of alternatives can be reduced due to their feasibility in meeting the users' needs. The chosen alternatives are, because of their feasibility, prone to be optimized by established engineering methods.
- Once optimized, final testing and validation of the production economics tells if the design has a good opportunity for becoming a competitive bioproduct on an existing market. This requires a close eye on the manufacturability of the alternatives, and their pricing and marketing possibilities. It is advantageous to perform economic evaluation interactively with optimization, so that the optimization parameters become those that best contribute to a favorable economy.

SWOT analysis (i.e., strengths, weaknesses, opportunities, and threats) is very useful as a "litmus testing" of the robustness of the design (Shinno et al. 2006). Along this path of work, the design converges into what should be the strongest alternative.

- During the development, potential design alternatives to the original product idea will initially diverge considerably. However, the alternatives become fewer when compared with the user requirements and economic prerequisites (Fig. 3.2b). Infeasible alternatives are expelled, making remaining alternatives converge to better opportunities to comply with the user requirements. Sometimes the outcome is unquestionable, while sometimes it may be a difficult matter of decision-making for the inventors, developers, and investors to find the most appropriate solutions that fulfil the business ambitions and targets for the product.

Is there a best methodological practice for designing in bioengineering? Or should different bioproducts or production systems influence the selection of methods?

At a holistic level, every bioproduct or production system can be described as a transformation process with inputs and outputs converted by functional systems. The transformation can be related to any bioproduct, whether it involves biological molecules or cells, information in and from analytical devices, or biotech services. This transformation process can be adapted to a variety of biological and technical functions. The functions can subsequently be exchanged with real components. These components will be possible to relate to material and energy consumption, and labor costs.

The approach has the great advantage of not taking it for granted that there is only one design alternative for reaching a design solution that complies with the users' needs.

This approach is particularly useful for design when biological systems are objects. The tools that are of most value are those that can elucidate the biological capacity in terms of selectivity (or specificity), reactivity per unit (volumetric or mass-related), longevity (stability or reproducibility), and availability (how easy the species of biomolecules can be accessed). These metrics serve to rank the biological system's capacity to fulfill the specific functional requirements of the design.

Design methodologies should look for diverse solutions. An alternative could be to ask if biological systems should be considered at all. Maybe the same functional outcome can be accomplished by non-biological means. For example, chemical reactions can sometimes carry out the same conversions as done in biological metabolic networks. If the number of reaction steps is few, classical reaction chemistry can perhaps provide better stability or reproducibility and at lower costs. Bioanalytical affinity systems can be replaced by molecular imprinted polymers, able to recognize target molecules for diagnostic or other analytical purposes.

From an industrial perspective, an attractive possibility is to redesign and reengineer existing products. Thereby, much design work can be circumvented. Perhaps production can be reused. Well-known cell lines with established protocols and already thoroughly investigated cell mechanisms can be utilized again, thereby reducing R&D costs and demand on regulatory testing. If old bioreactors, centrifuges, and chromatographic equipment can be reused, investments can be scaled down.

Another potential possibility is to reduce R&D by testing a new product directly on the market. Regulators demand testing and verification, allowing sales on a global market. However, regulatory thresholds have steadily increased in the protection of human health and welfare. Competition puts harder pressure on both the quality and price of new bioproducts. Investors have high demand for product development and do not accept failed launches. Thus, the market should not be used as a testing arena.

Alternatively, attempting to accelerate development by launching a new bioproduct directly into the market to bypass rigorous research and development (R&D) introduces severe risk. Regulatory agencies mandate exhaustive testing and validation protocols before permitting sales on the global market. Furthermore, these regulatory thresholds have steadily intensified to ensure the uncompromising protection of human health and environmental welfare. Concurrently, intense market competition exerts significant pressure on both the quality and pricing of novel bioproducts. Because capital investors demand highly reliable product development pipelines and rarely tolerate failed commercial launches, the commercial market must never be used as a testing ground.

3.3 Design Mission and User Requirements

The aim of the methodologies is that they should systematically substantiate and refine the inventive idea. The mission of developing the inventive idea must result in a product that complies with the actual needs and requirements of the intended users of the bioproduct.

With the term *design mission,* we include the work for carrying out the design of the product idea according to defined objectives of the final product. It requires adapting the idea in a realistic fashion according to user and market conditions. For example, the new inventive idea of a diagnostic device must, in its design, consider its manufacture as well as fulfilling the critical criteria for being an attractive product on the market. The design mission should also ensure this.

The primary aim of these methodologies is to systematically substantiate and refine the initial inventive concept. Developing an inventive idea must culminate in a bioproduct that directly complies with the empirical needs and requirements of its intended users.

The term *design mission* encompasses the entire scope of work required to translate a product concept into reality based on the defined objectives of the final product. This process requires adapting the initial idea realistically to align with both user and market conditions. For example, the design mission for a novel diagnostic device must simultaneously address manufacturing feasibility and satisfy the critical criteria necessary for market competitiveness. Ensuring this dual optimization is a core requirement of the design mission.

In every mission, it is paramount to distinctly clarify the design objectives. This is intertwined between the inventive idea and user needs. For bioproducts, the idea may emanate from a biological capacity that is to be exploited as well as meet the utility or needs of the presumed users. Obviously, one must ensure that these needs are known and thoroughly understood, evaluated, and considered. This insight is then used for carrying out the design of the idea into a functional final product.

The user concept is here seen in a wide sense and can be distinguished in the following groups:

- Users that will use the final product themselves (the end-users)
- Users that will provide the product to the end-user group (e.g., doctors, pharmacies, vendors of food and other consumer products)
- Users that will manufacture the product (workers/production managers of a manufacturing factory for the product)
- Users that expect to profit from the product (inventors in the product, owners of the company providing the product, the management of the company)

In this context, the user concept is interpreted in a broad sense and can be categorized into the following distinct stakeholder groups:

- *End-Users*: Individuals who will directly interact with and utilize the final bioproduct
- *Intermediary Providers*: Professionals and vendors who distribute or prescribe the product to the end-user population, including physicians, pharmacists, and consumer goods distributors
- *Manufacturing Personnel*: Plant operators, technicians, and production managers responsible for the physical fabrication and scale-up of the product within the manufacturing facility
- *Commercial Stakeholders*: Parties who expect an economic return from the product, such as inventors, corporate management, and equity investors

These categories of user groups have all their own needs and expectations that affect the design mission. Surely, the needs of the users may change over time for various reasons (new and better products with the same functionality, revenue too low for the investors, etc.) (Table 3.2).

Furthermore, it is necessary to understand what type of needs should be dealt with. These can be simplified into the following statements:

- Needs related to what the product should achieve; or, differently said, what functional manifestation should be achieved by the product.
- Needs related to values that the users prioritize.
- Needs that are either qualitative or quantitative. Thus, the users may be able to express different desires for the product's capabilities. In the best case, this is possible to express with a number or range that is measurable; other needs that are difficult to define, for example, usefulness for a practical purpose.

The next step is to prioritize the needs and requirements. The priorities should be related to a variety of needs and requirements: from the customers, the market, the

Table 3.2 Needs and requirements for a new bioproduct for those involved in its use and production

User category	Typical needs and requirements	Consequences for the design
End-users	High reliability, intuitive usability, cost-effectiveness, and convenient accessibility	Embed specific, high-performance physical and functional attributes directly into the product architecture
Distributors and intermediaries	Product trustworthiness, exhaustive validation testing, and high supply-chain reliability	Optimize storage stability (shelf-life), packaging dimensions, transport logistics, and comprehensive quality assurance protocols
Production operators and plant managers	Robust process control, straightforward product testing/quality control, and high capacity for automation	Simplify the manufacturing process layout, design easily controllable unit operations, and integrate automated monitoring loops
Company management	Low production costs, highly reproducible quality, and straightforward manufacturing logistics	Prioritize parameter optimization, robust scaling methodologies, and minimal manufacturing facility footprints.
Investors and corporate owners	High profit margins, minimized operating expenditures, and strong market competitiveness	Minimize manufacturing cost-of-goods-sold (COGS) and maximize product differentiation relative to existing alternatives

business activities, and combinations of these. The company activities encompass the manufacture of products, sales strategy activities, cost reduction, and short lead times. The ranking of priorities will depend on the company's focus. These priorities must hold a certain standard. Standards must be quantifiable and possible to assess. Ranking of these is decided by those who are expected to use the invention. The standards are reached by the elements that form the prerequisites for them. Neglecting to grasp the real user needs risks resulting in a failed design. This requires an interplay between the users/customers and the developers/producers.

3.4 Translating the Design Mission into Functionality

Once the user needs are established and prioritized, they must be framed from a functionality perspective (Pahl et al. 2007). The purpose of the functionalities is to generalize these needs and investigate all potential design options of interest. The aim is to identify these options in terms of what they can achieve.

Consequently, during the product formation phase, engineering priorities must center on end-user requirements rather than the underlying technology itself. If a scientifically sound inventive concept fails to address the specific functional needs of its target stakeholders, its prospects for market viability remain severely limited. A recurring risk in engineering design is that inventors overvalue commercial opportunities, neglect practical functional perspectives, and become overly captivated by

Table 3.3 Five types of bioproducts with varying expectations on functionality

Bioproduct	Product performance functionality	Desired functionality
(i) Therapeutic cell cultures	High tissue biocompatibility, strict analytical purity, and predictable in vivo efficacy	Rapid, patient-specific manufacturing turnaround and just-in-time delivery logistics
(ii) Biotherapeutic drugs	High clinical efficacy, established safety profiles, and robust formulation shelf-stability	Noninvasive or simplified administration routes, standard storage requirements, and convenient patient formats
(iii) Cultured food products	Optimality in organoleptic profiles (taste, odor, visual appeal) and high nutritional density	Extended shelf-life, minimal storage constraints, and straightforward culinary preparation/handling
(iv) Biological service systems	High analytical precision, low limits of detection, and robust reproducibility	Streamlined, user-adapted data reporting and rapid turnaround times for actionable results
(v) Diagnostic devices	High clinical sensitivity, analytical selectivity, and technical repeatability	Intuitive point-of-care usability, automated operation, and reliable reagent supply chains

the novelty of a technological breakthrough. Paradoxically, acquiring exclusive intellectual property rights and scaling up production for a standalone technology is relatively straightforward (Shinno et al. 2006); however, securing long-term market adoption demands an uncompromising alignment with user expectations.

Five types of bioproducts dominate in bioengineering (Table 3.3). Their unique functionalities explain this dominance: (i) Cells with unique biological capacities such as regenerative tissue cells and edible cells. (ii) Proteins or other biomolecules with therapeutic capacity to cure diseases. (iii) Cultured food products with better nutritional properties. (iv) A service organization providing reliable testing service of drug and food. (iv) A diagnostic tool able to measure fast and accurately disease-related targets.

Functional utility is highly context-dependent, varying significantly across product classes and end-use applications. While certain biological products maintain long-term market tenure, others fail to withstand competitive pressures. Retrospectively, product viability, or lack thereof, can be attributed to functional superiority relative to contemporary alternatives. However, these benchmarks are dynamic; the necessity to reconcile evolving functional requirements serves as the primary catalyst for innovation, driving the development of inventive solutions that navigate these shifting performance landscapes.

Consequently, defined functionalities represent the core elements of the engineering design process. They should ensure that the product reaches supremacy through a streamlined design from raw materials and other inputs to a functional product on the market.

In this context, conceptualization refers to the process of conceiving and elucidating the functional interplay that defines the final product. Each primary function can be analyzed as a discrete system, which in turn encompasses its own hierarchy of subordinate subsystems.

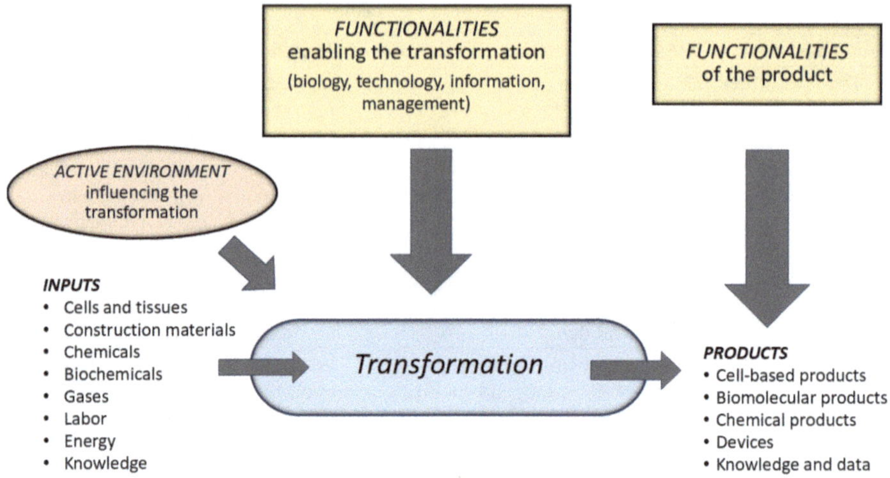

Fig. 3.3 The two functionality aspects should be considered in relation to the transformation process when designing a bioproduct: (i) the functionality of the production process and (ii) the functionality of the product itself

Thus, two perspectives of functionality must both be covered in the design (Fig. 3.3):

- The users' expectations on the functionality of the product they acquire
- The functionality that enables the transformation of inputs as raw materials and other components to become the final product

From an engineering perspective, it is critical to thoroughly investigate every dimension of system functionality prior to equipment selection. Designers frequently transition from functional definitions to process operations prematurely, mistakenly substituting abstract functions with specific unit operations and mechanical equipment within early-stage design solutions. This premature convergence can be systematically mitigated by strictly applying functional diagrams that are entirely devoid of the physical apparatuses intended to execute those functions. Focusing solely on *what* must be accomplished, rather than *how* it will be achieved, deliberately delays equipment selection.

Consequently, all essential product functionalities are comprehensively analyzed before being objectified into physical hardware. This approach establishes a disciplined, stepwise understanding, ensuring that technical gear and specific experimental or process procedures are introduced only in later design stages. These biological functions and unit operations can subsequently be configured into logical sequences that remain valid across multiple potential solutions using different physical objects. Ultimately, this structured abstraction allows design solutions to converge into a select few candidates that optimize alignment with end-user, market, and production requirements.

3.5 Conceptualization of the Design

The functionalities needed for driving the transformation of inputs of raw materials and other resources to the desired product can be diversified into technical functions, information functions, management functions, and human functions (Hubka and Eder 1988; Mandenius and Björkman 2011). These functions are realized by systems and subsystems that interact with the transformation process, independently or in consort, to transform inputs into the final product. This leads to a complex pattern of interplay between the systems.

To be understandable, the structure of these functional systems must be schematized (Fig. 3.4a). Such schemes should be further detailed by their interactions with the transformation.

When drawing the conceptual scheme, the prioritized needs should have a significant impact on its shape so that the needs decide the choice of functions and systems to be involved in the transformation. Consequently:

- The *biological systems* must have such functionality that the biological transformation needs can be reached.
- Also, the *technical systems* must have such functionality that these can handle the biological functions according to the expressed needs and targets.
- The *information function* must ensure that the product's capacity to reach the targeted needs is possible to observe.
- The *human functions* concern both the customers' requirements and practice but should also concern the requirements of the manufacturing personnel.
- The *managerial functions* coordinate and control the transformation according to targets. Especially in the food and pharmaceutical industry, it involves regulatory issues. Public laws and rules must be obeyed, and the design must consider this in the design of the new product and set its target values.

During the translation of an inventive concept into a viable bioproduct, the core biological functionality, along with the specific systems and subsystems required for its realization, remain paramount. Consequently, at this stage of the design process, it is highly advantageous to thoroughly investigate the biological systems and systematically analyze their interfaces with other functional engineering domains.

These complex interfaces can be analyzed in a structured manner using an interaction matrix (Fig. 3.4b). The *x*- and *y*-axes of this matrix map the various functional systems against the sequential transformation steps, highlighting the significance of each intersection. Crucially, interactions can occur in opposite directions; while one functional system may influence another, the reverse cross-coupling effect must also be evaluated. This requires a comprehensive assessment of the nodes on both sides of the matrix diagonal. For most bioengineering applications, it is sufficient to evaluate these matrix nodes using a three-tiered qualitative scale (e.g., critical, relevant, or negligible), although a higher quantitative resolution can be applied if necessary.

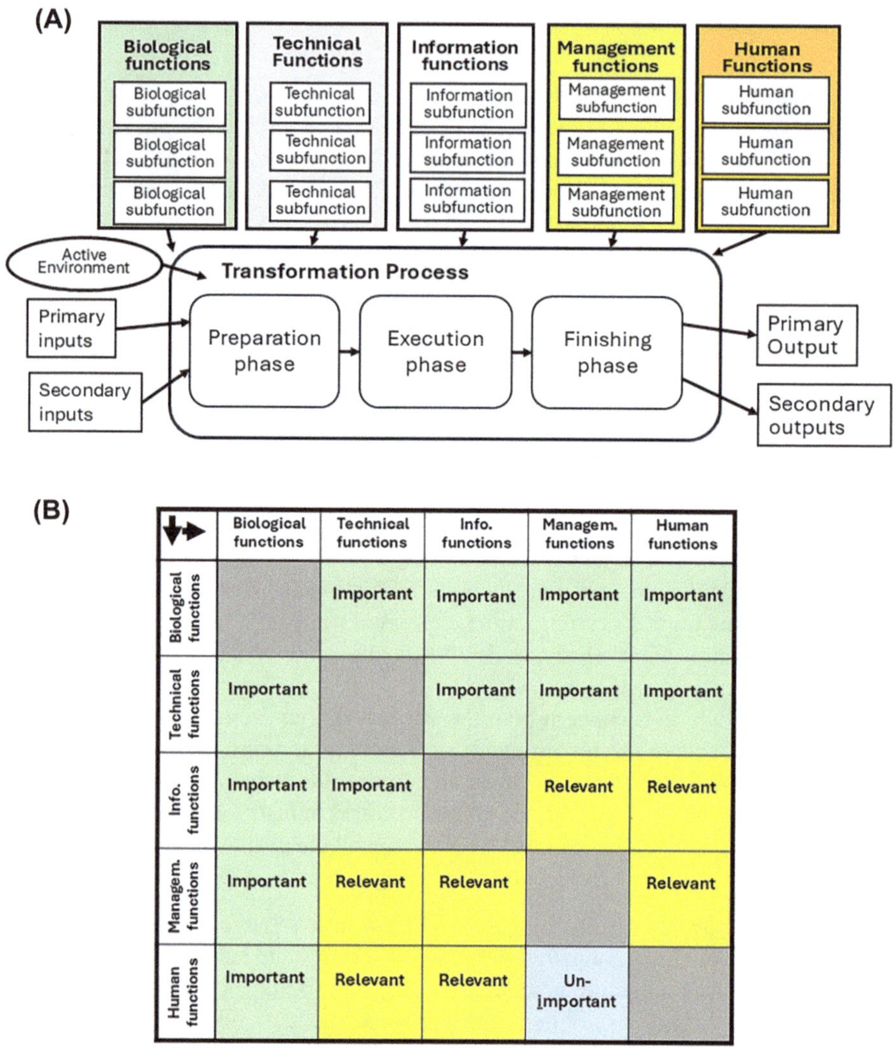

Fig. 3.4 (**a**) The transformation process, the inputs and outputs to and from it, and the functional systems and subsystems required. (**b**) An interaction matrix of functional systems, subsystems and transformation process. (**c**) Functional components arranged in alternative configurations

After studying the interactions, the conceptual analysis proceeds by identifying functional entities or components that are needed to carry out the transformation (Fig. 3.4c). At this stage in the design work, it is still the identified functional entities, and not real objects, that drive the transformation. The functions are configured in a

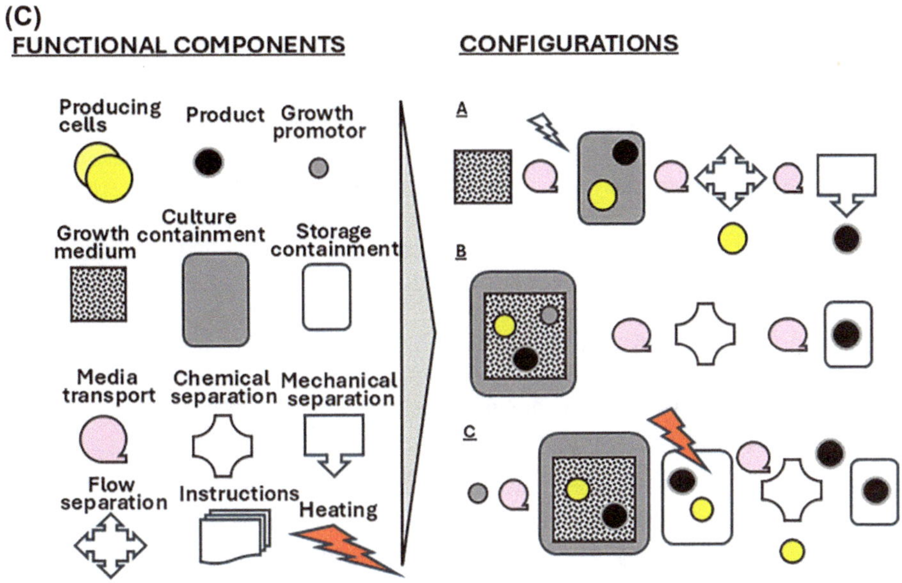

Fig. 3.4 (continued)

consecutive transformation sequence. There are many alternatives to configure the functions which the designers should investigate.

The alternative configurations are compared with the priorities and metrics of the users' needs. This indicates which sequences are most relevant at this level of design development.

The configurations that comply with the objectives of the design mission and the expressed needs are of interest to develop further. First at this stage, the transformation process can be turned into a schematic drawing with real objects. Each functional object can be replaced with more than one possible object, such as a biological unit, technical machine, or other technical device, for carrying out a function. For example, different cell types can exhibit the functionality of biological conversion; several containments of cell cultures can be used. An iterative procedure for modifying and reconsidering these choices is recommended.

The configurations that comply with the objectives of the design mission and the documented user requirements are selected for further development. At this stage, the functional transformation process can be translated into a schematic engineering drawing populated with physical components. Each abstract function can be mapped to multiple potential physical alternatives, such as a specific biological unit, mechanical machine, or specialized technical device.

For example, different cell types can exhibit the functionality of biological conversion; several containments of cell cultures can be used. Adopting a structured, iterative procedure to continuously modify, evaluate, and refine these physical choices is highly recommended to optimize the final configuration.

3.6 Improving Performance of Biological Systems

The outcome of bioengineering design depends heavily on effectively exploiting a biological system's inherent capacity to carry out the transformation process. However, identifying and deploying methodologies that can efficiently optimize the design of these biological systems remains a significant challenge. These methodologies should primarily strive to augment the host cell factory's metabolic potential, product yield, and overall process robustness (Fig. 3.5). It is not too difficult to foresee in theory how improved performance can be achieved, in relation to the objectives and functionalities of a bioproduct. What is not easy to anticipate is how such development efforts can be managed sufficiently well to lead to the desired performance outcome in a cost-efficient way.

There are primarily seven biotechnological methodologies and techniques that have the potential to enable this:

1. *Cell engineering* methods for modifying the whole cell's growth and metabolism, usually with the purpose of enhancing the productivity of the bioproduct. It is partly accomplished by using combinations of the techniques below (Pörtner 2021; Al-Rubeai and Naciri 2014).
2. *Protein engineering* methods for changing the peptide sequence to improve the function of the folded protein, for example, by stronger affinity, better catalytic activity, or higher stability. This leads to improved bioanalytical performance or product formation (Wong and Tee 2020; Bornscheuer and Höhle 2018).
3. *Genetic engineering* methods for changing the gene sequence and its translation to express a new peptide or a peptide with another amino acid sequence. The new sequence could introduce a new function of the cell, such as a new protein

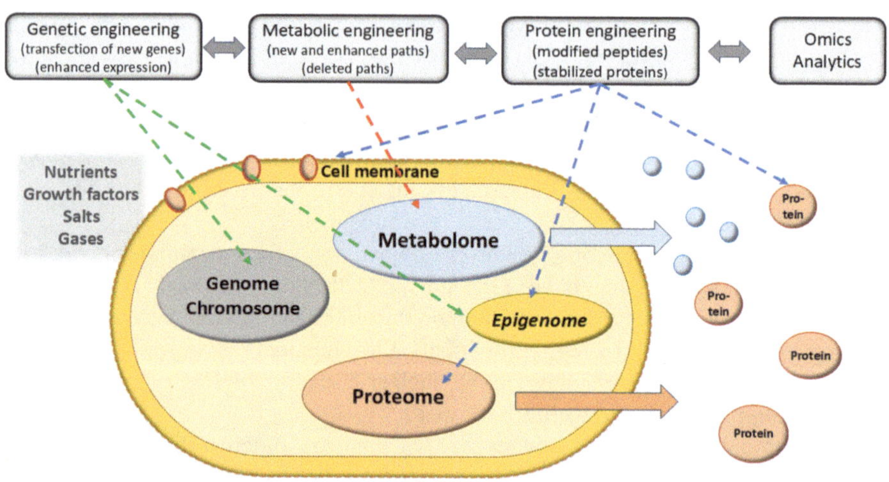

Fig. 3.5 Biotechnological core methodologies have the capability to enhance the capacity of biological cells in a variety of bioproducts; these are eminent tools for enabling successful designs

product, or modify the cell physiologically for enhancing productivity (Mann 2018; Jazayeri et al. 2018).

4. *Metabolic engineering* methods are based on applying previous methods for introducing new metabolic pathways or to speed up rates in bottleneck steps in a pathway. New product formation or enhanced productivity of existing pathways will become a result (Nielsen et al. 2021).
5. *Cell selection* by efficiently applying screening techniques will allow the selection of useful cell lines with favorable productivity of the product. The screening techniques can be used for natural as well as modified cell lines or strains. The impact on design is profound when a significantly more productive cell line is identified (Ahmad et al. 2015).
6. *Omics methodologies* for analyzing and monitoring biological and biochemical properties and activities. Omics techniques support the above methodologies as well as facilitate bioengineering design (Arivaradarajan and Misra 2018).
7. Access to *molecular libraries or cell repositories*, either commercially available or established in-house, by providing powerful resources for bioengineering design (American Type Culture Collection 1992; US National Institute for Medical Research 2023).

Generic engineering methods are especially interesting for bioengineering design due to their impact on the performance of biological systems and should be devoted to actions such as:

- Increasing specific rates of each cell in the biosystem
- Enhancing stability and reducing degradation of expressed product
- Developing better inducer and promoter systems in the used expression vectors.
- Adapting the expression systems to selected host cells
- Improving host cells in terms of stability of vectors and expressed products
- Improving secretion and excretion of expressed products from host cell organism
- Exploiting modification of product molecules by changing genome sequences

These bioengineering actions are preferably considered early in the design work and when comparing design alternatives. The actions are relevant to any kind of biosystem, whether it is a biosystem for biotherapeutics, recognition elements in diagnostic devices, assay methods applied for services, or integral parts of bioengineering instrumentation.

The decisions of the bioengineering designer should be guided by the following aspects:

- How can productivity be enhanced by refining the genetically engineered system?
- Which host cell should be selected for promoting productivity and culturing conditions?
- Which biological systems should be selected to limit the production costs?
- Which choice of host-vector system will be best for diminishing the downstream processing needs?

- How can product stability, including storage stability, be enhanced through better molecular genetic engineering modifications?
- Which host-vector can best meet IPR constraints?

All these aspects are directly or indirectly connected to the users' requirements and priorities.

In a business-driven design project, there is little time for developing the biological systems *per se*. In industrial design, the R&D often has to choose those "fruits that hang low" mainly to save cost and time.

Consequently, a core capability is to rapidly identify alternative biological host systems. Microorganisms and higher eukaryotic cells in their wild-type states provide an extensive natural repertoire of biochemical pathways for biological reactions and conversions. However, these natural platforms can be significantly augmented through genetic engineering to maximize product titers, yields, and volumetric productivity.

As a result, the primary methodological challenge lies in mobilizing advanced molecular and computational tools capable of identifying and enforcing the ideal genetic and environmental conditions for optimized biological performance.

3.7 Scaling Up Production

The potential for scaling up the production capacity of the designed bioproduct to the volume required by the market is of utmost concern for a foreseen commercialization (Mandenius and Björkman 2012; Harmsen 2013; Harnish and Ross 2022). Finding the best way to carry out the upscaling without compromising the functions and the quality of the product is pivotal.

To achieve this, several distinct upscaling approaches can be considered:

- Volumetric scale-up of the designed production process. Increasing the working volume of individual unit operations
- Using parallel production lines by performing the production process in several parallel lines.
- Increasing the capacity of the biological system to produce more per cell and time in the same production volume
- Improving the scheduling of the unit operations in the production line
- Optimizing the productivity in each unit so the volumetric productivity of the plant is increased

For each scale-up approach, there are pros and cons (Table 3.4). The cost of increasing the size of production equipment should be compared with the cost of an exchange for a biological system with higher specific productivity or the cost of optimizing the process. Combinations of approaches are possible. For example, the upstream stage can be volumetrically scaled up, and the downstream stage can be continued with several parallel lines (Table 3.5).

Table 3.4 Systems on functionality driving the design of the transformation into bioproducts

Functional system	Functionality of the system	Typical subsystems
Functional biological systems	Biological systems involved in the transformation into the bioproduct	Host cell platforms, enzymes, structural proteins, nucleic acids, and functional carbohydrates Active bioenvironments (e.g., tailored formulation media, growth factors, and metabolic buffers)
Functional technical systems	Technical systems involved in the biological systems or the biological systems' functions	System containment architectures (e.g., bioreactors, process vessels) Fluid dynamics and mass transport hardware (e.g., pumps, piping, impellers) Analytical instrumentation and process monitoring equipment
Functional information systems	Information critical for successful and safe transformation and the control of it	Information about product quality, performance of technical functions of transformation, impurities
Functional management systems	Functions for steering the transformation process by quality measures and regulatory claims	Legal frameworks, compliance documentation, and standardized operational guides (e.g., Good Manufacturing Practice, Good Laboratory Practice)
Functional human systems	Human functions for the transformation of the bioproduct	Qualified engineering, maintenance, and administrative personnel Ethical oversight boards, bioethics compliance protocols, and sustainability risk-assessment bodies

Table 3.5 Scale-up methodologies for bioproduction

Scale-up approach	Advantages (pros)	Disadvantages (cons)	Methodology
Volumetric scaling (*Larger unit dimensions*)	Lowers cost per unit volume Maximizes equipment capacity	Requires physical plant reconstruction Increases capital expenditure	Mass balance modelling
Parallel lines (*Scale-out/ numbering-up*)	Reuses existing asset designs Reduces engineering risk	Demands significant facility space Multiplies monitoring & control needs	Economic analysis Capacity modelling
Operational scheduling (*Time optimization*)	Optimizes existing asset footprint Avoids physical reconstruction	Increases labor requirements Complicates shift management	CAD scheduling programs Discrete event simulation
Biological optimization (*Yield enhancement*)	Utilizes existing facility footprint Minimizes hardware changes	Involves high R&D uncertainty Requires regulatory re-approval	Genetic cell reengineering Statistical optimization

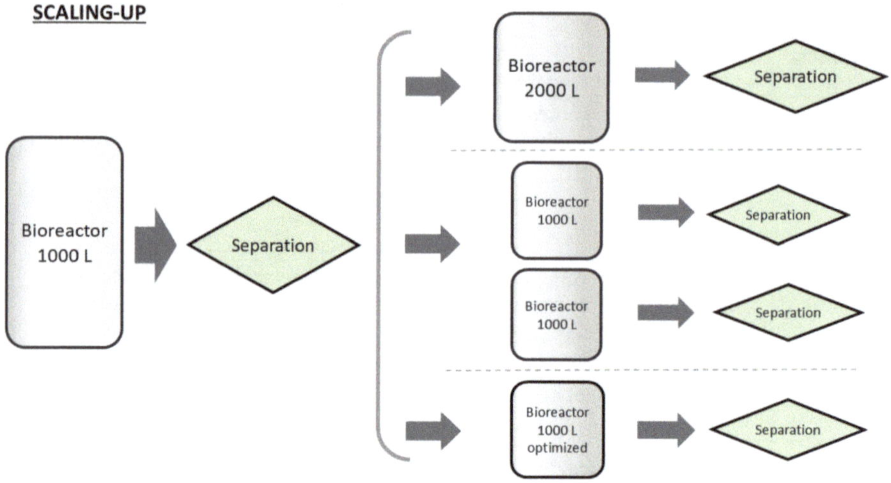

Fig. 3.6 Options for bioproduct scale-up: volumetric scale-up (increasing unit size), parallel scale-up (multiplying unit operations), and optimized scale-up (using factorial design)

It is attractive to systematically investigate the potential of scale-up by using mass balance-derived modelling for predicting time and volume effects in relation to cell density and product concentration. This can be both convenient and time-saving. With bioreactors or culture flasks, stepwise transfer to a larger scale is commonly applied (see, e.g., Design Case 3 in Chap. 5 where mechanistic modelling is used).

The primary objective of scale-up is to maximize bioproduct yield per unit of volume and time within the facility. The productivity metrics often vary. It could be the number of units, where units are directly volumetrically related to the product. For example, the number of units produced (e.g., chips, formulated tablets of a drug, ampoules with the drug).

The scale-up must cover several other parameters to be of value and to allow comparison of design alternatives. The volumetric measure could be translated to molecular masses of the product. This may concern raw materials, manufacturing equipment investments, transport capacity in the system, production time, and specified equipment or devices.

There are also more complex relations to the size of units in plants or numbers of sub-plants in networks or engagement of subcontractors. This can lead to various scale-up strategies and significantly impact production economy (Fig. 3.6).

There are a few other effects to consider for biological systems. When producing biologics, large-scale reactors are known to suffer from stress and reduced capacity when scale increases. Gradients of transfer of nutrients and oxygen are rate-limiting. Such effects are not typical for other production systems. These effects have their origin in the vulnerability of cells to gradients in the vicinity of the cell membrane and other interfaces where product molecules are passing through and influenced by retardations of reactions (Harmsen 2013). This will influence the production economy negatively, making it a critical design issue. However, a larger scale can also compensate for this.

3.8 Evaluating the Economics of Design Alternatives

Design options that remain viable following conceptual analysis and operational modelling must undergo a rigorous economic evaluation (Peters et al. 2003; Towler and Sinnott 2012; Ray et al. 2022). The primary ambition at this stage is to facilitate a comparative cost analysis among design alternatives, rather than to calculate the precise capital required for final implementation. Cost differentials between alternatives typically stem from variations in raw material consumption, manufacturing equipment specifications, facility footprint, and specialized labor requirements. Primarily, this evaluation delivers a preliminary assessment of the fixed capital investment needed to establish production, while offering a baseline estimate for realistic market pricing of the new bioproduct. Consequently, the core objective is to benchmark and rank competing designs based on economic feasibility, rather than to provide a definitive, granular cost accounting.

Some of the costs in the evaluation are annual and dependent on production volumes; others are initial purchasing costs for investment in equipment and installation of the equipment in the construction of the plant facilities (Kristiansen 2006; Petrides 2015) (Fig. 3.7).

In the economic evaluation of the design alternatives, it is also necessary to include all upfront R&D work that has been carried out for the development of the product. Especially for the kind of bioproducts that require extensive product and

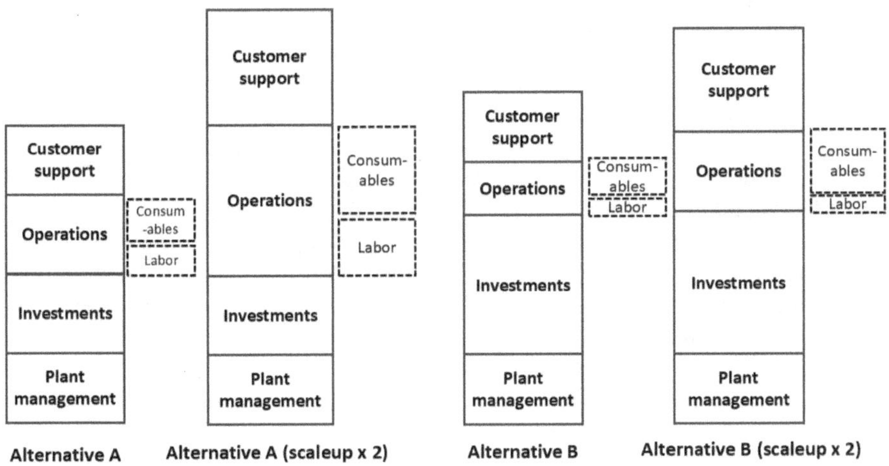

Fig. 3.7 Distributions of costs for two design alternatives showing which type of costs (operational costs, investment costs) dominates the design options

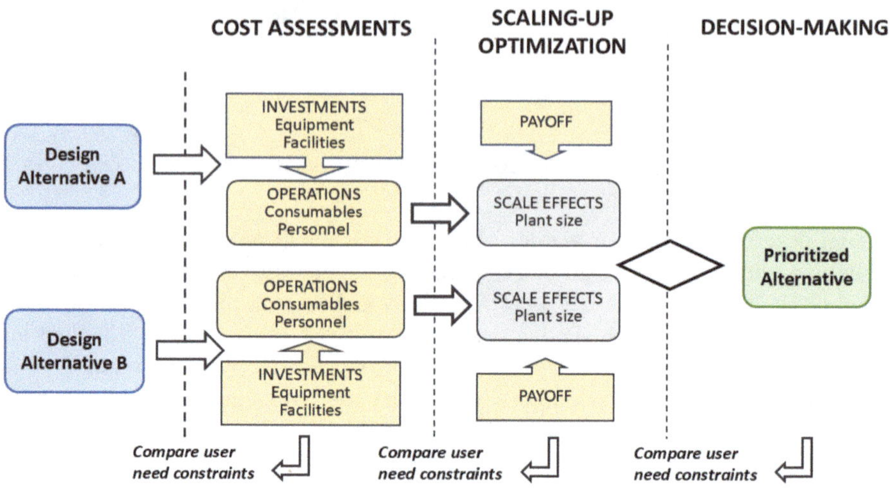

Fig. 3.8 Critical economic factors (investments, operational costs, optimization, and scaling effects) influence decision-making between two design alternatives

production development and testing, this is essential (e.g., in pharmaceutical development).

Extensive R&D will drastically increase the payback costs, which will affect the market price of the product. When considering subcontracting as an alternative to developing own in-house production lines for parts of the production, the cost structure could be substantially influenced.

A tricky part of the economic evaluation is to find ways to access reliable information about costs for equipment, raw materials, and other auxiliary costs. Useful information sources are open list prices, internal information, and educated guesses or price appreciations.

Labor costs are easier to estimate. Costs for installations, buildings, taxes, and plant management are estimated by using established multiplication factors (Kristiansen 2006).

The core objective of the economic evaluation is to make a realistic estimation of the net income, defined as the residual revenue generated after selling the product and deducting all manufacturing costs. This metric provides a qualified estimation of the economic viability and competitiveness of each design alternative (Fig. 3.8). The evaluation of production economics is further detailed in Chap. 4 and exemplified through the design cases presented in Chap. 5. While digital tools can streamline these evaluations and improve time efficiency if used judiciously, a standard spreadsheet program, equipped with financial functions (e.g., EXCEL), generally provides all the necessary functionality. However, more advanced specialized software packages can also offer significant utility (see Sect. 3.11).

3.9 Optimizing Design Solutions

Detailed designs derived from conceptual configurations can be optimized to improve performance. These optimization efforts can focus on either the bioproduct itself or its production process, helping teams reach specific design targets.

There are many ways to optimize design alternatives (Martins and Ning 2021; Glassey 2016; Sioshansi and Conejo 2017). While optimizing the biological system is highly important, optimizing non-biological components is just as critical for overall production economics (Table 3.6).

When optimization methods can combine those factors that maximize the capacity of the bioproduct and its production and determine their optimal values, optimization efforts are successful (Mandenius and Brundin 2008). Statistically based methods are appealing for this purpose (Brereton2003; Mandenius 2016). Also, structured and mechanistic models can significantly contribute to grasping the dependability of parameters. This is of value especially when parameters change over time or production volume (Nielsen et al. 2011; Doran 2013). There is an important distinction between optimizing the product itself, such as product size and amount of active substance, or optimizing the production conditions, such as process unit size, production flow rates, and production times. However, both are of interest in the design for optimizing the design alternatives (Table 3.6).

Table 3.6 Objects in the design of the bioproduct and its production realistic to be optimized

Objects for optimization	Rationale for optimization	Expected outcome
The biological system		
Production cell lines Media composition Feeding strategies Metabolic pathways	Maximize synthesis rates Minimize toxic byproduct Enhance nutrient utilization	Higher product titers Reduced waste Shorter cycle times
Production process units		
Downstream unit operations Process operating parameters Heat and mass transfer rates	Overcome bottlenecks Minimize step-by-step loss Reduce energy and buffer footprints	Elevated step yields Lower consumable costs Consistent product quality
Bioanalytical performance		
Analytical assay precision In-line monitoring tools	Ensure rapid, accurate quantification Minimize measurement error margins Detect process deviations early	Faster batch release times Reduced out-of-specification batches Robust process control data
Product stability		
Formulation buffer conditions Storage and handling temperatures	Prevent molecular degradation/aggregation Extend active shelf-life profiles Maintain therapeutic or functional potency	Lower product rejection rates Simplified cold-chain logistics Increased commercial viability

Optimization requires analytical resources and methods for biological, chemical, and physical parameters as well as substantial time for experiments (Brereton 2003). These can be expensive and may heavily burden the upfront R&D costs. Thus, optimization efforts should be limited and prioritized to bring down the development costs. The potential outcome of different optimization strategies is therefore an important decision. The initial design work does not necessarily have to include optimization experiments. However, it is of great value to identify and realize its potential effect on costs and performance for reaching the targeted objectives in the design mission.

3.9.1 Optimizing Designs Using Design of Experiments (DoE)

Design of experiments (DoE) is a preferred statistical methodology for production process optimization (Brereton 2003; Dong et al. 2008; Mandenius and Brundin 2008; Montgomery 2013). DoE is highly suitable for analyzing several of the optimization targets outlined previously and can be adapted to almost any optimization. Here, it has primarily the advantage that it could result in better performance of bioproducts and production processes (Mandenius and Brundin 2008). For bioprocess optimization, it has become common practice to use DoE for improvement of growth and production media. A typical culture medium has ten to twenty nutrient components for sustaining high growth and production rates (Mandenius 2016). For industrial cell cultures, that number may be even higher. Since some of the culture medium components are very costly, their impact on production expenditure is substantial (e.g., insulin, transferrin, specific growth factors).

Performing real experiments according to a DoE plan requires exclusive resources (e.g., culture equipment and analytical methods). The planning of DoE experiments takes relatively short time while the experimental work consumes substantial time and labor. A good plan reduces this. However, planning requires knowledge about media factors or other parameters and responses. Acquiring this knowledge may need some effort and must be carried out with good insights into the cellular systems (Table 3.7).

Executing a DoE requires a well-structured workflow (Fig. 3.9). Briefly, several factors likely to exert a high impact on the optimization target are identified, and realistic operating ranges are defined based on historical experience or baseline data (Montgomery 2013). These independent variables might include specific culture media components, bioreactor operating parameters—such as temperature, pH, and dissolved oxygen tension—or the critical operating parameters of a separation column (Dong et al. 2008; Knoespel et al. 2010). In the initial phase of experimentation, these factors are screened against relevant process responses.

The responses are typically related to the performance of the system. In a cell culture, this would normally be productivity or anything else related to the

Table 3.7 A selection of potential factors to be analyzed with DoE and expected outcomes

Factors to be optimized by DoE	Role in the designed bioproduct	Expected outcome of DoE
Culture media composition:		
Carbon and nitrogen sources Trace elements, growth, and differentiation factors Inducer agents Buffer composition	Influence the metabolism and physiology of the cell, resulting in shifts of rates and use of raw materials. Control actions by biochemical signaling	Increase in growth and expression rates. Increase in yields. Saving of raw materials
Culturing conditions:		
Time for induction	Optimize physical and chemical conditions in the culture. Modulate the access of nutrients, avoiding overfeeding and stress conditions	Increase in target productivity. Prolongation of growth and expression of target
Feed profile shapes		
Temperature profile		
pH and ionic strengths		
Chromatographic conditions:		
Elution media Column aspect ratios Flow rate	Interaction target and impurity Separation resolution Time for separation	Higher separation purity. Reduce separation time Production economics
Formulation conditions:		
Stabilizer and buffer	Best stabilizing effect	Better longevity of product
Diagnostic devices:		
Geometries, antibody/enzyme, and reagent conditions	Performance of reaction in device. Rate/range Consumption of reagents	Reduce size of device. Lower reagent costs

bioproduct's capacity. The purpose of the first round is to reduce the number of factors. In a second round of experiments, the most prominent factors are analyzed with more input information. The outcome is usually presented as a response surface as a 3D plot that shows the optimal conditions. For example, this could concern the composition of a culture medium or the procedure for carrying out the cultivation. Commercial software can be used to guide the designer in the DoE and for choosing suitable statistical calculation methods.

Consequently, it is reasonable to question the allocation of resources required for DoE optimization. However, a well-engineered experimental plan can be streamlined to minimize the total number of required trials. Furthermore, factorial experiments offer the advantage of increasing knowledge and understanding of both the bioproduct and its manufacturing.

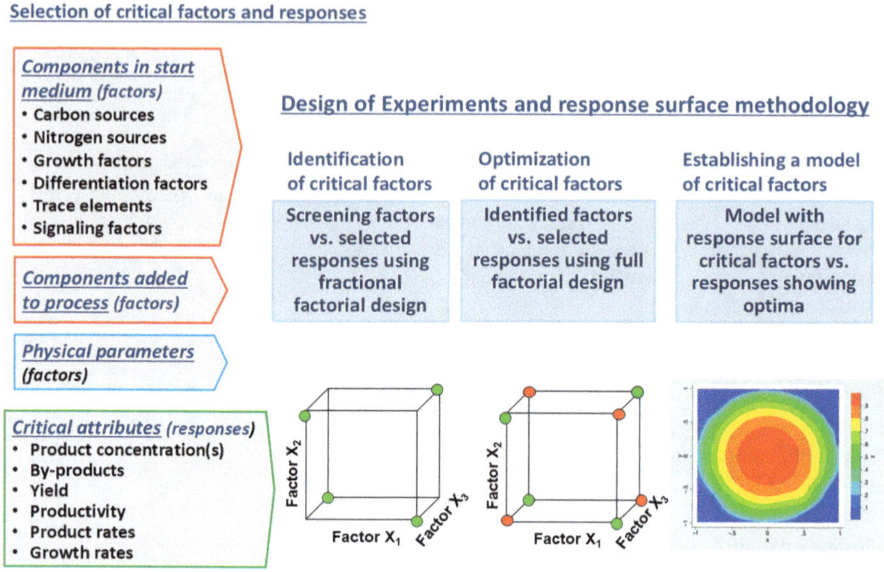

Fig. 3.9 Overview of sequential design of experiment methodological procedures, highlighting screening phases and optimization steps. (Permission from Mandenius 2016)

3.9.2 Applying Mechanistic Modelling to Bioproduct Design

Mechanistic and structured modelling, much like design of experiments (DoE), demands significant front-end effort and deep domain expertise (Nielsen et al. 2011; Doran 2013). Consequently, these resource-intensive approaches are best deployed after initial screening and ranking of design alternatives. At this advanced stage, mechanistic models serve to rigorously optimize the selected design pathways and maximize performance.

The ambition of the modelling is to further improve the outcome of the design. This could sometimes be marginal improvements but could often be significant. Consequently, one must first consider if mechanistic models really have a high potential for improving performance. A typical example is to investigate how much biological mass is needed for generating a biotherapeutic protein at a given time. Another example is to estimate the expression rates of a host cell culture during a certain period. A third example is to estimate the yield when separating cells from a culture under various centrifugation conditions. In the examples, modelling is possible if reliable equations for cell growth, expression rate, or centrifugation performance are known or can be formulated.

The actual value of the modelling is whether the model can be connected to the design in terms of productivity, and from that to production economics. From economic perspectives, the size of equipment, related to investments, and

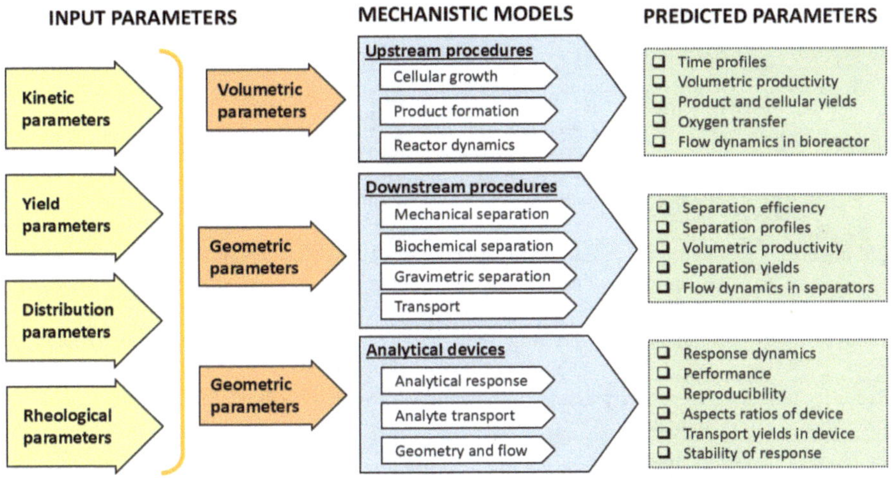

Fig. 3.10 Potential predictable parameters using mechanistic modelling for bioproduct design, where geometry, volumes, and operational efficiency directly impact the prediction of kinetic behaviors

consumption of raw materials and labor, related to operational costs, are of interest to minimize by modelling.

If the developed product is a device based on biological capacity, e.g., an analytical enzyme or antibody, the conversion rate in an assay would be related to the amount of biological agent, reaction time, and range of measurements. Parameters that can be translated to equations are then easy to simulate.

The model parameters must be close to reality to present meaningful results. This could be verified by tuning parameters versus real data. In the early phase of the design work, such experiments are not realistic due to the time needed to perform such experiments. More convenient is to search for literature data and use these as approximations. Within certain limits, that can suffice or at least give a better understanding of limits and constraints of a design solution.

The complexity of equation systems can vary considerably, and the number of descriptive variables can be extended to very large numbers, either dependable or parallelly acting variables of value for design decisions. In the design cases presented in Chap. 5, examples show how the conditions can vary and are coupled to the actual design case.

Mechanistic models of relevance to bioengineering design mostly comprise multiparameter spaces and several predicted measures (Fig. 3.10). Note especially that mechanistic modelling is not only commonly used for typical cell biology-related bioprocess and bioproduction systems but can also be used to model the performance of devices and instruments.

As illustrated, specific physicochemical parameters exhibit significant recurrence across diverse system architectures, regardless of their distinct functional roles. For instance, kinetic rates and product yields represent ubiquitous metrics across most

Table 3.8 Parameters to consider for mechanistic modelling with potential effects on design

Parameters	Role of parameters	Mechanistic model	Expected outcome
Culture time	Time for reaching targeted cell density	*Monod or extended models*	Assessment of culture to a given density of cells
Product time	Time for reaching targeted amount of product	*Luedeking-Piret or extended models*	Optimization of scheduling and productivity
Culture size	Giving the required volume for the targeted values	*Relation to volume in mass balance equations*	Optimized reactor size to production target
Recovery unit time	Reducing recovery time	*Unit operation equations*	Shorter recovery time
Recovery unit size	Unit capacity assessed by model parameters	*Descriptive unit operation equations*	Optimization of recovery unit sizes
hCell line kinetics	Showing variability of cells and productivity	*Determination of rate constants in models*	Optimization of size
Separation time	Column size, materials and operations	*Demanding modelling*	Shorter separation time in sequences
Purity of target product	Separation factors in relation to separation materials and operation procedures	*Kinetic models DoE may be a better opportunity*	Reduced impurity level
Time for analysis of an analyte	Time for performing analytical procedure	*Kinetic equations Michaelis-Menten equations*	Response time of analytical device
Concentration of analytical reagents	Assessing the amounts of reagents consumed per assay	*Kinetic rate equations for analytical reactions*	Consummation of reagents in assays and kits

bioprocesses; these serve as critical objective functions that must be maximized to ensure industrial viability.

Identifying immediate targets for mechanistic modelling can be challenging (Table 3.8). As with DoE, the most critical parameters are those directly impacting product economy, quality, and utility. These performance metrics comprise both variables and constants; however, constants are only stable under specific operating conditions and can often be transitioned into variables during process optimization.

In control engineering, models commonly describe the actions of control loops. In measurement engineering, models describe signal responses. When it comes to designing, the dimensions and time of the designed object become the prioritized modelling topics. That could be attempts to anticipate required volume for a process, time for reactions, influence of concentrations of acting cells, reactants, raw materials, elicitors, and nutrients. Luckily, these categories of parameters are often described in existing (bio)engineering science. They can easily be implemented as differential equations with appropriate constraints and variables (Doran 2013).

The fidelity of predictive models is fundamentally dependent on the quality of the underlying datasets. While primary data is ideally sourced from in-house experimental rigs or peer-reviewed literature, experienced engineers can often derive reliable heuristic estimates where empirical gaps exist. Given the complexity of these datasets, computational frameworks are essential for executing modeling protocols—particularly for characterizing unit operations such as centrifugal separation, membrane filtration, sedimentation, and bioreactor kinetics (see Sect. 3.11).

3.9.3 Exploring Other Optimization Frameworks

The industrial platform Six Sigma (6σ) provides engineers with several practical, readily available methods adapted for industrial applications (Pande et al. 2014). In industry, the 6σ platform has become a highly valued tool due to its versatility and convenience. It features wide applicability and provides clear avenues for implementing different statistical optimization techniques.

The 6σ platform is primarily used for process development (Six Sigma Official webpage 2025). Originally introduced by the Motorola company, the platform provides a comprehensive collection of statistical and related methods for structuring and analyzing production data. Often, the purpose is to identify the root causes of irregularities related to product quality (The Council for Six Sigma Certification 2025). The framework combines established methodologies, such as statistical process control, principal component analysis, factorial design, root cause analysis, and fishbone analysis. These methods are most effective for improving processes already in operation, where fine-tuning and optimal operating conditions can be systematically refined.

A major advantage of the 6σ platform is that it provides industrial practitioners with structured, proper guidance for implementation. By doing so, 6σ furnishes a convenient concept for training and collaborative process development in commercial environments.

The 6σ framework is constantly evolving and advancing. Multivariate 6σ, for example, highlights its resourcefulness for engineered systems where the number of production parameters grows overwhelmingly large (Ferrer 2021). This is frequently the situation for bioengineered products and complex production systems. Interestingly, novel methodologies such as machine learning and related computational methods are now being integrated alongside 6σ (Runosson and Cronemyr 2023).

From the perspective of this design guide, the integration of DoE within 6σ holds strong relevance for optimizing design alternatives. However, as a general and initial design tool, 6σ may suffer from the lack of an inherently structured approach for screening and analyzing early-stage design alternatives.

3.10 Validating and Testing Final Designs

Before a selected bioproduct design alternative can be implemented, its operational robustness and stability must be thoroughly validated. For industrial products, a preliminary validation dossier must be presented to regulatory agencies and control organizations for formal scrutiny (United States' Food and Drug Administration 2011; European Medicines Agency 2016). These regulatory bodies operate under strict national and international frameworks, which are frequently developed through collaborations between global harmonization councils and statutory authorities (International Council for Harmonisation 1995; European Medicines Agency 2016).

The pre-validation and testing of a product are normally carried out prior to the legislative validation. This becomes a needle's eye for new designs. In the pharmaceutical industry, validation must be approved in internal and external preclinical and clinical trials. For other bioproducts such as devices and instruments, process supply, commodity products, beta-site testing, or similar validation arrangements are applied.

The outcome of the pre-validation process may lead to redesigning parts of the product. This will add costs but also save costs in the subsequent legal validations and revalidations.

The final validation settles the format of the new bioproduct and its production to be implemented, as it will reach the customers on the market. Here, the customer priorities become real. For pharmaceutical products, revalidation is also mandatory.

Regulatory agencies and certification organizations accurately prescribe procedures for validation (United States' Food and Drug Administration 2011; European Medicines Agency 2016).

Importantly, the total costs for validation, especially in the event of negative outcomes, lead to redesign, which can vary significantly. Thus, in an economic evaluation, it is necessary to foresee this and have margins to cover such costs.

For the designer, it is necessary to understand the impact of validation. Design solutions must facilitate validation. This could be done already at the conceptualization stage.

A useful method to pre-validate a product and production design is the SWOT analysis. In this framework, the strengths (S), weaknesses (W), opportunities (O), and threats (T) of the design alternatives are systematically appraised and scrutinized (Shinno et al. 2006). This analysis is facilitated by using targeted checkpoints that align with typical bioproduct properties (Table 3.9). While not all checkpoints are relevant to every bioproduct, most can be specified further to suit the actual product under evaluation. Notably, a SWOT analysis for a new bioproduct is not static; it evolves over time, shifting dynamically alongside changing market conditions.

The benefit of SWOT analysis is its adaptability and versatility. It can focus on certain parts, for example, the production process only, supply networks, or business conditions. The design cases in Chap. 5 illuminate the variability of possibilities in the SWOT analysis.

Table 3.9 SWOT analysis checkpoints for bioproducts

SWOT checkpoints	Example of critical characters
Strengths	The product possesses robust intellectual property rights (IPRs). The manufacturing process is protected by strong IPRs. The product holds a unique position in the market. Production costs are minimal, enabling a competitive low market price. The product causes minimal environmental impact
Weaknesses	The product relies on numerous interdependent components. Many components must be sourced or purchased from external subcontractors. Product shelf life and storage stability are limited. The design contains an excessive number of integrated parts. Long-term service and technical support are becoming cost-prohibitive
Opportunities	Manufacturing can easily be relocated closer to key target markets. The product has strong potential for global distribution. The product can be readily adapted for entry into adjacent markets. The core product platform can be leveraged to develop derivative products. The existing production infrastructure can be utilized for similar bioproduct lines
Threats	Existing IPR protections and patents face imminent expiration. Competing or higher-value alternative products are entering the market. Shifting political regulations adversely impact production costs and sales margins. Biological components of the production strain or process are overly vulnerable. Bioproduct is highly susceptible to microbial contamination. Regulatory validation or revalidation dossiers are rejected

3.11 Utilizing Digital Design Environments

Digital tools are valuable assets for supporting design work. This section highlights their applicability for designing as well as some reasons for being cautious and restrictive in using them (US Food and Drug Administration 2025).

Most digital tools are intended for general engineering applications, while a few are dedicated to design and to bioengineering, some also with eminent utility for bioengineering design. The following categories of digital software tools are of particular interest:

- Computer-aided design software programs for drawing and compiling flow sheets, scheduling and simulations of design solutions
- Software programs for factorial design of experiments (DoE) and other statistical methods for optimization of products and production conditions
- Software programs for implementing simple or more advanced modelling to study critical parameters of the designed systems
- Software tools for economic analysis and evaluations

These tools are generally user-friendly and developed with deep insight into their potential applications (Table 3.10). Commercial software packages enjoy wide acceptance across academic and industrial engineering sectors and are frequently utilized in training both scientists and engineers.

Table 3.10 Useful digital tools for supporting bioengineering design

Digital tool	Utilities and advantages
SuperPro Designer, SPD™	Flow sheeting, batch scheduling, and economic calculations. (www.intelligen.com)
Gensym G2	A knowledge-based system for configuring manufacturing processes by object-oriented programming (www.gensym.com)
MATLAB with toolboxes	Implementation of mathematical equation systems. Extensive graphical commodities. Toolboxes for statistics, neural networks (www.mathworks.com)
Aspen Plus	Version for biological production available. An alternative to SPD™. (www.aspen.com)
Mathematica	An alternative to MATLAB with similar possibilities (www.wolfram.com)
"R"	An open-source program with wide possibilities (www.r-project.org)
SIMCA/MODDE	Statistical software for, e.g., PLS, PCA, and DoE (www.sartorius.com)
Scalable Simulation Frameworks (SSF)	Modelling platform, applicable to bioengineering design scale-up application (Wang et al. 2020)
MiniTAB	Alternative to Simca/Modde and SSF (www.minitab.com)
Modelica	Implementation of mathematical equation systems. Libraries for industrial application fields. An open-source program (www.modelica.org)

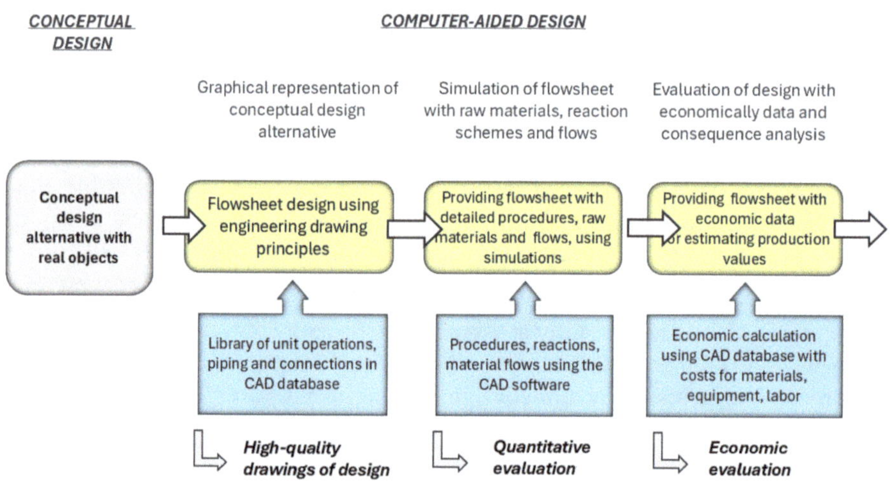

Fig. 3.11 Typical structure used in several computer-aided design software packages. The conceptual design alternatives can be tested at an early development stage with these and can, in some software, even include economic evaluation

Digital tools for industrial design: Digital tools should provide the industrial designer with functions that facilitate and speed up the development work in a structured manner (Fig. 3.11). This could especially concern:

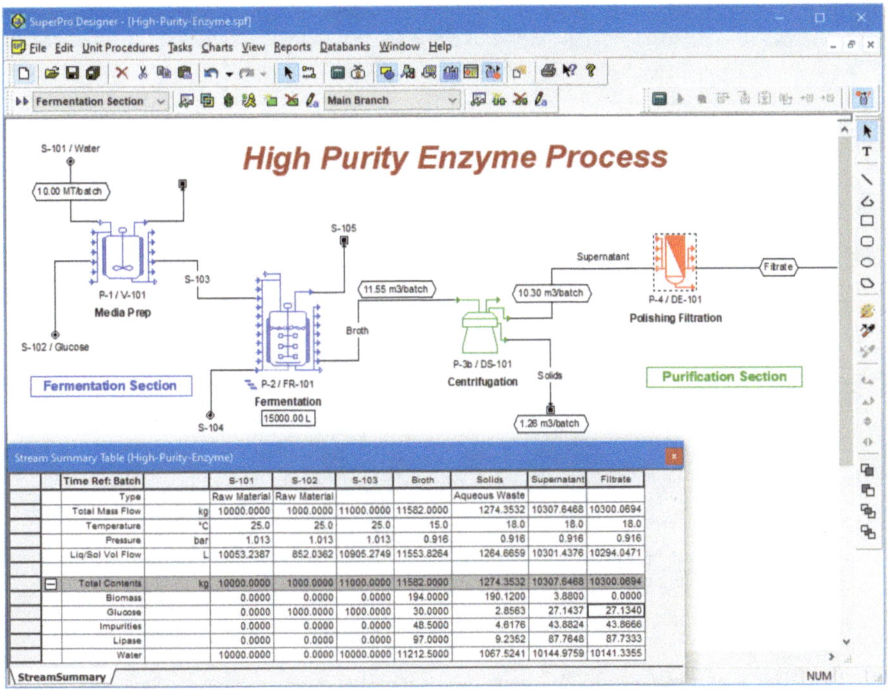

Fig. 3.12 The user interface of the digital software SPD. It uses dropdown menus with bioprocess unit operations. The screen for a part of an antibody production is shown (Reproduced by permission of Intelligen Inc.)

- To replace demanding manual design tasks with digitally aided procedures for flowsheet creation and system configuration. For example, specialized bioprocess simulation software, such as SuperPro Designer (SPD) or Aspen Plus, can perform automated flow sheeting and economic calculations. These platforms are designed for bioengineering workflows, frequently offering dozens of pre-configured upstream and downstream unit operations (Fig. 3.12). Additionally, users can typically program custom unit operations, such as automated assembly machinery or robotic interfaces, depending on project needs.
- To simulate and predict design performance using dynamic models or advanced computational methods. These tools evaluate variables such as alternative raw materials, fluctuating prices, piping network configurations, fluid flow rates, working volumes, and equipment properties. They can also integrate reaction stoichiometries and yield factors. Standard commercial software packages, including Aspen Plus and SuperPro Designer (SPD), possess these simulation capabilities to varying degrees, providing valuable computational support for detailing complex design configurations.

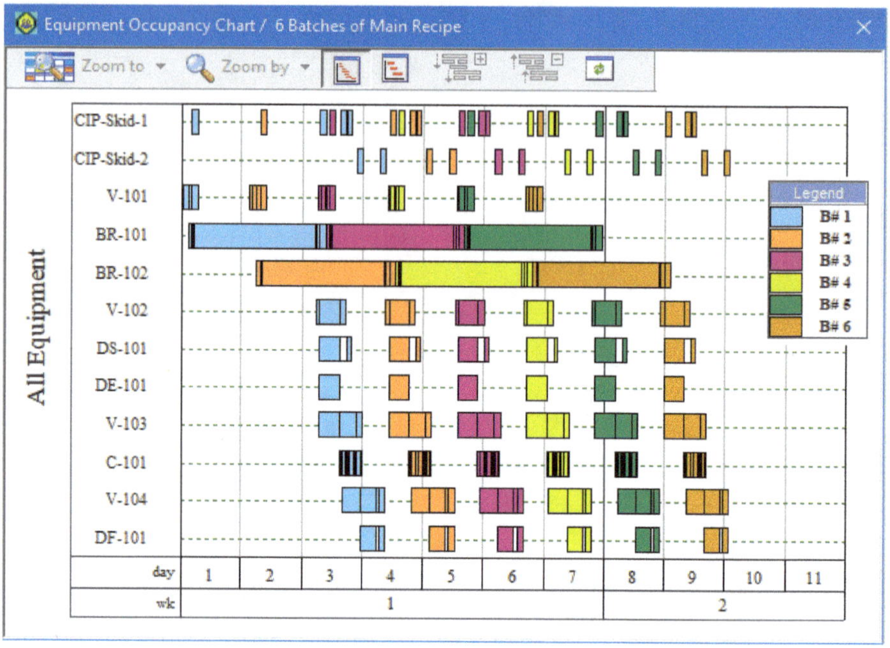

Fig. 3.13 The user interface of the digital software SPD when used for scheduling process operations. (Reproduced by permission from Intelligen Inc.)

- *To evaluate production economics, thereby supporting the decision-making stage when selecting between design options*. Production profitability is heavily driven by raw material, equipment, labor, and quality and safety control expenditures. Characteristics unique to bioengineered products include the expenses associated with cell line or strain acquisition, the variable costs of purification unit operations, and the subsequent recovery of biological compounds. Process scheduling and batch operations also exert a major influence on overall manufacturing economics (Fig. 3.13). Digital tools, such as Aspen Plus and SPD, include a variety of built-in functions to facilitate this type of cost assessment.
- Advanced computations require software programs with extended capacity and usually require a deeper understanding and knowledge of the programming language for the software. Typical design applications could be structured and mechanistic modelling with the purpose of optimizing design procedures and layouts. MATLAB, Mathematica, and Modelica are useful software that exemplifies this. Also, more widespread programs such as "R" and Excel have extensive possibilities to implement modelling applications require special acquaintance with these functions of the software.
- Several of the advanced software programs have specialized toolboxes that extend and tailor these programs' computations. The toolboxes usually provide an interactive formulation with ready-made symbols and display functions.

Simulink and Simulink with MATLAB, System Modeler with Mathematica, and Modelica and their libraries of user applications (Axelsson 2023).

Digital tools for statistical analysis and optimization. In general, statistical software is based on investigating how input data can be selected or adjusted to favor the parts of the design.

Usually, software has standardized statistical functions implemented; other software expects the user to develop the computation procedures for the purpose. Common statistical software programs have a high degree of versatility in this respect (e.g., MiniTab, MODDE, SIMCA, and “R”). These programs are partly also available through platforms such as 6σ.

Considerable time can be invested in statistical computation. Thus, one should be selective in choosing the objects for optimization with statistical software to avoid spending time and effort on something that does not always result in improvements of design work.

Risks associated with digital design tools. Effectively utilizing digital tools requires realistic expectations regarding their computational precision. Designers occasionally overestimate the accuracy of software performance metrics and predictive calculations. In addition to this primary concern, several specific risks accompany the integration of digital tools into bioengineering design.

First, deploying these tools too early in the design phase can cause engineers to become entangled in software technicalities. Digital applications should only be introduced with a clear intention that serves the overarching design objectives. When applied strategically, these tools yield more robust, well-founded results.

Second, software databases may lack real-time updates regarding raw material prices, equipment expenditures, labor rates, emerging technological innovations, shifting intellectual property conditions (such as new patents or changing ownership), and evolving regulatory legislation.

Third, computational software demands high-quality input data that can be difficult to acquire. This challenge applies directly to obtaining accurate product dimensions, kinetic rates, and financial estimates. Such data scarcity often creates a high entry barrier for digital analysis. To mitigate this threshold, utilizing validated literature databases can save valuable development time.

In conclusion, when these risks are managed, digital design tools enable engineers to accomplish more extensive evaluations with a higher degree of precision.

References

Ahmad HM, Rashid M, Rahman MU et al (2015) Ethical issues of biotechnology, possible risks and their management. J Biol Agricult Healthc 5(11):49–54. ISSN 2225-093X

Al-Rubeai M, Naciri (eds) (2014) Stem cells and cell therapy. Springer, New York. https://doi.org/10.1007/978-94-007-7196-3

American Type Culture Collection (1992) Catalogue of cell lines and hybridomas. The Collection

Arivaradarajan P, Misra G (2018) Omics approaches, technologies and applications: integrative approaches for understanding omics data. Springer

ASPEN Plus for bioprocesses (2025). https://www.aspentech.com/en/products/engineering/aspen-plus. Retrieved October 2025

Axelsson JP (2023) Design ideas behind bioprocess library for Modelica. In: Müller D, Monti A, Benigni A (eds) Proceedings of the 15th international Modelica conference 2023. https://doi.org/10.3384/ecp204

Bornscheuer UT, Höhle M (eds) (2018) Protein engineering, methods and protocols. Methods in Molecular Biology 1685. Humana Press/Springer Nature, New York. https://doi.org/10.1007/978-1-4939-7366-8

Brereton RG (2003) Chemometrics, data analysis for laboratory and chemical plants. Wiley, Chichester

DoE software (2025) (Modde, Sartorius). https://www.sartorius.com/en/products/process-analytical-technology/data-analytics-software/doe-software/modde. Retrieved October 2025

Dong J, Mandenius CF, Lübberstedt M et al (2008) Evaluation and optimization of hepatocyte culture media factors by design of experiments (DoE) methodology. Cytotechnology 27:251–261. https://doi.org/10.1007/s10616-008-9168-6

Doran PM (2013) Biochemical engineering principles, 2nd edn. Elsevier, Amsterdam. https://doi.org/10.1016/C2009-0-22348-8

European Medicines Agency (2016) European Medicines Agency's guideline on process validation for the manufacture of biotechnology-derived active substances and data to be provided in the regulatory submission. European Medicines Agency, London

Ferrer A (2021) Multivariate six sigma: a key improvement strategy in industry 4.0. Qual Eng 33(4):758–763. https://doi.org/10.1080/08982112.2021.1957481

G2 platform for process development and design. (Gensym) http://dev.gensym.com/platforms/g2-standard/. Retrieved October 2025

Glassey J (2016) Multivariate modelling for bioreactor monitoring and control. In: Mandenius CF (ed) Bioreactors, design, operation and novel applications. Wiley-VCH, Weinheim, pp 369–390

Harmsen J (2013) Industrial process scale-up. A practical Innovation guide from idea to commercial implementation. Elsevier Science, Amsterdam. ISBN 9780444627261

Harnish V, Ross S (2022) Scaling up compensation: five design principles for turning your largest expense into a strategic advantage. Forbes Books

Heinzle E, Biwer A, Cooney C (2006) Development of sustainable bioprocesses. Modelling and assessment. Wiley, Chichester

Hubka V, Eder WE (1988) Theory of technical systems, a total concept theory for engineering design. Springer, Berlin

International Conference on Harmonization (1995) ICH Quality guideline Q5C. Quality of biotechnology products. Stability testing, 5th edn. International Conference on Harmonization

Jazayeri SH, Amiri-Yekta A, Bahrami S et al (2018) Vector and cell line engineering technologies toward recombinant protein expression in mammalian cell lines. Springer

Knoespel F, Schindler RK, Luebberstedt M et al (2010) Optimization of a serum-free culture medium for mouse embryonic stem cells using design of experiments (DoE) methodology. Cytotechnology 62:557–571

Kristiansen B (2006) Process economics. In: Ratledge C, Kristiansen B (eds) Basic biotechnology, 3rd edn. Cambridge University Press, Cambridge, pp 239–252

Mandenius CF (2016) Design of experiments for development and optimization of bioreactor media. In: Mandenius CF (ed) Bioreactors, design, operation and novel applications. Wiley-VCH, Weinheim

Mandenius CF, Björkman M (2011) Biomechatronic design in biotechnology: a methodology for development of biotechnology products. Wiley, Hoboken

Mandenius CF, Björkman M (2012) Scale-up of cell culture bioreactors using biomechatronic design. Biotechnol J 7(8):1026–1039. https://doi.org/10.1002/biot.201100463

Mandenius CF, Brundin A (2008) Bioprocess optimization using design-of-experiments methodology. Biotechnol Prog 24:1191–1203. https://doi.org/10.1002/btpr.67

Mann R (2018) Genetic engineering and biotechnology. Callisto Reference. ISBN 9781632399205

Martins JRRA, Ning A (2021) Engineering design optimization. Cambridge University Press, Cambridge. https://doi.org/10.1017/9781108980647

Mathematica simulation software. Wolfram https://www.wolfram.com/mathematica/. Retrieved October 2025

MATLAB and MATLAB toolbox. https://www.mathworks.com/products/control.html. Retrieved October 2025

Minitab statistical software for industry and students. https://www.minitab.com/en-us/solutions/industry/academic/. Retrieved October 2025

Modelica software and tools for simulation and computation. https://modelica.org/tools/. Retrieved October 2025

Montgomery DC (2013) Design and analysis of experiments, 8th edn. Wiley, New York

Nielsen J, Villadsen J, Lidén G (2011) Bioreaction engineering principles, 3rd edn. Springer, New York

Nielsen J, Stephanopoulos G, Lee SY (eds) (2021) Metabolic engineering: concepts and applications. Wiley VCH. https://doi.org/10.1002/9783527823468. ISBN:9783527823468

O'Brian D (2019) Engineer 4.0: life science handbook for medical devices and biopharmaceuticals. Kindle. ISBN-13: 978-1795753340

Pahl G, Beitz W, Feldhusen J et al (2007) Engineering design, a systematic approach, 3rd edn. Springer, Berlin

Pande PS, Neuman RP, Cavanaugh RR et al (2014) The Six Sigma way: how to maximize the impact of your change and improvement efforts, 2nd edn. McGraw-Hill Education, New York. ISBN: 9780071497329

Peters MS, Timmerhaus KD, West RE (2003) Plant design and economics for chemical engineers, 5th edn. McGraw-Hill & Co, New York

Petrides D (2015) Bioprocess design and economics. In: Harrison RG, Todd P, Rudge SR et al (eds) Bioseparations science and engineering, 2nd edn. Oxford University Press, New York, pp 441–510. https://doi.org/10.1093/oso/9780195391817.001.0001

Pörtner R (ed) (2021) Cell culture engineering and technology. Springer, New York. https://doi.org/10.1007/978-3-030-79871-0

R software for statistical computing. https://www.r-project.org/. Retrieved October 2025

Ray SC, Chambers RG, Kumbhakar SC (2022) Handbook of production economics. Springer, New York

Runosson D, Cronemyr P (2023) Prediction of total quality performance. In: Proceedings of 26th Excellence in Services International Conference (EISIC)

Shinno H, Yoshioka H, Marpaung S et al (2006) Quantitative SWOT analysis on global competitiveness of machine tool industry. J Eng Des 17(3):251–258. https://doi.org/10.1080/09544820500275180

Sioshansi R, Conejo AJ (2017) Optimization in engineering, models and algorithms. Springer. ISBN 9783319567679

Six Sigma Official web page. Retrieved October 2025

Statistical software (SIMCA, Sartorius). https://www.sartorius.com/en/products/process-analytical-technology/data-analytics-software/mvda-software/simca. Retrieved October 2025

SuperPro Designer (design software). Product features. https://www.intelligen.com/products/superpro-product-features/. Retrieved October 2025

The Council for Six Sigma Certification. Official Industry Standard for Six Sigma Accreditation. https://www.sixsigmacouncil.org/. Retrieved 2025-10-03

The European Medicines Agency's scientific guidelines (2025) Quality guidelines. https://www.ema.europa.eu/en/human-regulatory-overview/research-development/scientific-guidelines/quality-guidelines. Retrieved October 2025

Towler G, Sinnott R (2012) Chemical engineering design: principles, practice and economics of plant and process design, 2nd edn. Elsevier, Amsterdam

Ulrich KT, Eppinger SD, Yang MC (2019) Product design and development, 7th edn. McGraw-Hill, New York

United States National Institute for Medical Research (2023) The human genetic mutant cell repository: list of genetic variants, chromosomal aberrations and normal cell cultures submitted to the repository, 4th edn. Camden, United States National Institute for Medical Research/ Legare Street Press. ISBN: 10-102149335X, ISBN-13: 978-1021493354

United States' Food and Drug Administration (2011) Current Good Manufacturing Practices (CGMP): Guidance for industry process validation: general principles and practices. U.-S. Department of Health and Human Services, Food and Drug Administration, Center for Drug Evaluation and Research (CDER), Center for Biologics Evaluation and Research (CBER), Center for Veterinary Medicine (CVM), Washington, DC

United States' Food and Drug Administration (2025) Computer software assurance for production and quality system software (guidance for industry and food and drug administration staff). U.S. Department of Health and Human Services, Food and Drug Administration, Center for Drug Evaluation and Research (CDER), Center for Biologics Evaluation and Research (CBER), Center for Veterinary Medicine (CVM), Washington, DC

Wang G, Haringa C, Noorman H et al (2020) Developing a computational framework to advance bioprocess scale-up. Trends Biotechnol 38:846–856. https://doi.org/10.1016/j.tibtech.2020.01.009

Wong TS, Tee KL (2020) A practical guide to protein engineering. Springer. ISBN-13 978-3030568979

Chapter 4
Bioengineering Design Training

This chapter provides advice on how to apply the fundamental principles and methodologies described in previous chapters in bioengineering design training. A structure for the training is presented where the student activities and tutorial actions are outlined. Guidelines for reviewing and appraisal of the students' performance and of the training program are suggested. Thus, the chapter is a bridge to the nine forthcoming design cases.

The presented training structure aligns bioengineering design with typical industrial requirements. It places high priority on industrial conceptual design thinking and efficiency of production economics. By that, the training model has broad application across a variety of products, encompassing the development of medical devices, services, and specialized equipment.

4.1 Training in Designing Bioproducts and Bioproduction Systems

Design training should be a rewarding and stimulating experience in applying basic and fundamental knowledge about the design of bioproducts in practice. Through such training, a genuine understanding of bioengineering is expected to be gained. A better apprehension of the constraints and possibilities of biosystems should be provided. Engineering proficiency should be developed for skillful realization of novel ideas and for seeing their practical implications (Doulougeri et al. 2024). This will span across physics, chemistry, biology, descriptive mathematics, analytical techniques, statistical methods, mechanics, and electronics. The main training challenge is to bring this together for conceiving the design of bioengineered bioproducts.

Engineering education frequently privileges extensive theoretical framework over practice. This imbalance tends to under-prepare students for the demands of

C.-F. Mandenius, *Bioengineering Design Methodology*,
https://doi.org/10.1007/978-3-032-33940-9_4

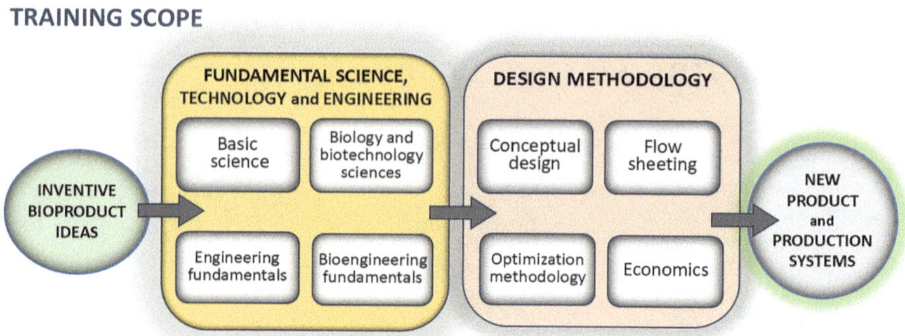

Fig. 4.1 The scope of training aims at developing the capability to translate inventive product ideas by fundamental scientific principles and methodologies into bioproducts

their future vocational life (Daly et al. 2012). Adding to this challenge, modern graduates must navigate within a global landscape characterized by rapidly shifting technological premises.

Tools are constantly improved and modified to facilitate engineering design work. Still, these novel tools are all, by necessity, derived from previous experiences and seldom achieve something authentically new. However, they contribute to shortening time and effort to reach similar endpoints. Training must have this in mind and avoid mixing up "tool technology" with fundamental thinking (Dym et al. 2005). The bottom line of a task is to remain in a timeless understanding and be able to find solutions, without focusing on new tempting tools.

Usually, engineering school education harnesses strengths in mathematics, physics, physical chemistry, reaction chemistry, basic biology, analytical methods, computer science, statistics, and electronics. To be meaningful, these subjects must be applied and practiced by understanding their actual values (Fig. 4.1).

At the first level, this can be done by showing valuable applications for society in each engineering subject. For example, in chemical engineering, about the chemical synthesis of pharmaceutical compounds or building chemical plants; in electric engineering, about the construction of motors and devices; in physical engineering, about power plants. In bioengineering, it is about utilizing biological reactions or systems to act or transform materials into new bioproducts or biologically derived information.

At a second level of training, it becomes meaningful to train students in practicing these capabilities with project-based assignments. From an AV tutorial perspective, this is demanding due to the difficulty of coordinating this in a consecutive didactic process. Often, it must be done with a teaching staff distributed in an organization that is not entirely shaped for the training.

Those conceptual tools and methodologies described previously will, if properly applied, serve this purpose excellently. This requires a systematic and structured approach in the design thinking and use of sketches, drawings, and computational means. Conceptual understanding becomes the glue for finding available means and materials for this. Our digitalized world allows us to do this more efficiently than before. But the underlying principles remain the same. Engineering has always been about handling information where new and alternative information may change the prerequisites for conceiving the creative design solution. The iterative character of the design process, now permitting cycles of rethinking to go faster, must also be trained accordingly to ensure that students can master the speed of modern design without losing sight of fundamental engineering logic.

4.2 Objectives of the Design Training

Bioengineering design training should be driven by three core objectives:

- To develop the ability to merge biological mechanisms into the design of bioproducts and production systems.
- To develop proficiency in understanding how general design methodologies are used in bioengineering design missions.
- To develop the ability to perform designs that align with production realities and business economics to successfully commercialize new bioproducts.

To support these core objectives, the training needs to incorporate three auxiliary objectives:

- To train the ability to design new bioproducts according to actual users' needs and to collect information from relevant or potential user groups likely to use or depend on the product.
- To train the ability to collect information from open sources of relevance for the design of new bioproducts and to collect and seek information by actively interacting with available expertise.
- To develop the understanding of how the designed bioproducts can be commercially protected by intellectual property rights and how existing intellectual property rights may limit the options for the design of new products.

These objectives all have well-defined training that is accomplished by several training means (Table 4.1). The means span across scenarios, training assignments, schemes for conceptualization, production economic frames, and optimization guidance.

Active interaction with industrial expertise plays an important role in providing realism but also moderation in the training.

The core of the design training for reaching the objectives is the actions carried out by the trainees. These actions are detailed in this chapter.

It is necessary to distinguish between objectives, means and actions. The chapter therefore also provides advice about evaluating the training organization itself, especially due to the outcome of the performance of trainees. In the eight design cases in Chap. 5, the objectives are concretely applied to modern bioengineered products.

Table 4.1 Objectives for training bioengineering students in bioproduct design

Training objective	Purpose of training	Means for the training
Proficiency in merging biological systems into the design	Exploit the biological perspective completely	Conceptual design mapping of the product idea
Proficiency in applying fundamental science and technology	Combining new ideas with scientific knowledge and applying established design methods	Conceptualization. Structured design work
Proficiency in integrating user needs into the design	Understanding how to integrate user needs from end-users and providers of products	Interviews, questionnaires, priority lists
Proficiency in using an economic perspective in the design	Ability to analyze the economic sustainability of the design	Structured economic analysis of investment and operational costs
Proficiency in open information sourcing	Finding shortcuts to better design solutions	Scientific literature databases, patent registries, and industry exhibitions
Proficiency in using info from knowledgeable expertise	Integrating specialized, exclusive, and relevant know-how	Direct outreach, interviews, and networking with experts

4.3 Structure of the Design Training

The training should be based on a frame that is convenient to use for tutorial guidance and student engagement. Such a frame must provide a solid structure for performing a highly qualified design training (Dym et al. 2005). In this guidance, the structure is realized through training scenarios. The training takes place within design assignments, supported by experienced tutorial management and industrial expertise, external information sources, reporting procedures, and performance evaluations (Fig. 4.2). The activities take place in dynamic flows of information and actions that mimic the reality of an industrial development environment.

In the nine design cases in Chap. 5, this framework is applied in the training. The framework allows a variety of training possibilities that pave the way for qualified development of engineers in industrial design.

Note that this bioengineering training could be involved in all parts of this structure. Still, the frame of the structure is general and applicable to all kinds of engineering design.

The details of the structure are described in the following, where the parts are explained.

4.3.1 The Training Scenario

Using scenarios is a well-proven training methodology widely applied in many areas (Della Volpe 2024). The ambition is to create a training situation as close as possible

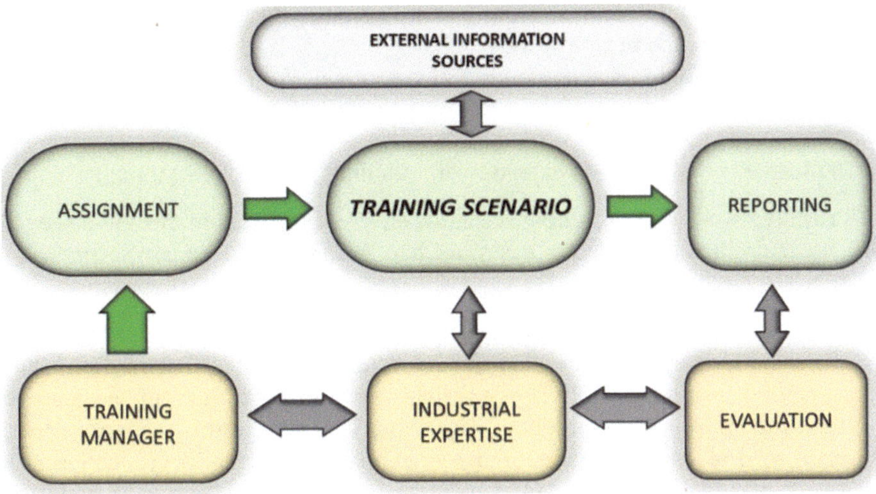

Fig. 4.2 The overall structure of the design training. The arrows indicate the flow of actions and information taking place during the training

to reality. In other fields of engineering, it is an established training approach in flight simulators, plant control operations, and emergency actions.

Creating training scenarios for engineering design requires much planning. Although the basic idea is similar, scenarios for design training have other frames, timescales, and purposes. This may change conditions, both with respect to applying design tools to process information, and to configuring design solutions. Also, the scenario model facilitates evaluating the training in a standardized fashion.

Several requirements for design training scenarios can be mentioned:

- The basic elements of the design training scenario are (i) an *industrial partner*, typically a company that produce bioproducts; (ii) a *design assignment* from the industrial partner to the trainees; (iii) an *industrial representation* from the assigning partner (industrial experts); (iv) a *design studio* with design tools; (v) *communication means* for the participants in the scenario; and (vi) a *group of trainees* that are to be trained in designing with the scenario as platform. The scenario should promote discussions on the results of design easily, making use of virtual drawing tables, and providing an opportunity to meet eye-to-eye.
- The scenario is based on an assignment description that describes the conditions for the scenario related to the scenario elements mentioned above. The representatives responsible for the description are the tutorial management together with the industrial experts.
- The design studio is the collection of digital and other tools for drawing, calculations, and modelling necessary for the design work.
- The scenario is not *one* locality. It is realized in communications between the participants (trainees, experts, tutors) using meetings, exchange of messages,

computer rooms, or other ways to access design software and other means for communication and design work.
- The scenario should strive to mimic real vocational life. This will facilitate seeing and distinguishing the borders of an assignment, a design task, the studio tools, and available methods.
- The scenario will typically extend over a training period of 1–3 months.

Basically, two types of training scenarios are recommended in this guidance and further exemplified in the design cases in Chap. 5. In Fig. 4.3, the two scenarios are illustrated.

(i) The group of trainees is a design team belonging to the assigning industrial partner. This partner can be a large biotech company, a smaller startup company, or any other organization where it is likely that there is a group of designers for the development of bioproducts. The trainees should, in this scenario, experience a virtual environment of the industrial management, production, and regulatory expertise that you expect in such organizations. The industrial expert(s) are responsible for acting as representatives for these units at the assigning partner (Fig. 4.3a).

(ii) The group of trainees is a design team belonging to a consultancy company. The consultancy company delivers design solutions to other companies. These other companies could be the kind of companies in (i) that would like an external partner's design solutions. The graphics highlight several important differences, for example, how the communication structures differ (Fig. 4.3b).

A few warnings and advice could be mentioned:

The tutorial management should establish rules for communication about the project work between the participants. For this, adequate tools could be provided, for example, templates and master tables, to visualize ideas and structures of solutions.

The pros and cons of the consultancy scenario are that the training team becomes a clearly defined unit versus the assigning company. One drawback is that in-house information must be acquired more actively from the assigning company.

The assignment can be directly related to an existing biotech company. However, the company can also be an imaginative "twin" to a real company with identical conditions and prerequisites that mimic a real industrial situation. The industrial experts are the recipients of the reporting from the assignees and take an active part in the evaluation of the project report.

4.3.2 The Team of Trainees

The training is carried out in a team of trainees. Thus, the ability to interact between individuals is an objective itself vital in the training. It is also the typical way to carry out project work in industry (Liu et al. 2015). For many apprentices this is not the

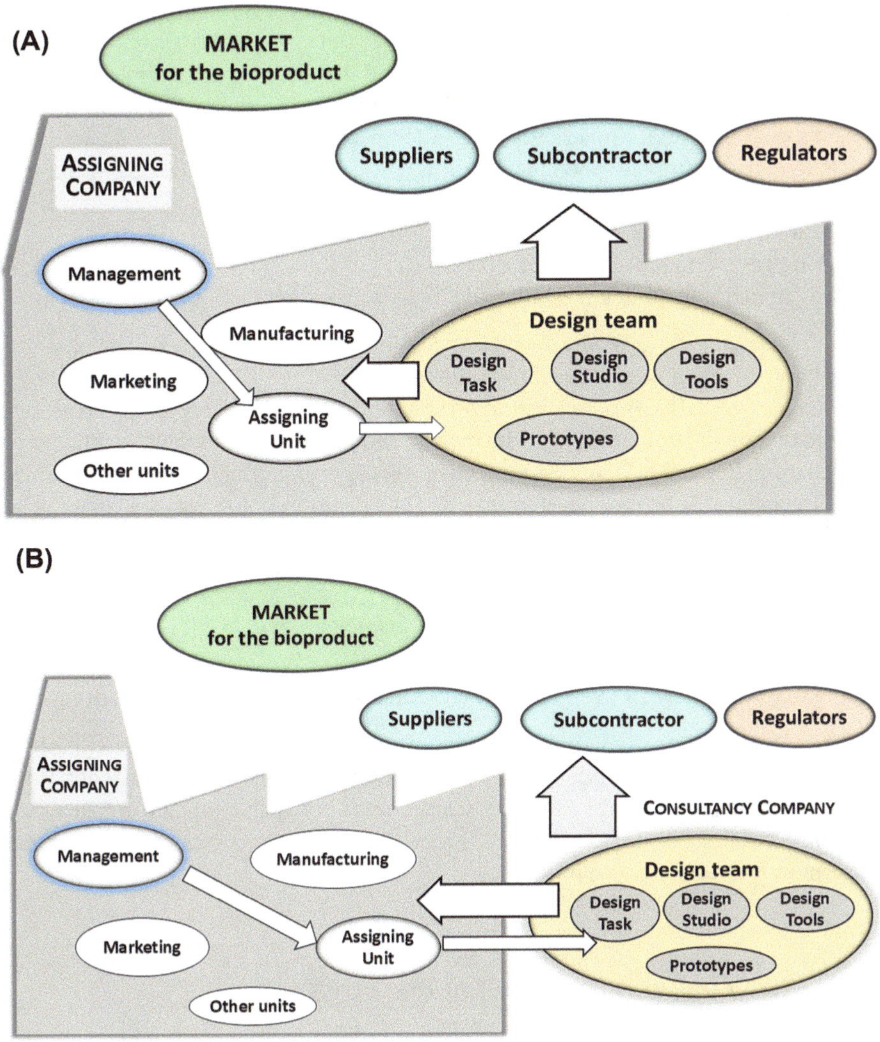

Fig. 4.3 Alternative organizational scenarios for the design training. (**a**) The trainees act as an internal design team (yellow) within a company (gray) producing and marketing the bioproduct. (**b**) The trainees act as an external consultancy firm (yellow) commissioned by a client company (gray) to deliver viable design solutions for the product. Arrows indicate interactions between team members and across the client company's organization

usual situation during education which tends to focus on individual performance rather than on the joint performance of a group or team. to be trained. The team members should have reached the right level of education and maturity for design work. During the training, they should, despite their background, be trained in fulfilling different roles, such as team leader, reporter, and negotiators of design ideas within the team.

For successful training, the composition of the team is a parameter that the training management can adjust. By knowing the educational background in terms of study direction and course curricula, a team with complementary backgrounds and competence can be formed. This will not only sharpen the strength of the team but also train the team members in interacting with people with varying backgrounds.

The trainees (students or other apprentices) in the design teams would ideally involve engineering students specialized in or with educational backgrounds in:

- *Modelling and programming,* with the role in the teamwork to take responsibility for the modelling of engineering systems.
- *Molecular and cell biology methodology*, with the role of providing aspects in fundamental molecular biology, its means, and methods. Note that the trainees are not being trained in running molecular biology experiments. But the trainees realize what results can be expected and what grounds for decision-making are within reach.
- *Statistics of biological and technical systems*, with the role of providing understanding of design of experiments and other statistical techniques. The main issue for the design training is to identify the kind of optimization tasks that are suitable. Thus, the design team should not carry out any experiments but be able to realize how to use statistics and what realistically can be improved by it.

Other backgrounds of value could be (i) food chemistry and biology, (ii) economics for *production*, or (iii) pharmacology and pharmaceutical technology. It is an advantage if the composition of teams varies between application cases. As is apparent from the list of backgrounds, the multidisciplinary competence of the team is essential for successful training.

4.3.3 The Design Assignment to the Team

The first event in the training is that the team members receive an assignment for the design of an industrial bioproduct. The assignment has three main purposes in the training:

- To define the industrial perspective of the scenario for the trainees.
- To describe what the objectives of the design mission are that the trainees are going to work with in the assignment.
- To relate the assignment to a qualified bioengineering context. Preferably, this is related to the state-of-the-art in biological science and biotechnology.

The assignment should be created by the tutorial management together with industrial experts. By that, the assignment will become sufficiently realistic from an industrial perspective and from current needs in product design. Importantly, the purpose and objectives of the product must be clearly defined from industrial and market perspectives.

4.3.4 The Role of the Academic Tutorial Management

The role of *academic tutorial management* is to take full responsibility for the design training. It could either be a course being a part of a curriculum at an engineering school, or a separate advanced course for selected students or professionals. The duties for the academic tutorial management are the following:

- To be the initiator of the training assignment. The formulation and description of the training assignment form the framework for the training. The management creates the assignment collaboratively with industrial expertise. This is a key aspect for the quality of the training and must be done with the necessary foresight into how the assignments are likely to develop.
- The tutorial management is responsible for putting together the members of the team of trainees. The educational backgrounds and versatilities described above about the team's competences should be a main concern for the tutorial management.
- During the training, the tutorial management supervises and provides guidance during the project work of the trainees in the team. The tutorial management preferably takes part in the team's project meetings. The tutorial management may take action to adjust the work of the team for its advancement.
- The management reads the intermediate and final reports from the trainees with support from the industrial experts.

The tutorial management is advised to apply a dynamic attitude in the training process and be prepared to improve the team's actions and, if motivated, introduce new conditions into the assignment.

4.3.5 The Role of the Industrial Experts

The industrial advisors are external specialists invited to support the training program. These individuals should possess direct experience in the product segment addressed by the project, ensuring a strong alignment with both the design assignment and the chosen training scenario.

The role and duties of the industrial experts are the following:

- To form, together with the academic training management, a realistic training scenario aligned with the experiences of the experts (Eris and Leifer 2003). The industrial experts should create the design assignment from their own experiences, knowing what is important and realistic. Especially, the experts can establish specific requirements grounded in realistic design goals, maintaining a responsive environment to address trainee inquiries and guide them through the complexities of the assignments.

- The industrial experts will act as representatives of the company in the scenario and be responsible for the assignment. They take part in meetings and discussions with the trainees.
- To be available for interviews and discussions with the trainees about conditions of the assignment in accordance with the training scenario. It is important to communicate with trainees so that a reality-based feeling is established in the training. This could cover production volumes, economic goals, actual costs, market-related conditions, and many other things.
- To read the interim and final reports from the team and provide industrially relevant feedback on their design solutions. By that, the industrial experts profoundly influence the project through these reviews. Typical demands for the reporting are as follows: (i) clarity of presentation by the team, (ii) highlighting of consequence analysis, (iii) understanding what is important in the deliverables, (iv) the notion of how to go ahead at various outcomes (in reality, between the review events/occasions), and (v) an understanding of what will happen post-assignment.

A few warnings should be mentioned:

Good guidance for teams of trainees by industrial experts is not always easy to achieve. Industrial experts sometimes tend to focus on other things than what is useful at the actual level of the trainees. It is the academic tutorial management's responsibility to ensure that adjoined experts are properly informed in advance about their role and level of training.

This is especially important when a project goes on over an extended time, easily leading to fragmented insights into the training achievements.

It is a risk that inexperienced training teams focus on detailed data that are not required for developing design solutions. This may result in requests directed to the experts for information about e.g., (i) negotiable prices of components, reagents, media and their dependence on quality and deliverability, and (ii) prices of critical equipment and relation to size and quantity. This must be responded to in a sensible way by the industrial experts.

4.4 Actions During the Training

The actions during the training can be divided into (i) those activities the trainees are expected to carry out within the frame of the scenario and the assignment and (ii) the tutor and expert actions for supporting the teamwork of the trainees in developing the assignment.

The trained team requires a structured action agenda. The agenda is delivered to the trainees prior to the training or when receiving the assignment. The main activities on the agenda focus on the following pillars:

- Applying basic design methodologies to the assignment.
- Analyzing and using available open information.
- Interacting with industrial expertise.
- Reporting to the assigner (the training manager, the industrial experts).

This results in two levels of training which should be distinguished. (i) The *trainees' level* where the students themselves act and structure their collaborative work within the design project under the leadership of one of the trainees, which should rotate. (ii) The *tutorial level* of the training where the tutors organize themselves with defined objectives and sharing of responsibilities and obligations in the training. These activities need careful consideration and planning.

The actions become the core of the training and must be well organized to attain a high quality. This must be based on a planned sequence of actions (Fig. 4.4).

The plan must have a specified expected outcome related to the training objectives. The actions of the team during the training are recommended to include the following ten steps:

1. Establish a *structure of the assignment* related to the assigner (e.g., a biotech company) showing (i) the relations to upfront research and development, (ii) the competence and the assigner's capability for development and production, and (iii) the assumed users and customers of the bioproduct.
2. Compile a *list of requirements* detailed into at least five prioritized requirements where each item is specified qualitatively or quantitatively with metrics relevant for the design mission.
3. Establish *a conceptual map* based on the assignment objectives and the above list showing the required transformation process for the design product. A map structure includes the stages of transformation and primary and secondary inputs and outputs with the functional systems required.
4. Conceive selected *preliminary configuration alternatives* of the conceptual map where the transformation process is detailed into functional unit operations showing inputs and outputs to each unit.
5. Compile a list of *patents or patent applications* relevant for the design alternatives that show opportunities or threats to the envisaged design and how these are relevant towards the requirements.
6. Conceive *detailed design drawings* for those configuration alternatives that best comply with the priorities and where real unit operations replace functional objects.
7. Present an *economic assessment of production costs*, distribution investment costs and operational costs. In the economic assessment, it usually suffices to include only the most expensive investments and the five most costly consumables. Importantly, the assessment must cover the estimates of plant installation, upfront R&D, labor, and marketing costs.

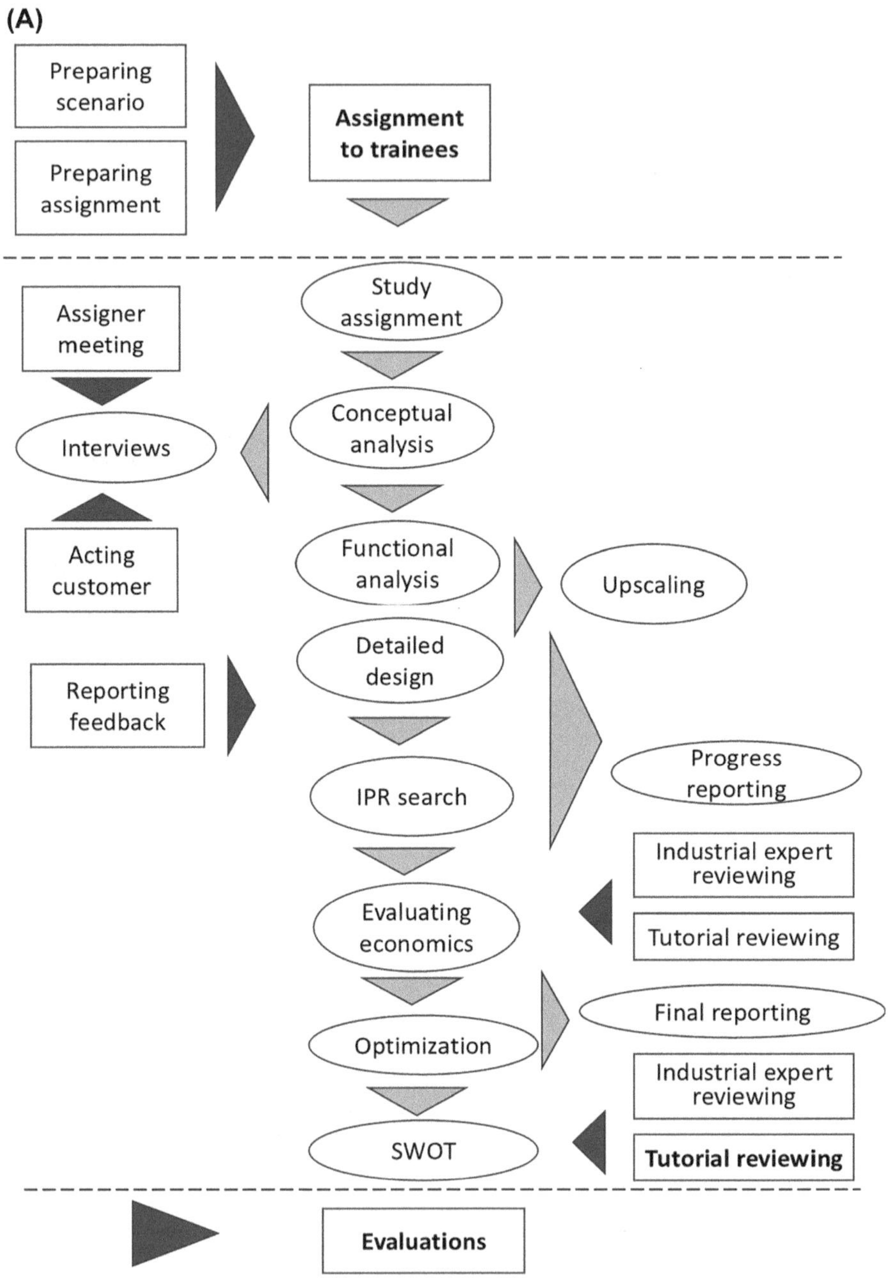

Fig. 4.4 (**a**) Flow of actions by the trainees in the training. (**b**) Bidirectional information exchange during the action between trainees and tutors. Trainees' flow of actions is shown in light gray, and tutorial flows of actions in light blue

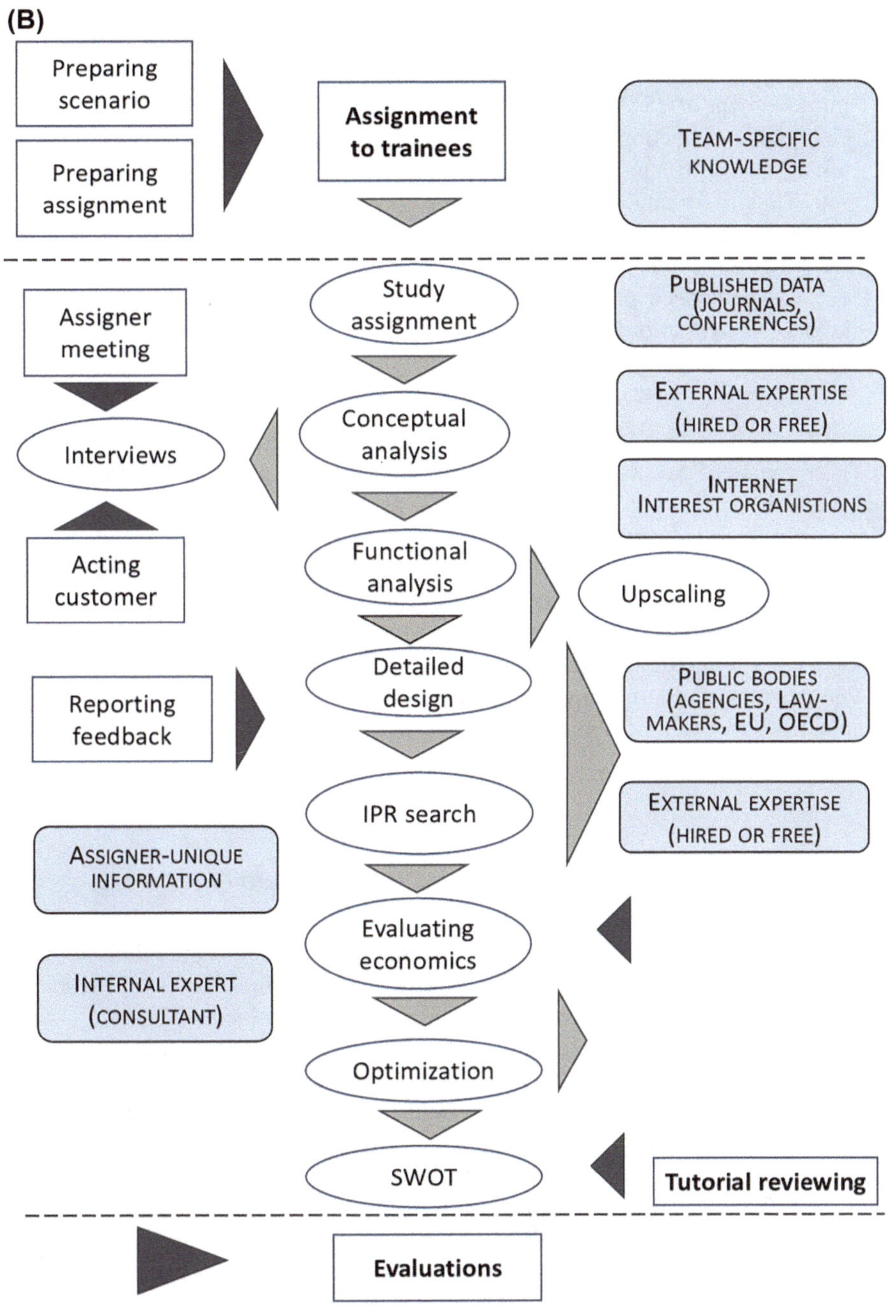

Fig. 4.4 (continued)

8. Provide an overview of the *five most relevant factors* that may contribute to improving the performance of the design. Identify the relevant responses to measure in a factorial experimental plan with the purpose of reaching an improvement of 25–50%.
9. Compile a collection of charts showing the *dynamics of the transformation* taking place in the designed transformation process based on mechanistic modelling with mass balance and kinetics. The charts intend to show the dependency on key parameters in relation to time for the design alternatives. Of particular interest are those parameters that affect the cost of production because of chosen plant volume, investment, raw material consumption, and labor, and by that influence the productivity of a plant or device or system.
10. Provide a summary of how the *users' requirements* are met in the final design alternative. The users' priorities should be visualized and economic factors and costs highlighted in relation to secondary alternatives.

These ten steps become the content of the final reporting to the assigner. Basically, the tables, drawings, and compiled lists also become the body of the reporting of the assignment. A short supplementary and descriptive text is needed. Typical engineering language, i.e., data, drawings, and diagrams, should constitute the essential content of the reporting. Standard engineering conventions in language and nomenclature must be used to enhance translingual communication, which is necessary in multinational companies.

The structure and strictness of the delivered reported material allow the tutorial management to evaluate the performance of the team more easily and provide sensible feedback.

4.4.1 Conceptualization of the Design Assignment

The use of conceptual thinking in functionalities should characterize the training.

As described in detail in the methodology chapter, the functions identified in the conceptual analysis should be replaced with real technical objects (Hubka and Eder, 1988; Ulrich et al. 2019; Jackson et al. 2024; Mandenius and Björkman 2011). This means that each function or subfunction, systems or sub-subsystems, will be realized with real technical units. It is a demanding step in the training and will require time to investigate, consider, and compare. Mostly, it will be a matter of technical performance and costs of the unit, thus, a trade-off between the unit's capacity and what is affordable. The assignment objectives and the user needs may constrain the choices (Table 4.2). An important part of the training is to withhold the decision about the real units until the requirements of functionality are completely clarified (Alonso-Rasgado et al. 2004). It is wise to implement this notion early, forcing the designer to have an open mind in these choices.

Especially in this step, the design solutions converge into a limited number of options. These options must comply with the intentions of the product idea, the

Table 4.2 Relationship between conceptual main functions, subfunctions and real objects

Main function	Subfunctions	Real units
Biological functions	Host cells able to produce	Access public cell bank. Subcontracting specialist company to make new cells. Using own proprietary cells
	iPSC able to differentiate and mature	Invest R&D of expression system. Buy systems. Develop culture conditions
Technical functions	Containment of cells	Bioreactors. Culture vessels. Incubators. Single-use units. Continuous culture system
	Techniques for observing cell actions	Optical sensors. Electronic sensors. Microscopes at line. QC lab. Immunology methods
Information functions	Information about cell state	Structure of cells. Expression of vectors. Rates. Purity. Impurities.
	Information about technical equipment operation	Sensors. Digital diagnostics. Using ML- and AI-derived information
Management functions	Procedures to control the plant's operation and quality	Adaptive controllers. Basic PID controllers. Offline test data
	IPR for the manufacture of the bioproduct	Employed patent engineer. Acquire others' IPRs. Applying for own IPR.
Human functions	Ethical compliance of plant to current public opinions	Green agenda. Expert audits. Employing an ethical officer
	Ethical conditions. Safety of employees	Warning systems. Training personnel. Using safe ingredients and biologics

assignment objectives, and the user requirements. During the initial evaluation phase, the design space expands into a broad array of diverging possibilities (Fig. 4.5). These options are then subjected to a series of rigorous filters, or hurdles, derived from (i) the specific constraints and objectives of the assignment, (ii) comprehensive user requirements, and (iii) a detailed appraisal of economic feasibility. Through this systematic winnowing process, the design is optimized until only a few viable, high-potential options remain.

In bioengineering, the availability of feasible biological systems is the most critical hurdles step. As the figure illustrates, this step is the natural starting point and probably most closely associated with the inventive idea. Next is to find plausible technical systems that can handle the biological systems. This may include a variety of technical systems, from mechanics, flow dynamics, heat container, and measurement and control techniques. Their varying feasibility diminishes the options.

The merged biological and technical systems should be optimized. The proneness to being maximized may change the order of feasibility of the design alternatives. The economic evaluation should decide which of these are most attractive from an industrially sound business perspective.

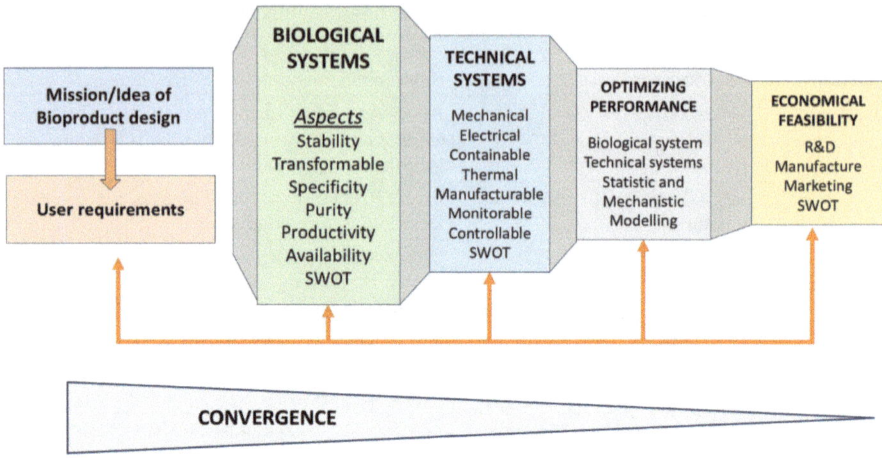

Fig. 4.5 Training is a consecutive array of actions driven by a set of conceived alternatives to converge into a preferred design. The tools contribute to refining and improving the design. Various aspects that the user requirement prioritizes. The convergence is correlated to the timeline

4.4.2 Actions for Detailing Design Alternatives

The next action is to provide a description of the technical implementation of the configuration. This must be detailed enough to allow an economic assessment of the cost to build and operate the plant for the intended production. This detailed design is implemented in technical drawings showing the significant operational units in the conceptual transformation process.

Important skills to be trained are the identification of the mechanisms of operational units and the ability to identify alternative units (Doran 2013; Heinzle et al, 2006; Mandenius, 2016).

Of importance is also to train the ability to scale the detailed design drawings. Initially, this can be preliminary or tentative outlines, i.e., possible to adapt and adjust to redesign once volumetric sizes are determined.

The training of the apprentices in drawing techniques for the transfer of functional systems and subsystems to process flow diagrams is a classical engineering skill. Rules and standards for technical drawings should be trained, especially if not practiced before by the trainees. At this stage of detailing the design, units are simply graphical boxes with input and output streams. The nine design cases in Chap. 5 exemplify typical layouts of diagrams.

It is to be noted that process flow diagrams are mostly used to depict unit operations in bioprocesses. Here, this extends the diagrams to depict processing flows in devices and testing service operations in design alternatives of a transformation process. Importantly, all graphical units are associated with material flows and costs for investments (in equipment and other facilities) and operational costs (labor, consumables). Thus, the units in the diagrams can also be, for example, detectors, analytical flow cells, testing procedures, and analytical instruments. The design cases in Chap. 5 show several such examples of diagrams (cf. Cases 1, 2, 5, and 6 for bioprocesses; Case 3 for testing service; and Cases 4, 7, and 8 for devices).

4.4.3 Evaluating Intellectual Property Opportunities of the Design

New bioproducts must be possible to protect by intellectual property rights (IPRs) to hinder other companies from marketing the same product design. Once a new product is available on the market, it can be copied or, to some degree, mimicked by competitors. The common way is to protect the uniqueness of the product by one or several patents. These patents should not infringe on other existing IPRs. Preferably, own IPR can be distinctly framed with claims that define:

- The unique structure (molecular, mechanical, or electronic) of the invented bioproduct that is not previously described in IPRs.
- Operative ranges of the new bioproducts.
- A unique principle of operation for the design of the bioproducts not previously described in any literature.

Patent databases provide what is previously inventive. Consequently, these databases are most valuable sources of information concerning other new inventive ideas and may inspire trainees to create new inventions. They are also good indicators for potential conflicts on the originality of ideas (Keswani and Possas 2024). It is easy to search for patent applications in patent databases (e.g., www.espace.com).

It is strongly motivated to carry out IPR searching once the conceptual options are prioritized (Table 4.3). If the IPR situation is unfavorable, reprioritizing is

Table 4.3 Useful information in patent databases and how to exploit the information

Patent information	Potential values of the information
Invention company	Reveals a potential competitor or a collaborator from which the IPR can be acquired
Patent claims	Shows the critical legal value of the patent. Shows the strength of the patent and what cannot be neglected
Application examples using the patent	May show relevant technical information that can be useful for your own design
Drawings of the patent	Shows the essence and quality of the idea. Check if it is really protected in the claims
State of patent	Shows the period the patent is legally valid
References mentioned in the application	Shows what the patent applicants considered relevant and what was previously protected

recommended. But the IPR search may also reveal valuable information about conceptual and technical matters that can provide cues to improving design alternatives. These can be of great value when the design configurations are detailed. Basically, methods already applied for patent applications are advised not to be reused or circumvented by the trainees in their own design.

4.4.4 Evaluating the Production Economics of Designs

The production costs for the design alternatives must be analyzed and compared. Bioengineers do not always have a thorough education in economics, which makes it an important part of the training. However, the principles of evaluation of production economics are not too difficult to understand and are thoroughly explained and exemplified in engineering literature (Peters et al. 2003; Kristiansen 2006; Towler and Sinnott 2012).

In the evaluation of the production economics of the design alternatives, one should be aware of the following difficulties:

- Information on actual costs for each raw material item and equipment unit is seldom easy to determine.
- A detailed design comes at a relatively late stage, and information about cost is desired early in the design work and takes time to find.
- Costs vary in a range that differs depending on location, timing, economic conjuncture, and world prices.
- Production costs in a typical manufacturing company are normally shared between several products, and it is not obvious how the cost burden should be distributed between products and their revenues.
- Most R&D costs occur and accumulate prior to the income from sales and are recurrently covered by income from a previous product.

These difficulties cannot be covered in the design training. However, it is important that uncertainties about these costs do not hamper creativity in the design work.

A convenient training approach could be to:

- Assess costs as a single stand-alone production and neglect compensation or adjustment from parallel or previous products.
- Provide the trainees with a list of standard costs for common raw materials, salaries, costs for facilities, typical equipment items such as pumps, tanks, bioreactors and separation columns, and centrifuges. This is to avoid spending too much time searching for prices for specific items.
- Let the industrial experts provide the trainees with critical costs, such as specialized equipment, patent application cost, etc.

A general cost structure for production of a bioproduct is helpful when starting the economic evaluation (Fig. 4.6 and Table 4.4). Certain cost items are critical; here

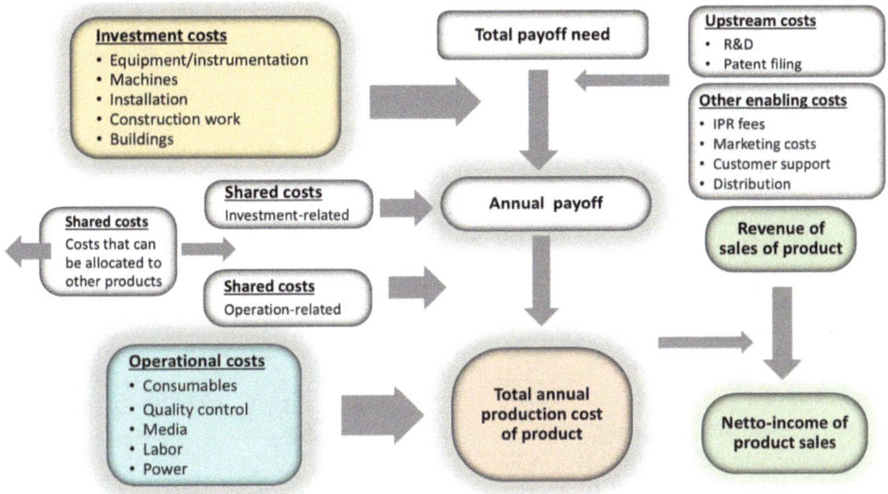

Fig. 4.6 Production economics flow when assessing the cost structure of a new design. Basically, the investments and operational costs could not exceed the revenue. But costs must also be seen in the total cost structure of the company, as the figure shows

the industrial experts usually must guide the trainees about what realistic cost levels are for an operating company. The kind of advice will mainly concern:

- How can the company reduce its procurement costs in a competitive market?
- How well can the company assess the most plausible sales price and, from it, appreciate the revenue?
- How much net income must the product generate for the company to keep the owners at bay concerning dividends and progress?
- How much of the costs can be shared with other products from their own company?
- How long payback time can be accepted?
- How much of the net income must be reinvested in new products or upgrading of existing products, including the present one?

The design team cannot easily judge these questions but needs to be aware of them and understand that production costs must be significantly lower than the sales price.

The general structure of the economic evaluation is shown in Fig. 4.6. The balance and flow of costs, income from sales, payback of investment, and upfront costs are important to relate to the actual design solutions to understand what critical parts of the design are.

When performing the evaluation of costs, it is convenient to use Table 4.4 as a template. The template is recommended to be divided into upfront costs, investments, auxiliary costs for the investments, operational costs divided into

Table 4.4 Organizing types of costs in production economy. General example

Costs with examples	Low estimate (kEUR)	High estimate (kEUR)
Investment costs for production		
Upfront R&D cost		
Internal product development	2000	3000
Subcontracted development	1000	2000
IPR filing	100	300
Total upfront R&D	*3100*	*5300*
Equipment and instruments		
Upstream equipment and instruments	1500	2500
Downstream equipment and instruments	1000	2500
Quality control instrumentation	500	100
Total equipment costs	*3000*	*6000*
Other equipment and instrument costs		
Construction and facility installation (× 0.9)	2700	5400
Buildings and plant areas (× 0.3)	900	1800
Planning and management (× 0.2)	600	1200
Validation	2000	4000
Legal costs (× 0.1)	300	600
Other investments costs	*6500*	*13,000*
Total investment costs	*9810*	*23,300*
Operational costs (annual costs or for quality-related costs)		
Consumables	600	800
Power for installations	100	200
Labor	2000	3000
Subcontractor reimbursement	1000	2000
Taxation of sale	200	400
Totaloperational costs	*3900*	*6400*
Operational costs (shared, upfront, or postproduction)		
Transportation of goods	100	200
Research and development	500	600
Management of sales	100	200
Total annual costs	*700*	*900*
Annual payoff of investment (5 years)	*18,000*	*36,000*
Total production costs	*64,000*	*109,000*

consumables, and other operational costs for salaries, building, maintenance, etc. For the annual operational costs, the annual payback of investments and upfront R&D costs are added in the template (depreciation) for a set period. For several of the cost items, it is recommended to use standard cost factors to assess typical costs appearing in all productions. Also, it is suggested to have two columns in that table, one for a low cost, and one for a high estimate.

It is essential that the economic evaluation maintains a level of precision that is appropriately scaled: it must be rigorous enough to rank design alternatives effectively, yet practical enough to support informed corporate decision-making without unnecessary complexity.

4.4.5 Actions for Optimization of the Design

The opportunity to optimize design solutions is a critical consideration following the economic evaluation. The objective is fundamental: determining whether strategic optimization can enhance a design's performance sufficiently to transform an otherwise non-viable concept into an economically feasible solution (Pahl et al. 2007; Ulrich et al. 2019; Heinzle et al. 2006; Mandenius and Brundin, 2008; Nielsen et al. 2011). Consequently, assessing optimization potential is a pivotal factor that directly influences the ultimate success of any design mission.

In a professional training context, the focus must be on developing the competency to disclose optimization possibilities and propose concrete corrective actions. Trainees must learn to systematically rank their options, identifying which specific components or parameters offer the highest potential for refinement and rigorously judging their anticipated technical effect and broader economic impact.

The tutorial role is to bring understanding for these purposes. Thus, it is not an exercise in carrying out any optimization methods but a training to identify where in the design there are potentials for optimizing the design solution. The main challenge is to predict the effect of optimization efforts or whether optimization at all will sufficiently improve the performance and economy of the design solution. Or, to consider if optimization needs to be carried out at all.

Basic methodologies for optimization are described in Chap. 3. A balanced discussion of their use, efforts, and experimental costs and efforts needs to be initiated at this stage. In industrial practice, several optimization tools are at hand. Mentioned in Chap. 3 are design-of-experiments, mechanistic modelling, and the 6σ platform. It is advised not to let optimization as such be too much of the purpose of the design training. The design training should instead be directed towards understanding and identifying the potential of optimization.

4.4.6 Using SWOT Analysis to Evaluate the Potential of the Design Alternatives

The previous chapter (Chap. 3) has stated the purpose of SWOT analysis. It is recommended to apply SWOT analysis as the final training action of a design mission (Shinno et al. 2006). The SWOT analysis then becomes the trained team's own appraisal and testing of the quality of their design solutions. The four perspectives in SWOT analysis, strengths, weaknesses, opportunities, and threats, are useful benchmarks for comparing the design alternatives. By testing the design alternatives in view of the strengths and weaknesses of their configurations, their economy, their opportunity to be optimized, or threats from IPR become helpful for ranking them.

The comparisons are preferably overviewed in a table (see Design Cases 1 and 2). This table also serves as an agenda for the internal discussion in the trained team, usually leading to revisions and new conclusions.

The SWOT analysis also becomes a useful frame for the reporting of the assignment, both for oral reporting and for a written final report.

4.4.7 Reporting Design Assignments

One of the training objectives is the reporting and documentation of the design results. This requirement encompasses written interim and final reports as well as oral reporting.

The reporting must be professionally addressed to the project stakeholder, which is typically represented by the "company" within the training scenario.

Importantly, reporting in a business context differs from academic reports, articles, or theses (Peters et al. 2003). Efficiency in providing the bottom line and rationale for a company decision is the purpose of the report. Therefore, the training must prioritize adapting to this purpose and go beyond the typical scientific report format (e.g., Introduction; Experimental methods; Results; Discussion; Conclusion; Acknowledgement; References).

A typical industrial reporting format is based on: (i) an executive summary, (ii) assignment (or project) objectives, (iii) frames and constraints, (iv) conceptual possibilities, (v) alternative solutions, (vi) economic consequences, (vii) potential improvements, and (viii) recommendations (Table 4.5). Thus, the information that is critical in a company's decision-making process is what must be highlighted in the report.

4.5 Other Aspects of the Design Training

4.5.1 Managing Project Timescales in Training

Training cannot be done in real time; the timescale must be compressed into what is realistic under the training conditions. Although this is caused by practical reasons, it also allows the tutors to adjust the training activities in the scenario favorably (Pahl et al. 2007; Ulrich et al. 2019).

Most design training is carried out over an extended time. Normally, this period is adapted to a course curriculum in a teaching program. Thus, it will be interrupted by other course activities, often with no connection to design training. The scenario time deviates from real time and can be interrupted as the tutors decide and find appropriate (Fig. 4.7).

Table 4.5 A preferred structure for reporting in industry with focus on business frames, outcomes, and consequences adapted to a design assignment

Item in report	Focus of item	Rationale for the assigner
Executive summary	The essential outcome of the assignment in short	The decision-makers should, in a short time, overview the basic outcome
Assignment preconditions	Description of the assignment from a design perspective	The assigner wants to be reassured that the design is correctly interpreted according to the assigner's incentives
Justification for inventive ideas	Brief recapitulation of the ideas and their business and customer relevance	The assigner wants to know this in detail (again)
Design methods applied in the study	Short description of the methodologies used in the design work	The assigner wants to appreciate the quality of the design work by the designers
Possible design options	Drawings and tables with explanations	The main structure and differences are what interest the assigner, not the details
Economic evaluation of design alternatives	State without details bottom line and structure of costs between alternatives	The assignee wants to compare the final costs for comparison with other business-related alternatives
Possibilities of future improvements	Explain how the designs can be optimized, efforts and cost for it	The rationale for future development is a priority issue in the decision-making
Recommendation to the assigner	Focus on the pros and cons of alternative designs and a conclusive final recommendation	The assigner should be able to draw business conclusions based on the recommendation

Thus, the training timescale is far from linear. The timescale cannot perfectly correlate with the path of the convergence arrow but with the consecutive order of events and actions. In training courses, this is both a challenge and an opportunity. The scenario play leader may interrupt time or accelerate time when convenient for tutorial reasons. This may easily lead to loss of realism.

Examples of typical discrepancies in time:

- Time for delivery of procurement costs. These delays are frequent and a reason for prolonging the design development. It is an irrelevant delay for training objectives that the tutors must try to circumvent.
- Time for building a plant for testing (pilot plant). This is a profound and obvious time delay counted in months and even years depending on size and workforce. It relates to construction and building costs, which should be understood and not neglected in the economic evaluation in relation to labor costs. It also influences the time-to-market negatively. Results from such tests and data can be provided by the tutorial management.
- Time for performing testing and delivery of test results. Results from such tests can be provided by the tutorial management.

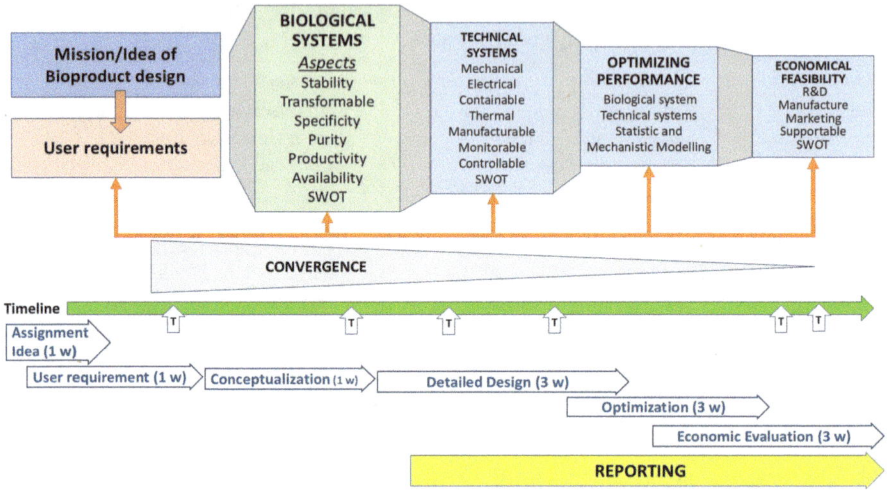

Fig. 4.7 The training activities are a consecutive order of actions that drive design alternatives to converge. The tutorial management must control the timeline within the available time frame of the training. The T-arrows indicate events controlled by the tutorial management to discontinue the timeline with complementary activities or conditions

- Time for validation. This is also a cost in the economic evaluation that must be considered. Results and costs from validations can be provided by the tutorial management.
- Time for regulatory response. This information can also be included in the scenario as an event changing conditions for the assignment. Regulatory responses can be provided by the tutorial management with short delays.

All the interruptions or delays may, if applied wisely, offer certain pedagogical advantages and may offer a dynamic to the training. By experience and knowledge about engineering realities, judgment, and imagination, specific training challenges can be introduced into a scenario.

It is important that these deviations from real time are dealt with properly. The tutors must carefully plan when accelerating or compressing the timescale in a realistically acceptable way with a pedagogical training perspective.

4.5.2 Adaptation to Vocational Training

If the trainees already have experience from vocational work, the design of the training should be adapted to what is relevant for their continuing training.

In Chap. 2, the need for vocational training was briefly mentioned. It is of growing concern in a rapidly changing industrial sector that professionals are regularly retrained and their knowledge and skills upgraded. Design engineering is

Table 4.6 Aspects of planning vocational training

Focus of training	Training advice	Expected outcome
New methodologies in bioengineering	Demonstrate new methods with concrete bioindustrial cases	Basic hands-on experience. Know-how for practice in industry
Rehearsing basic bioengineering	Mini courses with content based on participant background	Previous knowledge and skill recapitulated and refreshed
Databases for bioengineering	Demonstrate capacity of databases for bioindustrial needs	Provided insights into resources and an updated collection of links to novel database facilities
New equipment for bioengineering	Invite qualified vendors of new equipment	Better insights into novel equipment and instrumentation and their applicability
Design cases for using new methodology and equipment, software and databases	Use design cases in this guidance updated and modified for the background and needs of the participant	An up-to-date experience and knowledge about new design conditions and possibilities

certainly an example where this needs to be a high priority. It is, of course, costly to constantly employ new staff for this, while updating training and skills costs less to implement. Therefore, cost-efficient training of high quality can be a rewarding payback approach. However, vocational training must consider:

- The available time span for training is shorter.
- The need for dedicated focus on novelty should be a priority.
- The participants are experienced, sometimes very qualified, and have high expectations of the quality of the training.

Vocational training teams can be expected to be more heterogeneous than students in a university environment where preparatory courses often align with the content of a design training course. The participants' age distribution at universities is smaller. University teachers usually have limited experience of industrial life and business issues and are used to working under other conditions and other priorities.

It is advised to plan vocational programs meticulously according to these premises for a balanced content related to their vocational experience (Table 4.6).

4.6 Evaluation of the Training Performance

Three aspects of the training need to be evaluated: (i) the trainees' general performance of design, (ii) their performance of applying biology in the design, and (iii) the overall quality of the training program.

Table 4.7 Evaluation of the trainees' general performance

Challenges for training of bioengineers	Outcome of training	Principal means for training
Capitalizing the power of biological systems in engineering products	The ability to define more distinctly what should be expected from a biological system in a new solution	Specifications of the target metrics of the biological system to be considered and employed
Creativity for finding and evaluating new solutions based on biological systems	Ability to see how the user needs are conceived in new designs in a measurable way that addresses the user needs and the possibilities of biology	Employing conceptual design in terms of combining functionality versus configurations with biological parts
Adaptation of biological systems for engineering purposes	Ability to understand in what way the biological systems need transformation and adaptation to fulfill user requirement boundaries	Combining conceptual configurations with specifications and biological diversity (i.e., access to various biological systems)
Identifying economic bottlenecks in manufacturing/fabrication caused by the limits of the biological systems	Ability to understand the solution from an economic perspective and transform the design of biological systems accordingly	Employing CAD tools in which economic evaluation procedures are implemented in terms of biological sensitivity and risk analysis

4.6.1 Evaluation of the Trainees' General Performance

The primary focus is the general performance of the trainees, assessing both individual contributions and the collective output of the team (Table 4.7). Because design rarely follows a single "correct" path, evaluation criteria remain largely qualitative or semi-quantitative. Similar to academic defenses or professional certifications, a committee of experienced members is recommended to conduct these assessments. This evaluation encompasses the quality of teamwork alongside the growth of individual apprentices. Committee members should operate under clear guidelines to appraise and reflect on the following benchmarks:

- *Conceptual Alignment:* The ability to synthesize user needs with realistic cost constraints while identifying potential biological refinements. This includes conceptualizing the product in direct relation to identified requirements.
- *Technical Proficiency:* Effective use of design tools to investigate conditions rooted in engineering mathematics and industrial economics.
- *Collaborative Management:* Leveraging the diverse capabilities of team members, including the production of interim and final documentation via technical drawings and formal reports.
- *Predictive Analysis:* The foresight to identify requirements for experimental verification and the quantification of design alternatives. While physical experimentation may be limited in a training environment, trainees must demonstrate the ability to foresee and discuss these needs.

A few additional advice on the above can be:

- A formal tutor-trainee dialogue that explores the reasoning behind reported conclusions is helpful. This discussion addresses why certain results may be inconclusive, inaccurate, or biased—often stemming from a lack of exposure to real-world conditions. Evaluators note the balance between reliance on instruction and the trainee's critical eye toward subjective conditions (Eris and Leifer 2003).
- While the ideal metric is observing how trainees utilize these skills in their forthcoming vocational careers (Daly et al. 2012; Liu et al. 2015), such long-term tracking is often impractical or unrealistic. Nevertheless, engaging trainees in discussions regarding future professional application provides significant educational value.

4.6.2 Evaluation of the Trainees' Performance in Applying Biological Aspects

Once the evaluation of the performance of general design work is ready, the performance of dealing with the biological issues in the design should be assessed. This should concern exclusively the biological aspects and how this interplays with other systems involved in the design. Two aspects are the most relevant to evaluate (Table 4.8):

- The inventiveness of the trainees in finding solutions where the design exploits biology and biological systems and what actual outcome of the training is accomplished.
- The trainees' proficiency in navigating complex biological systems to pinpoint economic bottlenecks, followed by the strategic adaptation of those systems to better align with the commercial objectives and performance expectations of the new bioproduct. The evaluation is recommended to have a strong focus on robustness or durability of systems or products in relation to the intended lifetime of the bioproduct. The skill to do this within an acceptable production cost window that the market can accept shall be assessed.

4.6.3 Evaluation of the Training Program

Finally, the quality of the training curriculum must be systematically evaluated. This process entails auditing the performance of both the tutorial management team and the invited industrial experts, alongside assessing the overall educational efficacy of the training. The assessment focuses specifically on the following aspects:

Table 4.8 Evaluation of the trainees' performance in applying biological aspects in the design training

Challenges for training of bioengineers	Outcome of training	Principal means for training
Creativity for finding and evaluating new solutions based on biological systems	Ability to see how the user needs are conceived in new designs in a measurable way that addresses the user needs and the possibilities of biology	Employing conceptual design in terms of combining functionality versus configurations with biological parts
Adaptation of biological systems for engineering purposes	Ability to understand in what way the biological systems need transformation and adaptation to fulfil user requirement boundaries	Combining conceptual configurations with specifications and biological diversity (i.e., access to various biological systems)
Capitalizing the power of biological systems in engineering products	The ability to define more distinctly what is expected from a biological system in a new solution	Specifications of the target metrics of the biological system to be considered and employed
Identifying economic bottlenecks in manufacturing/fabrication caused by the limits of the biological systems	Ability to understand the solution from an economic perspective and transform the design of biological systems accordingly	Employing digital design tools in which economic evaluation procedures are implemented in terms of biological sensitivity and risk analysis
The quality of reporting	Ability to bring forward the bio-related message to the assigner in accordance with the objectives	Follow the template in Table 4.4

- How relevant and balanced the training and chosen scenarios have been for reaching the training objectives proposed in Sect. 4.2. Have all the objectives been achieved in the training? Have the training cases been composed so that the objectives have been possible to reach?
- Have the industrial experts been able to contribute to the training in relation to the conditions of the scenario? Have the industrial experts interacted with the trainees at the right level? Have the experts focused sufficiently well on the objectives in the assignment?
- Have the trainees been provided with relevant information? This could include information about technical matters in the description of the assignment, economic information about equipment and raw materials, and the assignee's business policy.
- Have the constraints in the assignment been realistic in relation to available training time and educational level of the trainees? Here shall be noted that these conditions differ considerably in academic programs and for vocational training.

- Has the gradient during the training period been adequate in relation to the assignees' prerequisites and advancement in the training?
- Have the user needs been presented to the assignees in a realistic way? Are the needs industrially relevant, and are they detailed enough, or should they have been better adapted to the training conditions?

References

Alonso-Rasgado T, Thompson G, Elfström BO (2004) The design of functional (total care) products. J Eng Design 15(6):515–540. https://doi.org/10.1080/09544820412331271176

Daly RS, Adams RS, Bodner GM (2012) What does it mean to design? A qualitative investigation of design professionals' experiences. J Eng Edu 101:187–219. https://doi.org/10.1002/j.2168-9830.2012.tb00048.x

Della Volpe V (2024) Scenario-based learning: an inclusive methodology. IOSR J Res Meth Edu 14:1–5

Doran PM (2013) Biochemical engineering principles, 2nd edn. Elsevier, Amsterdam. https://doi.org/10.1016/C2009-0-22348-8

Doulougeri K, Jan D, Vermunt JD, Bombaerts G et al (2024) Challenge-based learning implementation in engineering education: a systematic literature review. J Eng Educ 113:1076–1106. https://doi.org/10.1002/jee.20588

Dym CL, Agogino AM, Eris O et al (2005) Engineering design thinking, teaching and learning. J Eng Educ 94:103–120. https://doi.org/10.1002/j.2168-9830.2005.tb00832.x

Eris O, Leifer LJ (2003) Facilitating product development knowledge acquisition: interaction between the expert and the team. Int J Eng Edu 19:142–152

Heinzle E, Biwer A, Cooney C (2006) Development of sustainable bioprocesses. Modelling and assessment. Wiley, Chichester

Hubka V, Eder WE (1988) Theory of technical systems, a total concept theory for engineering design. Springer Verlag, Berlin

Jackson A, Barrella E, Bodnar C (2024) Application of concept maps as an assessment tool in engineering education: systematic literature review. J Eng Educ 113:752–766. https://doi.org/10.1002/jee.20548

Keswani C, Possas C (2024) Intellectual property issues in life sciences disputes and controversies. Taylor and Francis Ltd

Kristiansen B (2006) Process economics. In: Ratledge C, Kristiansen N (eds) Basic biotechnology, 3rd edn. Cambridge University Press, Cambridge UK, pp 239–252

Liu ML, Liu NT, al Ding CG e (2015) Exploring team performance in high-tech industries: future trends of building up teamwork. Technol Forecast Social Changes 91:295–310

Mandenius CF (ed) (2016) Bioreactors: design, operation and novel applications. Wiley VCH, Weinheim

Mandenius CF, Björkman M (2011) Biomechatronic design in biotechnology, a methodology for development of biotechnological products. Wiley, Hoboken

Mandenius CF, Brundin A (2008) Bioprocess optimization using design-of-experiments methodology. Biotechnol Prog 24:1191–1203. https://doi.org/10.1002/btpr.67

Nielsen J, Villadsen J, Lidén G (2011) Bioreaction engineering principles, 3rd edn. Springer-Nature, New York

Pahl G, Beitz W, Feldhusen J et al (2007) Engineering design, a systematic approach, 3rd edn. Springer Verlag, Berlin

Peters MS, Timmerhaus KD, West RE (2003) Plant design and economics for chemical engineers, 5th edn. McGraw-Hill & Co, New York

Shinno H, Yoshioka H, al Marpaung S e (2006) Quantitative SWOT analysis on global competitiveness of machine tool industry. J Eng Design 17(3):251–258. https://doi.org/10.1080/09544820500275180

Towler G, Sinnott R (2012) Chemical engineering design: principles, practice and economics of plant and process design, 2nd edn. Elsevier, Amsterdam

Ulrich KT, Eppinger SD, Yang MC (2019) Product design and development, 5th edn. McGraw-Hill, New York

Chapter 5
Design Cases for Training

The scope, purpose, and pedagogical value of the following design cases are explained here. Tutors should view the design cases as flexible blueprints rather than rigid instructions. They should be modified and adapted by instructors to meet specific curriculum needs, programmatic goals, and varying student skill levels. By adjusting constraints like timelines, brief scales, or target audiences, tutors can seamlessly integrate the design cases into their existing course structures to maximize student engagement and learning outcomes.

5.1 Applying Design Training in Design Cases

The previous chapters have described the fundamentals and methodologies for bioengineering design. In the following nine design cases, these fundamentals and methodologies are exemplified, trained, and realistically applied. The training focuses on conceptual design methodology, modelling, and economic evaluation.

- *Mechanistic models* are primarily used to outline and dimension a design. They help determine necessary upscaling and the size of the equipment required for operational procedures. By predicting the relationship between physical size, biological capacity, and production targets, the mechanistic models help trainees decide if a biological system is a viable alternative. This facilitates critical "go/no-go" decision-making, as seen in Chap. 5 cases.
- *Statistical models* refine outcomes by setting ranges for key design parameters. By identifying potent factors in relation to observable responses (as detailed in Chap. 3), trainees can evaluate potential improvements. Even with limited data, these tools help determine if a target, such as a 25% yield improvement, is realistically attainable.
- *Economic models* assess whether a design is viable under current market conditions. While math is often straightforward, these models require time and accurate

C.-F. Mandenius, *Bioengineering Design Methodology*,
https://doi.org/10.1007/978-3-032-33940-9_5

cost data. Trainees must learn that extreme precision is not always necessary; a confidence level within 20%–40% is often enough to discard unfavorable alternatives early on. The goal is to treat these as a basis for decision-making rather than a simple mathematical exercise.

- *Conceptual analysis* envisions innovative solutions for customer requirements. Where the users' needs help prioritize design features to ensure the final product fulfills its core mission. Specified metrics are used to translate the user needs into concrete goals for the design team.
- *Practical frameworks* comprising computer-aided design for technical drawings and detailed configurations, *structural templates* as tools for organizing operations, material flows, labor, and unit dimensions, and *reporting routines* based on standardized communication protocols to streamline teamwork and prevent information redundancy.

Each case involves an imaginary company that assigns a specific commission to a team of trainees. These "fictive" companies are named after their specific sector (e.g., *Biopharma*) and present substantial challenges ranging from new product development to the refinement of production systems.

5.2 Selection of Cases

The purpose of these design cases is to demonstrate how the fundamental principles of bioengineering design (Chap. 2) and design methodology (Chap. 3) are applied to real, concrete design missions. All nine design cases are rooted in industrial applications within the life science sector, where biology is central to the final product.

Each assignment assumes an early stage of product or production development. Therefore, the deliverables should provide recommendations and principal design solutions grounded in realistic technology and production economics.

The cases follow a uniform outline. First, a design assignment is presented from a fictional company. Directly related to an existing or new product, the assignment is given to a hypothetical design team. The trainees form this team to solve the problem under the guidance of tutors and industry-experienced experts. The exact scenario for the trainees is described in detail for each case. The trainees operate either as an independent team within a consultancy firm or as an R&D unit within the client company (cf. Fig. 4.3).

The nine cases represent typical existing products, and the fictional client companies are named to identify their specific bioindustrial sector. While basic company profiles are outlined in the scenarios, several real-world biotech companies closely mirror these setups. All assignments require the application of essential design methodologies. For each case, a recommended approach is presented and highlights its critical aspects.

The cases span various sectors of the biotech industry: biopharmaceuticals, food, instrumentation, biomedical devices for healthcare, and biotech contract services.

Depending on the sector, specific elements are emphasized. For instance, regulatory frameworks are critical when designing both food and drug products as well as their manufacturing systems.

As shown in the table, end-users play a pivotal role in the design process. Similarly, the client company must be able to manufacture the product in an economically viable manner. Typically, these companies need to assess business opportunities, requiring highly reliable data to inform their investment decisions. At this early stage, exploring alternatives and conducting risk assessments are vital—concepts that these design cases clearly illuminate.

Thus, considering the customer perspective is essential. Customers often exist at multiple levels. The client company is the immediate customer of the trainees. In turn, the client company delivers products to its own customers, who may serve another tier of consumers entirely. This chain is clearly illustrated in Case 3 (the zebrafish platform): (i) the zebrafish service company is the assigner to the trainees, (ii) the service company sells its drug evaluation services to major pharmaceutical corporations, (iii) these pharmaceutical companies develop and manufacture drugs for hospitals and pharmacies, and finally, (iv) these providers deliver the medication to the ultimate end-user: the patient.

The nine cases cover:

- Biotherapeutic products
- Cell-based products
- Diagnostic products
- Biomedical products

Although the core innovation is rooted in biological systems, all product applications integrate other relevant, cutting-edge technologies. These include continuous single-use production, biosimilar chemistry, microfluidics, advanced bioanalytics, biomaterial composites, and sensor technology. By combining these technologies, these biological concepts can be realized as truly innovative, marketable products.

5.3 The Design Cases and Their Training Purpose

The guidelines in Chaps. 2, 3, and 4 are all in one way or another applicable to most design missions. The nine design cases presented in Chap. 5 show this for quite different kinds of missions—products ranging from biomolecules, foods, instruments, and production systems of biological origin. The nine design cases are:

1. Design of production of a human growth hormone biotherapeutic biosimilar with increased efficacy (Case company: *Biopharma*)
2. Design of an integrated end-to-end continuous process for monoclonal antibodies against non-Hodgkin lymphoma (Case company: *Biotherapeutica*)
3. Design of service production with a zebrafish model (Case company: *Drug Technologies*)

4. Design of a microfluidic device with tooth cells and liver cells for testing of oral drugs (Case company: *Biochip Engineering*)
5. Design of a production of ventricular cardiac cells from stem cells (Case company: *Global Biopharma*)
6. Design of a functional food with stem cells (Case company: *Food Bioentrepreneurs*)
7. Design a point-of-care diagnostic biosensor for SARS-CoV-2 testing (Case company: *Diagnostic Incorporated*)
8. Design of a bedside blood glucose testing device for diabetic patients (Case company: *Medtech Sensorics*)
9. Design of a novel hemodialysis device for kidney replacement (Case company: *Dialytica*)

The names of the companies in the case scenarios are fictive but indicate their business ambition. These cases cover drugs, food constituents, commodity products, and diagnostic devices. Although they vary significantly in market reach, customer base, production scale, and underlying biological systems, they are all approached with the same design principles and methodologies as described in the previous chapters. The sequence of methods and tools remains consistent across all scenarios.

The nine design cases present significant challenges in applying general design methodology and integrating it with bioproduct design—specifically regarding biological constraints, bioengineering requirements, and biology-oriented user needs (Tables 5.1 and 5.2). Below, the main and secondary training challenges are summarized.

Table 5.1 General design challenges in the case studies

Design case	Main design challenge	Secondary design challenge
Case 1: Biosimilar growth hormone production	Scale-up of biosimilar production	Ensure therapeutic safety and economic scale-up
Case 2: Continuous therapeutic antibody production	Design a continuous end-to-end production	Integration of single-use (disposable) units
Case 3: Zebrafish model for drug evaluation	Robotizing testing service production	Implementing digitalization in the service production
Case 4: Microfluidic device for drug testing	Integrating stem cell and microfluidic technology	Adapting service to advanced customer needs
Case 5: Ventricular cardiac cells for cell therapy	Production of personalized product	Economic scale-up
Case 6: Cultured food production	Achieving economic production of cultured food	Developing animal-like food characteristics
Case 7: Diagnostic SARS-CoV-2 device	Mass production of a diagnostic device	Integrating and managing subcontracted production
Case 8: Glucose sensor for diabetic care	Mass production of a low-cost diagnostic sensor	Designing reusable devices for home-based testing
Case 9: Design of a hemodialysis system	Meeting customer needs in a medical device	Analyzing the trade-offs between novel design and cost

Table 5.2 The bioproduct design challenges in the case studies

Design case	Primary bioproduct challenge	Secondary bioproduct challenge
Case 1: Biosimilar growth hormone production	Expressing a biosimilar human growth hormone	Achieving purity levels for medicinal release
Case 2: Continuous therapeutic antibody production	Expression of antibody in a continuous process	Combining biocomponents in single-use operations
Case 3: Zebrafish model for drug evaluation	Designing a drug testing service platform	Ensuring high predictivity and in vivo response
Case 4: Microfluidic device for drug testing	Operating sequential iPSC-derived tissue (tooth/liver)	Delivering pharmacologically relevant data
Case 5: Ventricular cardiac cells for cell therapy	Controlling production of iPSC-derived cardiac cells	Ensuring high functionality of ventricular cells
Case 6: Cultured food production	Managing stem cell-derived myoblasts	Utilizing bioprinting with three components
Case 7: Diagnostic SARS-CoV-2 device	Biorecognition of infective viral structures	Achieving selective viral biological detection
Case 8: Glucose sensor for diabetic care	Integrating biosystem compactness and sensitivity	Reaching sufficient stability and reproducibility
Case 9: Hemodialysis system for blood purification	Bioengineering of an engineered medical device	Ensuring biomedical performance in blood purification

Chapter 6
Case 1: Cost-Efficient Production of a Human Growth Hormone Biosimilar

6.1 Assignment: Background, Description, and Objectives

This assignment aims to design a new production process for a human growth hormone (hGH) biosimilar product that is going to replace a previous hGH product (Smith and Thorner 2000). The biotherapeutic indication for the biosimilar human growth hormone (hGH biosimilar) is the same for patients with growth hormone deficiency (Collett-Solberg et al. 2019; Czepielewskia et al. 2019). The biosimilar process is expected to lower the production costs with unchanged productivity and quality.

The assigner, *Biopharma*, is a pharmaceutical company that, for several decades, has been one of the leading providers of hGH for pediatric treatment of severe growth retardation in children (growth hormone deficiency, GHD). The disease is caused by a monogenetic deficiency of the gene for native hGH (22 kD), which is secreted in the pituitary gland in the brain and controls a cascade of growth factors in the endocrine system of the body (Mustafakulov et al. 2024). Deficiency causes severe effects not only on stature but also on internal malfunctions of vital organs in the body. Treatment by daily injections of the hormone at an early age reconstitutes growth to a normal body stature. The pharmaceutical is distributed in the arterial blood vessels through hGH solutions and is a lifelong therapy. The original drug from *Biopharma* has been produced by recombinant gene technology using a bacterial host cell.

With the purpose of improving drug efficacy in patients, hGH productivity during bioprocess-based production, and the quality of the final purified hGH product, the R&D of *Biopharma* has devoted considerable effort to developing a new hGH drug with higher pharmacological efficacy, higher expression rate per recombinant cell, and fewer side-products. The new hGH structure has been attained by extensive protein engineering, resulting in a target molecule with a remaining active site but with considerably lower molecular weight (11 kD). The new peptide structure is less prone to forming variants (oxidized, forms, and oligomeric forms), which simplifies

C.-F. Mandenius, *Bioengineering Design Methodology*,
https://doi.org/10.1007/978-3-032-33940-9_6

product purification. A host-vector system has been developed where the host (an engineered *E. coli* strain with hGH-degrading proteases deleted) has also been developed. The ownership of the new host-vector system is protected through intellectual property rights (IPR) acquired by the company (e.g., Bao et al. 2022).

Biopharma has decided to assign its own process R&D team to design an efficient production process for its new biosimilar hGH product. The following objectives and criteria should be met by the R&D team:

- Two design alternatives for the production of the biosimilar hGH (hGH) shall be delivered. The design alternatives are expected to be based on the hGH biosimilar developed by *Biopharma, which* shall be produced at a level of 8 kg per year. The designs must exploit novel production technology for producing at least 8 kg of biosimilar per year.
- The design alternatives must result in a hGH biosimilar product with the same quality profile as requested by the regulatory authorities for the presently produced hGH.
- The new design alternatives must reduce the production costs by 50% compared to the present hGH production.
- The design alternatives should be possible to protect as intellectual properties and not infringe on other IPR not owned by Biopharma. The designs should aim to reduce the number of operation units/steps in the plant compared to the plant for the existing product; (ii) decrease the total plant volume, leading to lower investment cost; (iii) decrease consumption of raw materials in all steps of production; and (iv) ensure the shortest possible production time for the complex production.

Biopharma has added the following specific caveats to the assignment:

- Additional IPR filing for a new production will be carried out by *Biopharma*. This will create an additional upfront cost of 100 kEUR and a yearly cost of 10 kEUR, which is to be included in the cost analysis of the alternatives.
- *Biopharma's* costs for preclinical research on the new biosimilar construct, including preliminary preclinical testing, should be included in the cost analysis and amount to 800 kEUR (United States Food and Drug Administration 2025).
- The payoff period for the investments must not exceed 5 years.
- To make a fair cost analysis of the new hGH biosimilar production, the investments for the present production of hGH shall be levelled to today's costs with the same payoff time.

6.2 Training Scenario for the Assignment

For the design training of students or other trainees, the training scenario should preferably be based on the following prerequisites:

- The trainees are assumed to be a PR&D team within *Biopharma's* own process development organization. Preferably, they form a team of 5–6 individuals with backgrounds in cell biology, biopharmaceutical technology, bioengineering, process design, and bioanalytical technology.
- The trainees have access to computer-aided design (CAD) tools, simulation and modelling tools for bioprocess design and calculations, as well as software for design of experiments (DoE) and process economic calculations (see also Sect. 3.10). For mechanistic modelling, the trainees have access to a MATLAB program with appropriate toolboxes or similar modelling programs. If the trainees have extensive prior knowledge about modelling, they may use such experience.
- The trainees are in close contact with *Biopharma's* management, marketing, procurement, and quality units. These are represented by tutorial industrial experts who are prepared to provide detailed information about the company's present in-house production, process laboratories, equipment, and other facilities. By that, access to *Biopharma's* competence in fermentation, cell culture, and protein separation technologies becomes available. The company's in-house expertise and intellectual property rights (IPR) know-how are available as well. The industrial experts share *Biopharma's* medical and marketing plans with the trainees to help them solve the assignment. They also provide necessary details about investment and production costs for the present hGH production.
- *Biopharma* has previous extensive experience in collaborating with subcontractors for providing microbial strains, cell lines, and small-scale manufacturing equipment. This experience is provided to the trainees by the tutorial experts.
- The trainees report to *Biopharma* with progress and final reports. The results should be delivered orally and in written reports and include transparent production cost estimations for the design. The typical time frame for the assignment is in the range of 3–4 months. This can be shortened if a lower demand for reporting is expected. Deliverables are expected to be concise and succinct and follow typical industrial standards (see also Sect. 4.4.7).

6.3 A Recommended Design Approach for the Assignment

6.3.1 Structuring the Assignment and Requirements

From the assignment description and the background of the *Biopharma* company, the conditions and general structure of the assignment are given (Fig. 6.1). As described and shown in the figure, many of the upfront activities have already taken place, and other business preconditions are settled. This includes the work with identifying a potent production system for the biosimilar hGH with methods for selecting host organism, vector system, cultivation, recovery, and formulation (Harrison et al. 2003; Doran 2013; Mann 2018; Pörtner 2021; Jagschies et al. 2017). The sales to the customers of the product are a job for the company's marketing people, and they are responsible for assessing the size of the market and

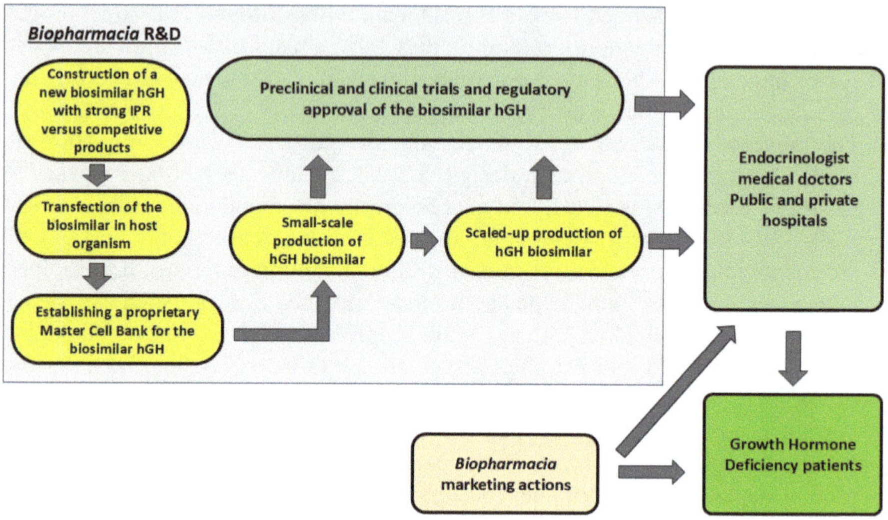

Fig. 6.1 The overall structure of Biopharma's development, production, and distribution of biosimilar hGH (red, yellow, and green). The assignment is focused on the production issues (yellow)

the product price (as given in the assignment). Thus, according to the assignment objectives, the assigned design mission should focus on the following issues:

- To consider how *Biopharma*'s new hGH biosimilar can be produced more efficiently by using state-of-the-art process technology and automation
- To identify what equipment and units are suitable and economically possible to use in design alternatives for the hGH biosimilar production
- To design process configurations that comply with the *Biopharma* annual production target and other production criteria
- To exploit the possibilities to optimize the steps in the new production process

By discussing with key stakeholders within *Biopharma*, especially marketing and production experts and potential users of the hGH product, especially clinicians and patients, important conditions for the design work can be established. These discussions should result in a list of well-defined requirements, with target specification metrics and priorities for the production and distribution of the hGH biosimilar product (Table 6.1). For the clinicians and patients, prioritized requirements concern efficiency and safety, availability, and price. For the company, the priorities are production costs, net income, and quality assurance of the biosimilar.

The patients' and the company's requirements on the use and production coincide. For example, efficient production has a direct influence on the price and deliverability of the product.

The discussions should be done eye-to-eye with *Biopharma*, primarily to clarify and detail the goals and constraints of the assignment and transform this information into metrics or other target specifications.

Table 6.1 Requirements, specifications, and priorities from patients for production

Requirement	Target specification	Priority
Patients and clinicians using the growth hormone biosimilar		
The price to customers should be lower than competitors' products	10% less than competitors' hGH products	Very high
Patients shall access disposable syringes for easy self-administration		Very high
Shelf-life of hGH biosimilar shall allow patients to store the drug at home	>1 year	High
Biopharma's production		
Production cost should be low compared to sales price	<20% at a production of 1 kg/yr. at a price of X EUR/g hGH	Very high
Impurity level in released hGH, should be lower than FDA demands	FDA accepts <0.600% impurity of adverse hGH form	Very high
A twofold increase in production should be possible with minor investments	From 1 kg hGH/yr. to 10 kg hGH/yr. Reinvestment <15%	Very high
Customer/clinician requirements should be met	¾ of requirements	High
Automation should be high, and personnel intensity minimized	Operator team should be less than three operators	High
Production time for one production cycle should be low	<1 week	High
IP protection should guarantee no infringement and be easy to protect	IPR should cover at least 80% of production line	High
Plant size at lowest production shall be reduced	Bioreactor <1000 L at 1 kg hGH/yr	Medium

Mostly, a company is well-informed about the specific customer needs from its marketing organization. *Biopharma's* economy and production people could easily quantify their requirements in terms of economic figures such as production costs and investments, quality criteria, product shelf-life, and market price level. Also, legal constraints can easily be precisely defined.

The customers' requirements for efficacy and safety are normally well-known. Certain aspects are unique and must be carefully and correctly specified. Experienced medical experts or pharmacologists should therefore confirm these target values. This will, in the case of the new hGH biosimilar, especially involve drug stability, clearance, toxicity limits, side-product levels, dose per time, and administration of drug. The formulation format may require daily injections and auxiliary convenience products for that. These issues are important managerial functions for the design and need to be considered when conceiving design alternatives.

6.3.2 Conceptualization of the Assignment

By making a conceptual map based on the objectives in the assignment, the requirements and target values from internal users and customers (clinicians and patients), the overall scope of the design mission is conceptually described. From the map, identification of design alternatives complying with the assignment's criteria should be carried out. By distinguishing the biological, technical, information, management, and human functions that are needed, well-structured outlines for the production of the hGH biosimilar can be worked out (Fig. 6.2). The assignment objectives and expressed requirements can easily be associated with the functional categories (Pahl et al. 2007; Mandenius and Björkman 2011; Ulrich et al. 2019).

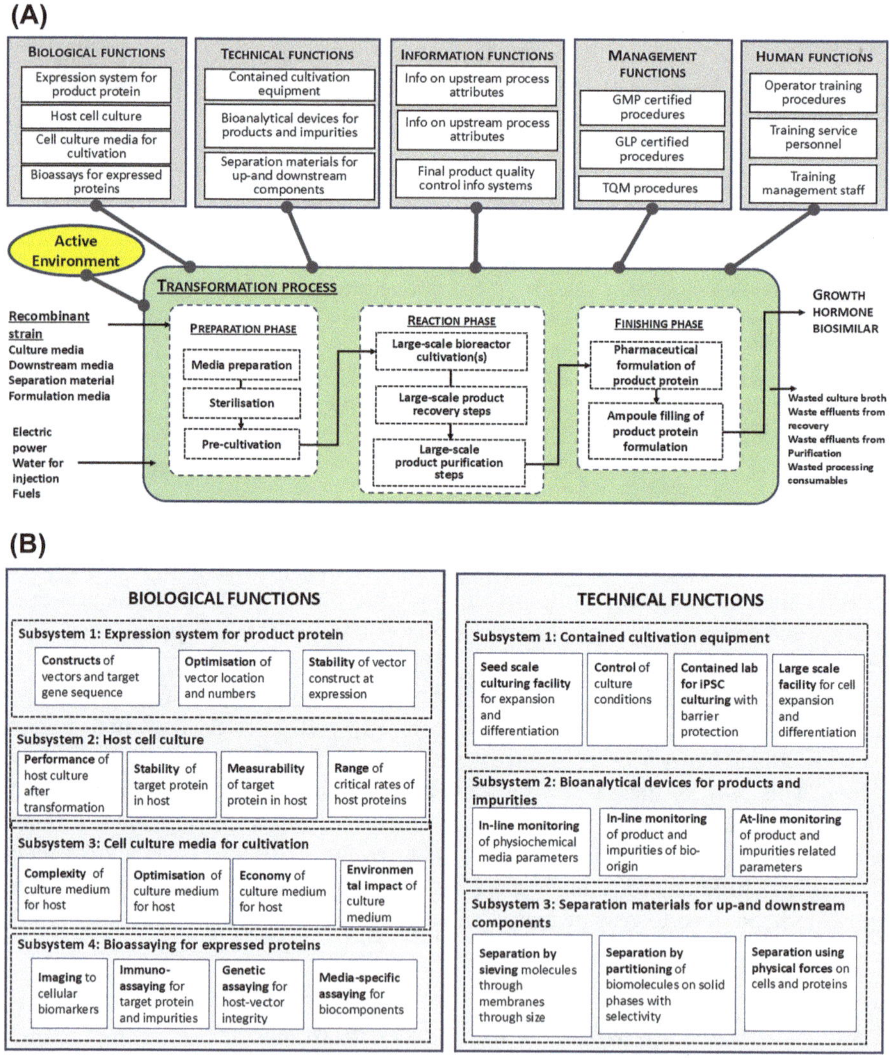

Fig. 6.2 (**a**) The functional mapping for a hGH biosimilar production process. (**b**) The biological and technical systems with subsystems in detail

Certainly, many of the assignment objectives depend on the biological and technical functions, such as the capacity of the biological system, the biological environment, and the technical functions for cultivation and separation. Most of the biological functions are on a biomolecular level that requires biological competence to understand (Jagschies et al. 2017). High priority has the efficiency of exploiting the capacity of the biological production system, i.e., the cell's capacity to express the product protein in a correctly folded form (Mann 2018). Purity and stability of the protein product are the top priorities. The map includes a competent host-vector system based on critical pharmacological parameters such as product stability and longevity, dose per patient and day, efficacy, and safety measures. These must in the design alternatives be related and compared with cellular productivity, volumetric conditions, purity needs, market volume, and the size of the production plant. The host-vector system is therefore a critical design issue. *Biopharma* has devoted much effort to this, and their IPRs play a major business role here. Also, the capacity of the host cells to grow with the gene for the hGH biosimilar can be optimized with the culture media.

Several of the objectives involve information management and human functions, e.g., production surveillance, quality control, plant operation by humans, and the needs of clinicians and patients.

These requirements connect to production economy and market price for the product per mass unit. With better performance of all these metrics, a better production economy and market price could be attained.

Human functions involve the clinical doctors and the patients. Their requirements interplay with the biological and technical systems. The safety of the delivered product has direct implications on the design of the production process, especially on the purification steps. The higher the demands, the more elaborate processing is required, which results in a surge of production costs, due to investments and consumables. The patients and clinicians wish to use the delivered product as long as possible and under conditions not requiring freezing, and the drug should be convenient to administer.

The information systems and human management systems can be detailed in several subsystems. Their impact on the design may be considerable. For example, a high complexity of technical systems will require a more extensive education and training of personnel involved. Management systems in the pharma industry are known for their demanding documentation and inspection routines from authorities. Also, requirements of quality management affect design and choice of biological and technical systems.

Economic consequences of these factors are sometimes neglected in design work. Here, e.g., FDA and other authorities will scrutinize hGH process documentation and demand elaborate validation of a new plant design.

The transformation process in the conceptual map may seem close to a conventional flowchart diagram (Pahl et al. 2007). The description of input of raw materials, fuel and power, and outputs of product and by-products, as well as secondary products and waste (Petrides 2006).

However, the transformation diagram is more than typical process flowcharts as it also brings in a preparation phase and a finishing phase. Product longevity and stability are created in this phase. An important reason for taking this wider scope is that many of the cost-intensive parts of the process are in the preprocessing and after-processing in the production train. If these are not involved when creating and analyzing design alternatives, cost estimation will suffer markedly.

In this case, preparation of media and handling of cell banks of host-vector culture are costly, time-consuming steps, as are testing of the final product with all quality control-related analytics and engineering.

The technical systems involve physics and mechanics, and chemical engineering. This will open up many alternative technical and biological solutions. The interactivity of these systems and the transformation process is complex (Fig. 6.2b). To anticipate inadequacies that may occur is not easy, but structuring interactions facilitates it a lot.

Basic configuration alternatives for reaching the objectives and targets should be considered. Here, four configuration alternatives (A to D) are conceived (Fig. 6.3).

From this simple but logical reasoning, it is obvious that the alternative with upstream processing in combination with a few or even a simple downstream purification step could be the most attractive design solution.

The design development should be thoroughly dedicated to the objectives of the assignment and priorities of Table 6.1, where pre-cultivation steps are to be decided, and types of bioreactors and recovery units are to be chosen. These kinds of questions require more consideration.

6.3.3 Detailed Design of the Selected Configurations

Two of the configurations in Fig. 6.3 (configurations C and D) are selected for the design of new production methods of the hGH biosimilar. Configuration A is identified to comply with today's production of hGH and, therefore, included in the design as a benchmark. In Fig. 6.4, these three production processes are detailed with existing or potentially possible steps and process units.

Today's production of hGH (i.e., a non-hGH biosimilar protein) is based on a batch process where the hGH is expressed intracellularly and remains inside the host cells during the cultivation (Fig. 6.4a). The cells are subsequently harvested and transferred to a storage tank. The cell broth is, by centrifugal pumping, passed to a homogenizer unit where the hGH proteins are released. The disrupted cells remain in the broth, which is collected in a second stirred storage tank. The broth is then passed to a tangential microfilter, where cell fragments are removed from the filtrate, while hGH and other soluble components and micro-fragments are recovered by the microfilter for further purification. These components are captured on an ion exchange material in a chromatographic column and gradually released by using a salt gradient. The pooled eluent with the hGH is purified in (i) a second ion-exchange column, (ii) a size exclusion column, and (iii) a hydrophobic interaction column. The

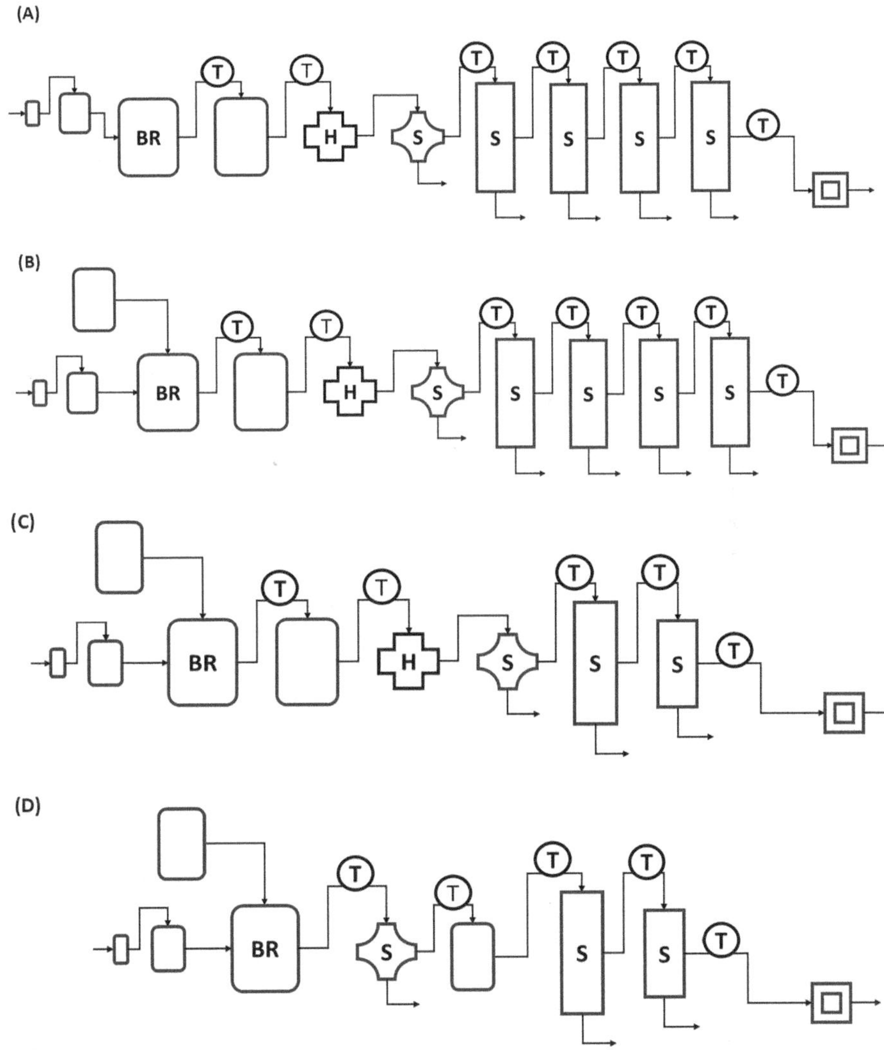

Fig. 6.3 Four possible configurations from the conceptual map. (**a**) A configuration adaptable to the present production of hGH. (**b**) A configuration where the upstream part is changed for controlled feeding. (**c**) A configuration according to B where the downstream part has been compressed to fewer steps. (**d**) A configuration according to C where the product is separated from the broth differently

purified hGH is diafiltrated, lyophilized, and filled into ampoules. The yields in each of these nine steps after the batch bioreactor are averaged to 80% (in total 13%). This means that the annual target value of 16 kg hGH (note that the molecular weight of 22 kD is twice that of the hGH biosimilar, 11 kD) requires that 124 kg hGH must be expressed in the bioreactor culture. The cycle time will be long due to the many steps, and the manual procedures will require considerable labor.

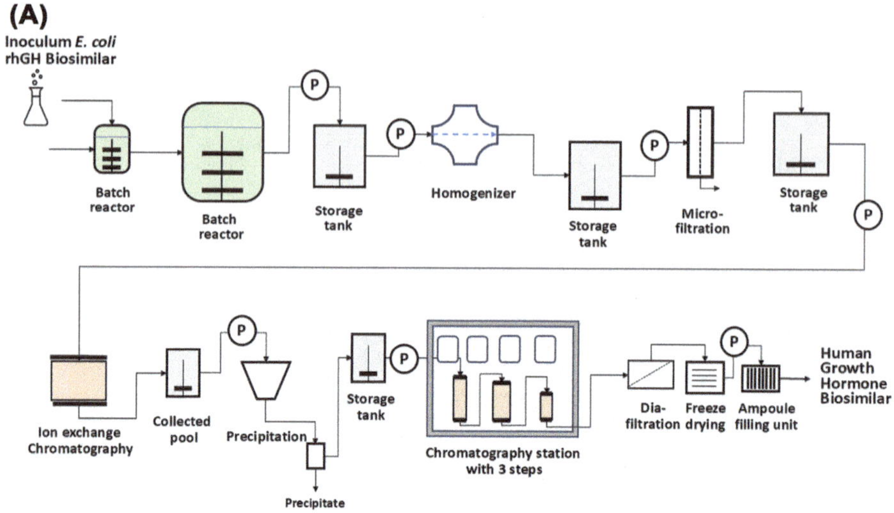

Fig. 6.4 Production alternatives for the biosimilar hGH. (**a**) The design of today's batch process. (**b**) The design alternative based on fed-batch with intracellular expression of the hGH biosimilar. (**c**) The design alternative based on fed-batch with extracellular biosimilar expression

In the design derived from configuration C, the cultivation expressing the hGH biosimilar is carried out in a fed-batch bioreactor. This will allow a higher cell density at a growth rate near the maximum specific growth rate for the host-vector system (Fig. 6.4b). As in the previous batch process, the cells must be disintegrated by a homogenizer, followed by further purification. The four columns in configuration A are replaced by one ion exchange column and one affinity chromatography column. The other steps are unchanged. The yields in each of these seven steps after the batch bioreactor are averaged to 82% (in total 25%). The exchange from a microfilter to an ultrafilter and a shorter time cycle for the process contribute to the higher average yield. This means that the annual production target of 8 kg requires that 32 kg of hGH biosimilar be expressed in the bioreactor culture. The shorter time-cycle results in increased availability of the equipment and probably also less need for operation and labor. For the fed-batch operation, automation is feasible. However, the exclusive specific affinity chromatography material must be developed, which requires additional R&D work and expenditures for specific ligands. Several of *Biopharma's* objectives in the assignment and in the requirements expressed by the users are met, such as a smaller size of the plant, higher annual production, automation, and the potential to reduce total production costs.

In the design based on configuration D, an improved host-vector system for the hGH biosimilar is assumed, where the hGH biosimilar is expressed directly to the culture medium. This will require additional R&D effort by *Biopharma* and result in higher upfront costs that must be paid back from the net income. It will, however,

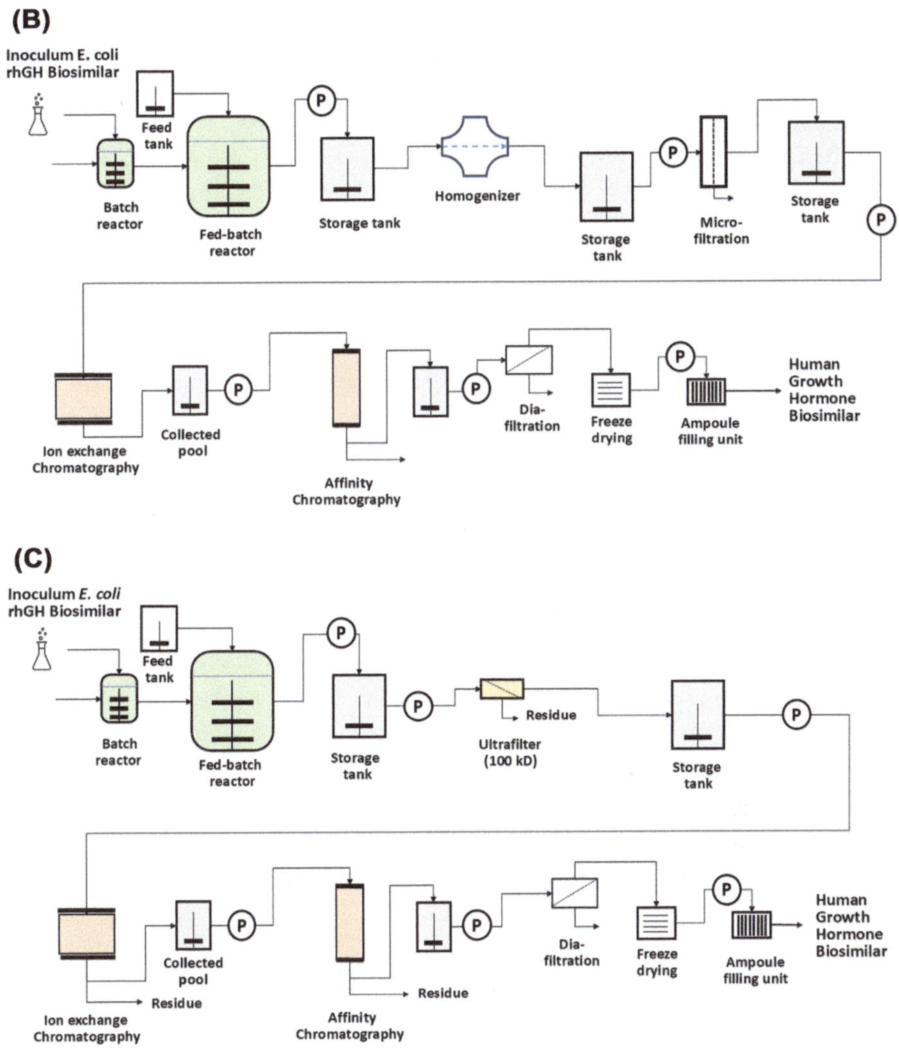

Fig. 6.4 (continued)

substantially simplify production and have significant prospects for improving yields (Fig. 6.4c). The homogenizer is replaced by an ultrafiltration unit with a cutoff close to the molecular size of the biosimilar product. Volume can already be reduced here and the size of the two chromatographic steps. Thus, the yields in these six steps after the fed-batch bioreactor are on average assumed to be 88% (in total 46%). This means that the annual target value of 8 kg hGH requires that 17 kg hGH biosimilar is expressed in the bioreactor culture. In this design, a shorter process cycle results in increased availability of the equipment and probably also less need for operation and labor. Automation is feasible for the fed-batch operation as well.

Equipment sizes are based on standardized production capacity figures. This should be scaled precisely in the design work by optimization of growth and culture conditions. As suggested in Sect. 6.4, this should create a potential for higher productivity in the two design alternatives.

Different host-vector systems are compared in terms of growth properties and productivities of hGH, accessibility of host-vector systems, media compositions, and the need for PR&D efforts. The success of maximizing the productivity of hGH should pave the way for reaching *Biopharma's* economic targets for the hGH biosimilar production.

It is of particular interest to investigate the strengths and opportunities of potential alternative host-vector systems, e.g., from current patent applications, techniques for transfection of the hGH biosimilar gene, and the possibility to optimize expression and cultivation regime.

The consequence of using more advanced separation materials will affect the expenditure and operational needs. Thus, the use of a more exclusive affinity purification column must be replaced more frequently, making the operation more expensive.

It is likely that both alternatives are suitable for the same host strain. The biological subsystems, involving selection of strains, optimization of the expression, and optimization of the cultivation media, are preferably established with optimization techniques as described below. The sizing of the units in relation to biological capacity could be investigated by mechanistic modelling. The sizing to the capacity of downstream steps can be roughly assessed from chromatographic material properties in relation to the productivity in the upstream and recovery stages.

6.3.4 Production Economics of the Selected Designs

The two new design alternatives detailed in the previous section are in this section evaluated for their production economics in relation to *Biopharma*'s objectives in the assignment. The alternatives are referred to as *intracellular biosimilar production* and *extracellular biosimilar production* and are benchmarked to *Today's hGH production.*

The aims of the economic evaluation of the design alternatives should be:

- To make a comparison of the investment and operation costs for the two detailed design alternatives
- To compare how these alternatives cope with the economy for the existing production process
- Assess how successful optimization of the production could potentially cope with the production target

To make the comparison fair, today's production is evaluated based on its cost for rebuilding today's plant with new units.

The investment and operational costs for production are assessed and analyzed as recommended by using established evaluations (Kristiansen 2006; Petrides 2006; Peters et al. 2003; Ray et al. 2022).

In a first assessment of economic conditions, it could be concluded that:

- There are opportunities to maximize productivity in the culture stage of the two design alternatives. A more efficient expression of hGH biosimilar in the host-vector systems will increase productivity.
- Downstream processing with fewer steps results in higher total yields. If the average yield is 80%–85% in each step, the effect on productivity improves the total yield in the order of 20%–30%. If the yield is enhanced by using more advanced chromatography to 90%, the gain is >40% in production yield. The two-step separation shortens the cycle time by 30%–50%, where a win in productivity follows.
- Higher yields allow scaling down the size of reactors, tanks, and columns. Alternatively, the plant can be used for a shorter period of the year or be available for scaling up production at a later stage.

Certainly, this favors the two design alternatives, but it will also require additional development. These costs must not drain the net income or risk a higher pricing of the product to the patients and clinics.

The investment and operational cost items are assessed based on these premises (Table 6.2). When justified, equipment investment costs are reduced to a smaller size. When justified, operational costs for raw materials and labor are reduced in the same way.

The cost for installing and operating the two plant alternatives is compared. To this are added other estimated costs as set by *Biopharma*, the estimated R&D efforts, and the payoff of investment costs. The total costs are overviewed for the two alternatives and compared with today's hGH production calculated as advised.

The total estimated production cost for both alternatives is within the targeted values. Obviously, the most favorable alternative is the extracellular biosimilar production process. This is mainly due to the reduced size of equipment, which is partly mirrored in the operational costs. The estimated total costs for today's process clearly favor the implementation of a new plant, especially if R&D costs could be kept under control. This is the case for both design alternatives.

At this stage of the designing, the estimated costs are not very accurate and can, by a deeper evaluation, reach a higher accuracy. Surely, many of the cost items will depend on procurement and local conditions and will change over time.

It should be emphasized that the production economics can be further improved by optimization of cultivation procedures, culture media composition, productivity, and yields in the process steps, which will have direct consequences on the required size of the plant. This will influence the production economy considerably.

The distribution of costs for alternatives is of profound interest to consider (Fig. 6.5). This is of interest if further scale-up of the biosimilar production is a

Table 6.2 Economic comparison of alternatives to today's process

Type of costs	Today's process (kEUR)	Intracellular biosimilar (kEUR)	Extracellular biosimilar (kEUR)
Investment costs			
Upfront R&D for production			
Host-vector system	300	200	300
Separation materials/ligands	100	250	250
Quality control methods	100	50	50
Total upfront R&D for production	*500*	*500*	*600*
Equipment and instrumentation			
Bioreactors (incl media tanks)	400	200	200
Separation units (incl. Auxiliary units)	550	150	150
Quality control instruments	50	50	50
Upfront production development			
Total equipment and instrumentation	*1000*	*400*	*400*
Additional expenditures			
Installation of equipment (×0.5)	500	200	200
Project planning (×0.3)	300	120	120
Taxation (×0.1)	100	40	40
Buildings (×0.3)	300	120	120
Validation of installation and methods	200	100	100
Total additional expenditure	*1300*	*580*	*580*
Total investment costs	2800	1480	1580
Operational costs (8 kg/year)			
Consumables for production			
Consumables upstream (raw mat)	200	50	50
Consumables downstream (media)	200	50	50
Consumables quality control	50	50	50
Total consumables for production	450	150	150
Additional operational expenditures			
Labor in production facility (incl. QC)	500	200	200
Renting of buildings	100	50	50
Taxation	30	30	30
Annual IPR expenditures	100	100	100
Management	100	70	70

(continued)

Table 6.2 (continued)

Type of costs	Today's process (kEUR)	Intracellular biosimilar (kEUR)	Extracellular biosimilar (kEUR)
Total additional expenditures	*830*	*450*	*450*
Total operational costs	1280	600	600
Annual payoff of investments (for 5 years)	*560*	*300*	*320*
Total annual production cost (8 kg)	**1840**	**900**	**920**
Production cost 1 g hGH biosimilar (EUR)	230	113	115

concern for *Biopharma* (Harmsen 2013). Basically, it should result in a decrease in the share of the investment in the costs.

6.3.5 Patents or Patent Applications that Could Endanger the Designs

A new production process for hGH biosimilar is dependent on IPR protection. Therefore, it is important to have a detailed knowledge about patents and patent applications that describe production systems that are on a new production system for a specified product. A search for IPRs for the hGH biosimilar from competing companies is therefore of great use to ensure that the suggested designs are not trespassing into other IPRs and that the process system to be used and that *Biopharma* has a good opportunity to file its own IPR applications. This will be important for avoiding legal conflicts (Keswani and Possas 2024).

Several IPRs of relevance for the assignment, where the focus is on biosimilars and fusion of hGH proteins, have been filed (Table 6.3). At least eight such IPRs may partly challenge the proposed production design:

- Structural feature of the hGH biosimilar with serious effect on its functionality (Karim et al. 2022)
- Method of purifying the hGH (Rasmussen et al. 2010)
- The use of hGH that is PEGylated (Rasmussen et al. 2025)
- The use of hGH that is glycosylated (Bolt et al. 2012)
- The use of hGH fused with immunoglobulin-IgG-Fc (Wei et al. 2021)
- The use of hGH fused with human serum albumin (Wenhui et al. 2023)
- The use of fused epitopic hGH (Alila et al. 1999)
- Composition for hGH fusion protein (Cha et al. 2019)

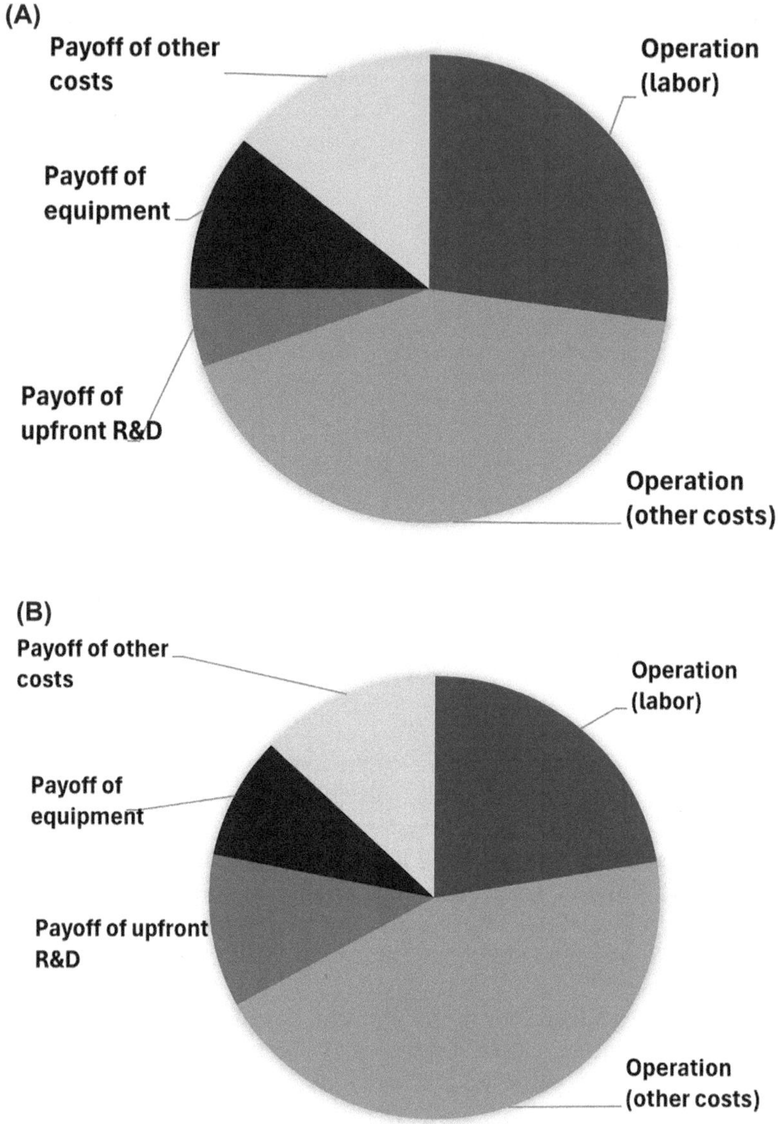

Fig. 6.5 Distribution of costs at scale-up of hGH biosimilar production

Biopharma must ensure that they control the IPR situation either by owned rights or licensed rights. They must also perform a risk analysis for potential new filings of similar IPR.

Thus, from a design perspective, it is profoundly important to know when implementing a new process design that the process is not affected by infringements or other potential threats to protect their hGH product production and marketing. The

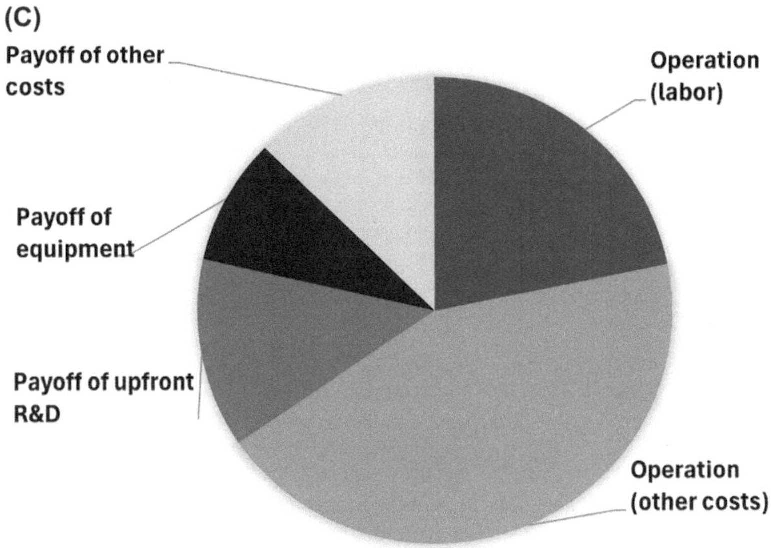

Fig. 6.5 (continued)

eight patents listed in the table are those that are considered to have the highest actuality in these respects. With this prerogative, the recycled alternative is still a robust choice for the new hGH expression system and its large-scale production of hGH.

It is important to evaluate (i) how the potential of the patent is a function of the cost structure of the design, (ii) if other ownership of IPR may change the situation, or (iii) if there is space for improvement related to the content of other IPR.

6.3.6 Optimization of Growth Hormone Biosimilar Production

In the objectives, it is emphasized that optimization should be employed to reach a competitive production process (Rezaei and Zarkesh-Esfahani 2012; Martins and Ning 2021). With the extended complexity of the proposed configurations, these options are many. The optimization strategy could be to select a few parameters judged to be the most appealing for optimization, without extensive consumption of resources and time. As all optimization is accompanied by experimentation or elaborate modelling work, it is advisable to identify approximately not more than five of these and carry them out with precision. (Table 6.4).

Table 6.3 IPR situation for recombinant growth hormone products

Patent title (owner)	Protection/description/claims	Inventors (year) appl. no.
Long-acting hGH compositions (Pfizer)	Pharmaceutical compositions comprising a long-acting hGH, and their use in growth-related disorders, methods of making, dosage forms, and uses thereof. In another aspect, disclosed herein are methods of treating growth-related disorders by administering the pharmaceutical compositions	Karim et al. (2022) WO2022197963A1
Purification of recombinant hGH by affinity chromatography resins (Novo Nordisk)	Purification of growth hormone polypeptides, e.g., hGH. Process utilizing an affinity resin comprising solid phase material having immobilized with low-weight synthetic ligands	Rasmussen et al. (2010) WO2010055135
Pegylated hGH compounds (Ascendis)	A chemically modified hGH is prepared by attaching a transient linker which comprises polyethylene glycol. The chemically modified protein may have a much longer lasting hGH activity than that of the unmodified hGH, enabling reduced dose and scheduling opportunities	Rasmussen et al. (2025) AU2014200350
N-glycosylated hGH with prolonged half-life (Novo Nordisk)	The present invention relates to novel hGH variants with one or more N-glycans. The hGH variants comprise an amino acid sequence which includes at least one N-glycosylation motif (N-X-S/T) from mutations not in the wildtype hGH	Bolt et al. (2012) WO2009156511 or US 2011/0118183 A1
Recombinant hGH Fc fusion protein, application, and engineering cell strain of fusion protein (Anhui Anke Pharma)	The hGH Fc fusion protein contains hGH, a flexible peptide linker (L), and a human IgG Fc fragment. Also disclosed are an activity determination method of the fusion protein and a host cell capable of expressing the fusion protein	Wei et al. (2021) CN112661858
Conjugate of rh HSA and recombinant hGH and preparation method thereof (Wuhan Healthgen)	A stable long-acting GH which is formed by coupling recombinant human serum albumin and recombinant hGH as raw materials through a linking group	Cha et al. (2019) EP4623935 A1

(continued)

Table 6.3 (continued)

Patent title (owner)	Protection/description/claims	Inventors (year) appl. no.
Pharmaceutical composition for treating GHD containing hGH fusion protein (Genexine)	A method for administering a hGH fusion protein (GX-H9) for treating GHD. Specifically, the present disclosure relates to a pharmaceutical composition for treating GHD, which comprises a hGH fusion protein (GX-H9) and a pharmaceutically acceptable carrier, wherein the fusion protein (GX-H9) is administered once a week	Cha et al. (2019) WO2009156511
Fused somatotropin epitopic peptides that potentiate GH activity (Pfizer)	Composite somatotropin peptides comprising somatotropin epitope amino acid sequences, and fusion proteins thereof, useful in potentiating GH activity. Also disclosed are vectors and host cells useful in their recombinant production of such molecules	Alila et al. (1999) US5889144 A1

Table 6.4 Optimization opportunities for production of growth hormone biosimilar

Object of optimization	Expected outcome	Applicable optimization technique
Expression system in applied recombinant strain with induction time	Increase in specific production rate	Factorial design of experimentally available parameters
Parameters in bioreactor	Increased growth rate of cells	Factorial design of selected parameters
Culture media composition	A favorable media composition for production and media cost	Factorial design of components
Chromatographic operation parameters	Improved separation performance affecting size and yield	Factorial design of critical parameters
Chromatography media composition	Favorable media compositions of several media to be used	Factorial design of components in media
Effects of recycling rates	Effects on productivity, size, and time of plant units	Mechanistic modelling
Assessment of processing time due to critical design parameters	Improvement of annual production, scheduling of plant	Mechanistic modelling

Design of Experiments for Optimizing biosimilar Production The design can be improved by using design of experiments to optimize the conditions in the up- and downstream steps for reaching a higher hGH biosimilar titer.

Table 6.5 DoE optimization of upstream hGH process

Object of optimization	Factors in DoE plan	Responses to measure
Culture media composition	Carbon source, nitrogen source, vitamins, metal salts	Cell density, cell viability, biosimilar titer, biosimilar rate, growth rate, yield of cells per substrate, yield of biosimilar per substrate
Cultivation conditions	pH, temperature, oxygen profile, impeller speed, baffle shape, inoculum size, inoculum density	Same as above
Expression of hGH	Induction time, inducer concentration, inducer profile	Same as above

Several options are at hand (Mandenius and Brundin 2008; Montgomery 2013; Brereton 2003). The culture media composition may be changed to increase the productivity of the hGH biosimilar by speeding up growth of the host cells. Yield factors for cell growth and the biosimilar expression per raw materials can be improved. The biosimilar yield can also be improved by optimizing the induction time and amount of inducer.

In the downstream process, several alternatives optimization by DoE can be considered. The chromatography steps are dependent on the separation material's performance due to loading capacity, binding strength, and kinetics. Costs for the material and the media are also of relevance to consider. Similar performance parameters can be identified for the filtration operations.

A variety of combinations of DoE factors and responses for the kind of parameters can be studied (Table 6.5). It is up to the designers to select and prioritize which sets of DoE factors are likely to lead to high impact. Here, it is suggested to focus on the composition of culture media and culture conditions, including induction of expression.

All designs should follow standard DoE procedures as described in Chap. 4, preferably with reduced factor experiments at two or three levels.

Optimization of the Growth in the Fed-Batch Bioreactor Producing the hGH biosimilar by Mechanistic Modelling Mechanistic modelling of the biological properties of the host-vector system of the hGH biosimilar can contribute to enhancing productivity. By setting up mechanistic models based on mass balances and kinetic equations and simulating these with time under a variety of assumptions such as media concentration, reactor volume, and feeding rate, the most favorable operation conditions can be established (Wang et al. 2003; Nielsen et al. 2011; Doran 2013). The model equations describing bioreactor production of the hGH biosimilar product would be:

$$dX/dt = \mu_{\text{host}} + X_{\text{host}} + F_{\text{in}}/V_{\text{bioreactor}} \cdot X_{\text{host}} \tag{6.1}$$

$$dc_{\text{biosim}}/dt = q_{\text{biosim}} \cdot X_{\text{host}} \tag{6.2}$$

$$dc_{\text{media}}/dt = F_{\text{in}}/V_{\text{bioreactor}} \cdot c_{\text{feed}} - F_{\text{in}}/V_{\text{bioreactor}} \cdot c_{\text{media}} - q_{\text{media}} \cdot X_{\text{host}} \tag{6.3}$$

$$dV_{\text{bioreactor}}/dt = F_{\text{in}} \tag{6.4}$$

$$\text{Prod} = V_{\text{bioreactor}} \cdot c_{\text{biosim}} \tag{6.5}$$

$$\mu_{\text{host}} = \mu_{\text{hostmax}}(c_{\text{media}}/(c_{\text{media}} + K_S) \tag{6.6}$$

$$\mu_{\text{host}}/q_{\text{media}} = Y_{\text{host/media}} \tag{6.7}$$

where X_{host} is the concentration of host cells (e.g., *E. coli*); c_{media}, the concentration of the limiting media component; q_{biosim}, the specific rate of expression of the biosimilar; μ_{host}, the host cells' specific growth rate; $V_{\text{bioreactor}}$, the volume of the bioreactor; and F_{in}, the feed flow rate of nutrient media with the concentration c_{feed}. The specific uptake rate of nutrient media is q_{media}. *Prod* is the total production of biosimilar in the reactor.

The growth follows Monod kinetics (Eq. 6.6), where μ_{host} is the maximum specific growth rate, K_S is the saturation constant for the limiting medium component, and $Y_{\text{host/media}}$ is the yield between biomass and media.

These parameters can be adjusted and constrained as relevant for the cultivation and the strain.

Three examples of simulations with the model show how cultivation conditions influence the production of the biosimilar (Fig. 6.6).

The *first example* (simulation diagram in Fig. 6.6a) shows the growth of the host organism and expression of the hGH biosimilar in a batch bioreactor. The amount of hGH biosimilar in the bioreactor is simulated over time while reactor volume, host cell, and expression kinetics are varied. The time for reaching the production target under the given conditions can be influenced by changing the seed concentration and the kinetics of the host cell.

In the *second example* (simulation diagram in Fig. 6.6b), the bioreactor is fed with nutrients that follow a preset feed rate profile. Other conditions are the same as in the batch. It shows that the total production of biosimilar can be increased. Again, with the model, it is easy to apply to other feed profiles, rates, and feed concentrations with the purpose of influencing the growth of the host organism and the extracellular expression of hGH biosimilar product. The simulation shows how different feeding profiles influence the formation of hGH biosimilar by controlling the feeding to the growth rate. The effect of control is significant for the level of products formed and demonstrates the potential of maximizing productivity in the upstream stage. It shortens the production cycle time and allows tighter scheduling of procedures in the process.

The *third example* (simulation diagram in Fig. 6.6c) shows how the kinetics for cell growth of the host organism and the expression of hGH biosimilar can be promoted by using host cells with more favorable specific production rates. It demonstrates the value of either developing the expression system of the host strain

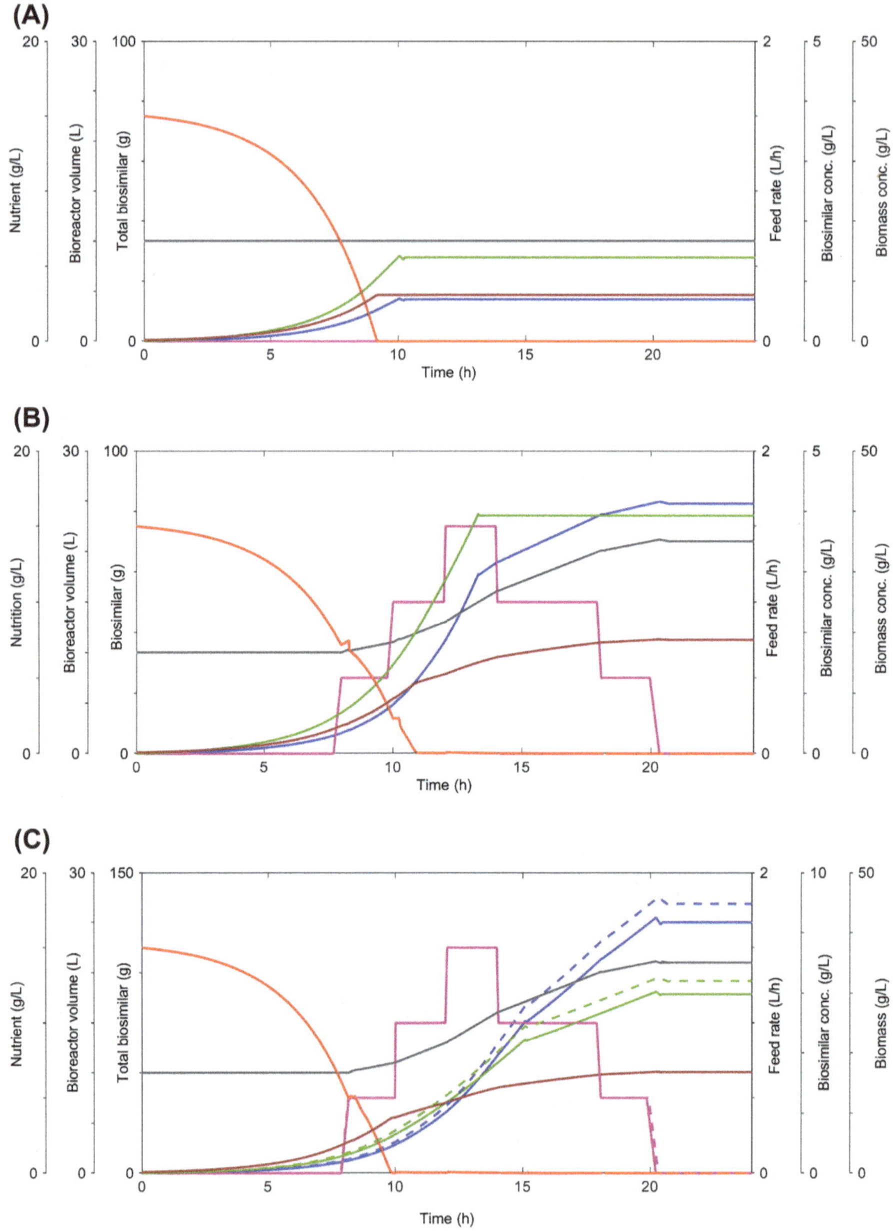

Fig. 6.6 Cultivation of hGH biosimilar. (**a**) Production in a batch bioreactor. (**b**) Fed-batch bioreactor production with a step-wise changing feed profile. (**c**) The same feed profile with improvements of growth and expression kinetics. The dashed line represents a strain with a 10% higher expression rate

or the environmental conditions in the bioreactor. These comprise both the composition of the medium (chemical composition of the medium) and the physicochemical conditions in the bioreactor (e.g., temperature, pH, oxygen tension).

Note that in the simulation Fig. 6.6c, the production of biosimilar in the bioreactor is 130–140 g after 20 h. Assuming a total yield of 45%–50%, this results in a production of 50–70 g per 3 days. This should be comparable with the annual production target of 8 kg purified product. In the simulation example, the reactor size is 500 L. The simulation helps in deciding the scale of the plant for reaching the annual target.

6.3.7 SWOT Analysis of the Selected Designs

After the evaluation of potential configurations, outlining of design alternatives, assessments of their production economy, analyzing the IPR situation, and considering optimization possibilities, it is advisable to perform a SWOT analysis (Shinno et al. 2006). The SWOT analysis should be carried out with the assignment objectives in focus as well as the user requirement priorities. This is carried out with the priorities in mind. Those issues that seem most relevant to consider and have a strong impact on the prospects for the design alternatives should primarily be of interest to analyze. Here, it is especially relevant to look at the quality of the produced hGH biosimilar, the size and scalability of the plant, and the production economy. Certainly, other issues can also be included. In the SWOT analysis, intracellular

Table 6.6 SWOT analysis comparing the two intra- and extracellular design alternatives

Priority criteria	Intracellular Alternative	Extracellular alternative
HGH biosimilar quality (stability, impurity)	*Strength*: Probably higher *Weakness*: Homogenization releases more impurities *Opportunity*: – *Threats*: QC very high	*Strength*: Less impurities; easier quality analysis *Weakness*: None *Opportunity*: Less impurities give higher quality vs others *Threats*: Instability in expression
Plant size and scalability	*Strength*: Higher density *Weakness*: None *Opportunity*: Fast to scale up *Threats*: Authorities disagree	*Strength*: Cell debris removed before purification *Weakness*: Expression too low *Opportunity*: Fast scale-up *Threats*: IPR too weak
Overall Production Economics	*Strength:* Compact process is more economically *Weakness:* High investment costs *Opportunity:* Automation can reduce costs and enhance quality *Threats:* Competitors have lower production costs and use low-salary countries for production	*Strength:* Compact process is more economically *Weakness:* Even higher investment costs and IPR costs *Opportunity:* IPR protects expression method *Threats:* Competitors have lower production costs and use low-salary countries for production

and extracellular alternatives are compared (Table 6.6). It should be emphasized that, at least at this stage, the analysis is entirely qualitative as accurate quantitative data is not yet at hand. Still, it serves the purpose of bringing to attention issues which are worth spending more time on in the design work. In summary, the SWOT analysis seems to favor the extracellular alternative if the development of such a host-vector system can be successfully accomplished.

6.4 Conclusive Suggestions for *Biopharma*

Based on the design alternatives as described above, several suggestions can be given to *Biopharma* for the production of a new hGH biosimilar product:

- *Biopharma* is recommended to build a completely new plant for the production of the hGH biosimilar. The process should use fed-batch cultivation followed by fewer and more efficient downstream steps for recovery and purification. Such a design would reduce operational costs and increase the productivity of the hGH biosimilar product.
- To further maximize the production capacity, *Biopharma* is recommended to develop a host-vector system that expresses the hGH biosimilar directly into the culture medium. This will significantly facilitate the recovery and purification of the product and enhance the production economy.
- These recommendations will reduce several operational costs, including labor costs, facility space, raw materials, and quality analysis. They will also reduce the size and number of units in the process.
- The intracellular as well as the extracellular production method can be further optimized by factorial design and mechanistic modelling. Examples of optimization goals are to improve growth and expression by varying the composition of the culture medium and optimizing the feeding procedure of the fed-batch bioreactor.
- The economic objectives in the assignment will be reached with both design alternatives.
- The quality criteria will realistically be met in the purification steps, especially by the affinity chromatography step.
- Of the two design alternatives, the extracellular expression alternative is the most favorable, due to fewer impurities.

Other advantages could be mentioned:

- Personnel intensity can be reduced or remain unchanged for larger production volumes.
- Due to the smaller size of the process for the same production target, the process can more easily be moved to another location.
- The design of the plant is general and possible to adapt for other products.

Some risks should be mentioned that affect the choice of alternatives:

- The new designs require substantial investment in equipment, plant construction and installations. This cost must be controlled to limit the payback time or market price.
- The new designs, their validations, and adaptation to new host-vector systems require additional early process development work, especially for an improved expression system and for affinity ligands.
- The hGH biosimilar product and its production should be protected by strong IPRs without infringing on the competitors' IPRs.

6.5 Tutorial Perspectives on the Assignment

The trainees have a range of challenges to approach in this assignment that may need advice and support from the tutors and industrial experts. The challenges are the following:

- To realize that the growth and expression capacity of the host-vector system are decisive for finding a design that reaches *Biopharma*'s production target.
- To realize the value of reducing the steps in the process to maximize the productivity of the hGH biosimilar.
- To configure design alternatives under the frames given in the assignment's objectives and users' expressed requirements.
- To judge how the scale of costs in the design alternatives influences the net income from the hGH biosimilar product.
- To integrate all requirements with their target metrics in the conceptual analysis, and from these develop design alternatives that exploit state-of-the-art bioengineering and optimization techniques.

The assignment is especially suitable for developing the following bioengineering skills:

- Ability to overview and compare alternative costs of equipment and consumables and other auxiliary costs such as costs for R&D and IPR during the design work.
- Understanding how size of production and time influence the production target.
- Transforming this notion into basic computational models that allow immediate testing of critical design parameters, such as growth and expression rates, concentrations, and volumes.
- Gaining experience in doing this in a design teamwork without becoming trapped in negotiating issues of minor relevance within the PR&D team.
- Ability to see the possibility to improve or refine productivity in relation to raw material inputs and maximizing productivity by optimization and modelling methods.

The tutorial support for the training should especially contribute to the understanding of the following:

- That all the elements of Fig. 6.1 are required for a good result and outcome.
- The relation between drug efficacy, produced amount of hGH biosimilar, and scale of plant.
- The impact of the biological capacity (specific productivity of the host-vector system) and the scale on production volume (annual amount of product).
- The value of performing a critical SWOT analysis.
- The impact of others' IPR and the necessity of an IPR strategy.

References

Alila HW et al (1999) Fused somatotropin epitopic peptides that potentiate GH activity. Patent Application US5889144 A1

Bao G, Guo L, Shen Y et al (2022) Growth hormone fusion protein and preparation method and use thereof. Patent Application WO2023123776A1

Bolt C, Kristiansen E, Boel TV et al (2012) N-glycosylated hGH with prolonged half-life. US 2011/0118183 A1

Brereton RG (2003) Chemometrics, data analysis for laboratory and chemical plants. Wiley, Chichester

Cha J-E et al (2019) Pharmaceutical composition for treating GHD containing hGH fusion protein. Patent Application JOP20170044 (B1)

Collett-Solberg PF, Jorge AAL, Boguszewski CS et al (2019) Growth hormone therapy in children; research and practice, a review. Growth Hormon IGF Res 44:20–32. https://doi.org/10.1016/j.ghir.2018.12.004

Czepielewskia MA, Garretb SAC, Vencioc N (2019) Efficacy and safety of a biosimilar recombinant hGH (rhGH Cristalia) compared with reference r-hGH in children with growth hormone deficiency (CERES study): a randomized, multicentric, investigator-blind, phase 3 trial. Growth Hormon IGF Res 48–49:29–35. https://doi.org/10.1016/j.ghir.2019.07.003

Doran PM (2013) Biochemical engineering principles, 2nd edn. Elsevier, Amsterdam. https://doi.org/10.1016/C2009-0-22348-8

FDA (2025) Development of therapeutic protein biosimilars: comparative analytical assessment and other quality-related considerations (guidance for industry). U.S. Department of Health and Human Services, Food and Drug Administration, Center for Drug Evaluation and Research (CDER), Center for Biologics Evaluation and Research (CBER), Center for Veterinary Medicine (CVM), Washington, DC

Harmsen J (2013) Industrial process scale-up. A practical Innovation guide from idea to commercial implementation. Elsevier Science, Amsterdam. ISBN 9780444627261

Harrison R, Tood P, Rudge S et al (2003) Bioseparation science and engineering. Oxford University Press, New York

Jagschies G, Lindskog E, Lacki K (2017) Biopharmaceutical processing development, design, and implementation of manufacturing processes. Elsevier, Amsterdam

Karim F et al (2022) Long-acting hGH compositions. Patent Application WO2022197963 (A1)

Keswani C, Possas C (2024) Intellectual property issues in life sciences disputes and controversies. Taylor and Francis Ltd, London

Kristiansen B (2006) Process economics. In: Ratledge C, Kristiansen B (eds) Basic biotechnology, 3rd edn. Cambridge University Press, Cambridge, UK, pp 239–252

Mandenius CF, Björkman M (2011) Biomechatronic design in biotechnology: a methodology for development of biotechnology products. Wiley, Hoboken. https://doi.org/10.1002/9781118067147

Mandenius CF, Brundin A (2008) Bioprocess optimization using design-of-experiments methodology. Biotechnol Prog 24:1191–1203. https://doi.org/10.1002/btpr.67.
Mann R (2018) Genetic engineering and biotechnology. Callisto Reference. ISBN 9781632399205
Martins JRRA, Ning A (2021) Engineering design optimization. Cambridge University Press, Cambridge, UK. https://doi.org/10.1017/9781108980647
Montgomery DC (2013) Design and analysis of experiments, 8th edn. Wiley, New York
Mustafakulov M, Uralov A, Ahmedova S et al (2024) HGH produced with recombinant DNA technology. BIO Web Conf 130:04009. https://doi.org/10.1051/bioconf/202413004009
Nielsen J, Villadsen J, Lidén G (2011) Bioreaction engineering principles, 3rd edn. Springer-Nature, New York
Pahl G, Beitz W, Feldhusen J et al (2007) Engineering design, a systematic approach, 3rd edn. Springer Verlag, Berlin
Peters MS, Timmerhaus KD, West RE (2003) Plant design and economics for chemical engineers, 5th edn. McGraw-Hill, New York
Petrides D (2006) Recombinant human insulin. In: Heinzle E, Biwer A, Cooney C (eds) Development of sustainable bioprocesses. modelling and assessment. Wiley, Chichester, pp 225–240
Pörtner R (ed) (2021) Cell culture engineering and technology. Springer Nature, New York. https://doi.org/10.1007/978-3-030-79871-0
Rasmussen JE et al (2010) Purification of recombinant hGH by affinity chromatography resins. Patent Application WO/2010/055135
Rasmussen N et al (2025) Pegylated recombinant hGH compounds. Patent Application MX20160016855 20101027
Ray SC, Chambers RG, Kumbhakar SC (2022) Handbook of production economics. Springer Nature, New York
Rezaei M, Zarkesh-Esfahani SH (2012) Optimization of production of recombinant hGH in *Escherichia coli*. J Res Med Sci 17(7):681–685. PMID: 23798931; PMCID: PMC3685787
Shinno H, Yoshioka H, Marpaung S et al (2006) Quantitative SWOT analysis on global competitiveness of machine tool industry. J Eng Design 17(3):251–258. https://doi.org/10.1080/09544820500275180
Smith RG, Thorner MO (2000) HGH, research and clinical practice. Humana Press. ISBN 9781592590155
Ulrich KT, Eppinger SD, Wang MC (2019) Product design and development, 7th edn. McGraw-Hill, New York
Wang L, Ridgeway D, Gu T et al (2003) Effect of process parameters on heterologous protein production in *Aspergillus niger* fermentation. J Chem Technol Biotechnol 78:1259–1266
Wei L et al (2021) Recombinant hGH Fc fusion protein, application and engineering cell strain of fusion protein. Patent application CN112661858 (2021) CN115400076
Wenhui Y, Yang D, Dong L et al (2023) Conjugate of recombinant human serum albumin and recombinant hGH and preparation method thereof. Patent Application EP4623935 (A1)

Chapter 7
Case 2: Design of an Integrated Bioprocess for a Therapeutic Monoclonal Antibody

7.1 Assignment: Background, Description, and Objectives

The aim of this assignment is to develop a continuous production process for a biotherapeutic monoclonal antibody. The monoclonal antibody (MAb) is going to be used for treatment of non-Hodgkin's lymphoma (NHL) in combination with an established oncogenic drug (Yazawa et al. 2005; Luo et al. 2022; Sapkota and Shaikh 2025). The goal of the assignment is to design the large-scale production for the antibody with a continuous end-to-end process.

The assigner, *Biotherapeutica,* is a minor biotherapeutic company in a research park adjacent to a life science-oriented university. The company employs 80 experienced and well-educated scientists and engineers with up-to-date backgrounds in biotechnology and pharmacology.

Biotherapeutica has recently developed a unique method for screening monoclonal antibodies targeted at specific cell structures, such as tumors and other malignant cells. Although other life science companies have similar methods for screening, *Biotherapeutica's* method shows better performance in the discrimination of oncogenic cells (Karlsson et al. 2021). The screening method is protected by intellectual property rights (IPR), making competition from other companies unlikely.

Using their screening method, *Biotherapeutica* has been successful in developing a monoclonal antibody specific to non-Hodgkin's lymphoma, which is one of several severe blood cancer diseases that inflict millions of individuals worldwide with profound healthcare costs (Singh et al. 2020; Patel et al. 2021). Preliminary clinical studies with the antibody have shown good results when using the antibody in combination treatment with an established oncogenic therapeutic drug, Rituximab™, for combating malignant lymphoma glands (Plosker and Figgitt 2022; Karlsson et al. 2021). Based on these results, the company plans to start commercial production of the NHL-antibody.

Decisive for this has been *Biotherapeutica's* estimation of the market for the NHL-antibody product. When using the combination treatment regime, an annual

C.-F. Mandenius, *Bioengineering Design Methodology*,
https://doi.org/10.1007/978-3-032-33940-9_7

global market of 500,000 patients has been predicted. The ambition is to reach a production capacity that can provide the main part of that market with their biotherapeutic monoclonal antibody and to cooperate with an established provider of Rituximab™.

The antibody has been produced at a small laboratory scale for clinical studies. For a scale-up to commercial production, an efficient production bioprocess is desired.

In commercial production, *Biotherapeutica* wishes to use state-of-the-art production techniques with single-use bioprocess equipment in an integrated end-to-end process (Jungbauer and Hammerschmidt 2017; Zhang et al. 2015; Agarwal et al. 2016). With this aim, they have assigned their own process R&D team to develop a new competitive production process for large-scale production of the NHL-antibody based on the following objectives and criteria:

- Three design alternatives shall be delivered by the process R&D unit where (i) *Biotherapeutica*'s unique screening technique is exploited and where (ii) an efficient host-vector system is identified in which the NHL-antibody's gene sequence can be transfected into a robust production cell line.
- The design alternatives should strive to accomplish an integrated end-to-end continuous processing although the continuity concept may be limited to parts of the process.
- The design must allow an annual production of 200 kg purified and formulated NHL-antibody. This production goal is assumed to cover 20% of the global market need (estimated by *Biotherapeutica* to be 100,000 NHL-patients per year).
- The design alternatives should ensure that critical quality criteria of the NHL-antibody product are reached. The purity of the formulated product should exhibit at least the same purity as in *Biotherapeutica* clinical studies to meet regulatory safety demands. This includes efficiently negating the risk of viral contamination.
- The designs must allow an increase in the annual production to 600 kg per year to meet an assumed increased market share of the NHL-antibody product.
- The assessments of the production costs of the three alternatives shall estimate investment and operational costs at an annual production of 200 kg NHL-antibody. Investments should be expected to be fully depreciated within 5 years of sales of the product. The production cost for the formulated product must not exceed 25% of the estimated sales price. *Biotherapeutica* has estimated a market price of 100 €/gram NHL-antibody. This price is 50% of the present market price for Rituximab™.

Biotherapeutica has added the following specific caveats to the assignment:

- Intellectual property rights (IPR) must ensure exclusive access to production methods, but IPR costs should not exceed 5% of the total investment.
- The design must comply with current Good Manufacturing Practice for novel bioprocessing technology.

- Subcontracting for specific tasks for cell line development, cell line purchase, procurement of specified bioprocess equipment, or other specific bioengineering tasks can be considered. Such investment or operational costs must be accounted for.

7.2 Training Scenario of the Assignment

For the design training of students or other trainees, a scenario should preferably be based on the following prerequisites:

- The trainees belong to a process R&D team at *Biotherapeutica* (cf. Fig. 4.3a in Chap. 4). They should form a team of 5–6 individuals with backgrounds in cell biology, biopharmaceutical technology, process construction and bioanalytical technology.
- The trainees have access to CAD tools, simulation and modelling tools for bioprocess design and calculations, as well as software for DoE and process economic calculations (see also Sect. 3.10).
- The trainees are in close contact with *Biotherapeutica*'s management, marketing, procurement and quality units. These are represented by the industrial tutorial experts that are prepared to provide detailed information about the company's present facilities and in-house production and process laboratories and equipment. By that, they access *Biotherapeutica's* background competence in cell culture technology and monoclonal antibody screening techniques. The company's in-house expertise and IPR know-how are available as well. The tutorial experts share *Biotherapeutica*'s medical and marketing plans with the trainees to the degree necessary for solving the assignment.
- *Biotherapeutica* has experience collaborating with subcontractors for cell lines and small-scale manufacturing equipment. This experience is available for the trainees through tutorial experts.
- The trainees shall provide *Biotherapeutica* with progress and final reports. The results should be delivered orally and in written form. The typical time frame for the assignment is in the range of 3–4 months. This can be shortened if lower demand for reporting is expected. Deliverables should be concise and succinct and follow typical company standards (see also Sect. 4.4.7).

7.3 A Recommended Design Approach

7.3.1 *Structuring the Assignment and Establishing User Requirements*

From *Biotherapeutica's* description of the assignment, its objectives, and background, a general structure can be conceived (Fig. 7.1). Several upfront activities have already taken place at the company, and other preconditions are settled. This includes the work on identifying the NHL-specific antibody using *Biotherapeutica*'s screening technique. The company has already decided that the production should be as continuous and integrated as possible and that a formulated NHL-antibody product should be the endpoint of their production. The marketing and sales to the customers of the product are the responsibility of the company's marketing people, as is the coordination with the supply of Rituximab. The marketing unit of *Biotherapeutica* is also responsible for assessing the size of the market and the product price (as given in the assignment and further explained by the industrial tutorial experts). Thus, the design tasks and challenges are the following:

- To identify a host cell line for expressing the NHL-specific antibody that is suitable for continuous production
- To identify equipment and operation units suitable for continuous operation that are accessible and economically possible to use in the design
- To consider how and to what degree continuous production can be accomplished
- To design process configurations that comply with *Biotherapeutica* production criteria

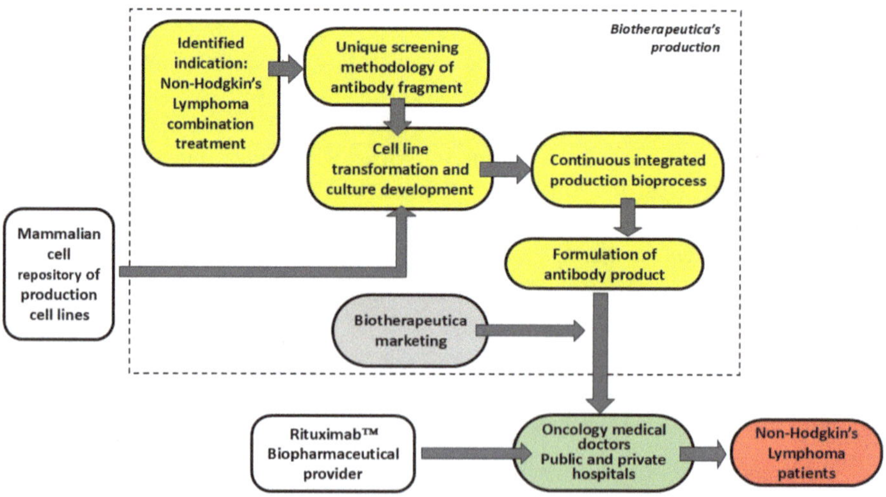

Fig. 7.1 Structure of Biotherapeutica's activities related to the NHL-specific antibody. The essential parts of the assignment are indicated in yellow

- To assess the economy for the production alternatives and compare these with *Biotherapeutica's* ambitions of production targets and costs
- To assess the scalability of the alternative designs for a larger production volume
- To ascertain that the design alternatives comply with regulatory requirements

Biotherapeutica has limited the costs for IPR and subcontracting. However, the preliminary costs are assessed from open or advised information.

The precise cost estimates are at this stage not as important as their relative levels. It may also be assumed that for a process R&D unit within the company, individual item costs are mostly known.

To decide upon a suitable host cell line should allow the use of established transfection techniques. Such cell lines are typically known and available from public or commercial cell banks or previously acquired by *Biotherapeutica.* A vector system in a CHO cell host with stable and robust cultivation properties seems like a realistic choice. Thus, costs are associated with licenses to use the cell lines for large-scale production, to carry out transfections, and to bank the transfected cell line.

Continuous integrated bioprocessing is well described for mammalian cells (Agarwal et al. 2016; Jungbauer and Hammerschmidt 2017). Importantly, the intellectual property situation must be thoroughly considered and rights perhaps acquired from others.

To reach the objectives in the assignment, optimization should be considered once a feasible detailed design is settled. That could preferably be done using statistical experimental design and mechanistic modelling.

Before conceiving the design alternatives, a deeper understanding of user needs is necessary. Users are here both users inside the company, especially those involved in production, but also marketing people responsible for sales with qualified insights into what medical doctors expect. This is done through discussions and interviews with experienced coworkers in the company, external technical expertise, and with the assigners. This should also include the customers, which in this case primarily are medical doctors who are going to prescribe and use the product clinically for the treatment of cancer patients with non-Hodgkin's lymphoma.

Table 7.1 includes specifications for each need or requirement, either qualitative or quantitative. The specified needs are then ranked based on their criticality, importance, or urgency. These figures should be agreed with the assigner, the management of *Biotherapeutica*. It should be possible to check recurrently during the design work that these needs are met.

7.3.2 Conceptualization of the Assignment

Based on the objectives, user requirements, priorities and specifications, a conceptual map should be established where functional needs for production of an NHL-specific monoclonal antibody are conceptually conceived and analyzed

Table 7.1 Biotherapeutica's requirements, priorities, and target specifications

Requirement	Target specification	Priority
Patients and clinicians using the NHL-therapeutic antibody		
The price for the NHL-antibody should be lower than comparable products	>10% lower price	Very high
Adverse side effects in patients should be so low that the product is trustworthy	Adverse side effects should comply with FDA requirements	Very high
Product shelf-life at customers should be high	The shelf-life of NHL-antibody ampoules should be >1 year	High
Quantities for average treatment should be delivered immediately	The range of 1500–2000 mg per patient and treatment	High
Clinicians should be well-informed about product quality	Annual market meeting for clinicians	Medium
Biotherapeutica's marketing unit		
Ratio of production costs versus market price should be low	< 10% at an annual production at market price of 100 EUR/g	Very high
IPR should assure the market position of the NHL-antibody	IPR should cover at least 80% of production	Very high
The formulation of the NHL-antibody should support the product's market attractiveness	A convenient formulation of the NHL-antibody product in compliance with patient and clinician requirements	Very high
The production of NHL-antibody should be possible to scale with the market needs	Upscaling from 500 to 2000 kg/year in 3 months should be possible	High
Biotherapeutica's production unit		
Throughput due to continuous production should be increased considerably	Throughput should be increased twofold	Very high
Impurities in released NHL-antibody should, with margin, be below FDA demands	Level of impure antibody form should be <1.2%	Very high
The size of the production plant shall be minimized to reduce cost and environmental impact	Plant size should be <50% of today's bio-plant	High
The production should be highly automatized to reduce personnel intensity and allow day-and-night operation	>50% of units are automatized Operator teams are ≤three operators	High

according to the principles described in Chap. 3 (Ulrich and Eppinger 2019; Mandenius and Björkman 2011) (Fig. 7.2).

The *transformation process* in the map shows a continuous bioprocess for NHL-specific antibody expression. The biological and technical functions of the map are open for exploiting state-of-the-art bioprocess technology, including the use of single-use equipment. Focus is, however, at this stage only on functionality.

The *biological functions* include (i) the NHL-specific antibody expression system, (ii) the nutritional conditions of the culture and its expression capacity, and (iii) the capture of the antibody product from its impurities. These functions encompass opportunities for different genetic constructs and host-vector systems, compositions of culture and production media, and various filtration and chromatography systems.

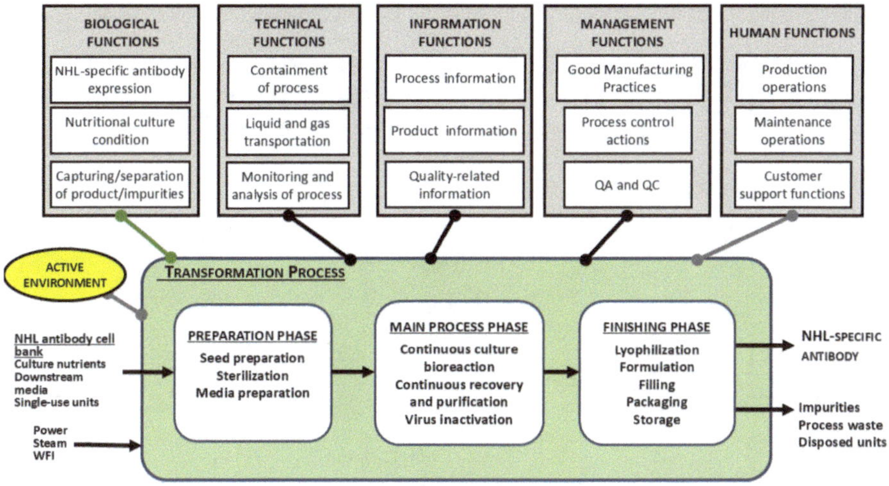

Fig. 7.2 Conceptual map of the production of NHL-antibody in a continuous end-to-end process system with single-use equipment

The preceding concerns will be to select these functions in compliance with the specified objectives in the assignment and user needs. What is important is that all functions that are involved in these are included. The design methodologies and tools for improving the biological system and its subsystems accounted for in Sect. 3.6 are relevant to apply (Pörtner 2021; Al-Rubeai and Naciri 2014).

The *technical functions* in the map emphasize (i) the containment of the process, the transportation of media to, in and from the process, and (ii) the functions for monitoring, surveillance, and analysis of such parameters that are essential to process and product information. The functions should be furnished for continuous end-to-end processing with single-use equipment.

The *information functions* assure access to information about the process and (ii) product and its quality. All these information categories related to the assignment objectives and user specifications with metrics and limits. The analytic methodology options for gaining this information are many. The subfunctions could be detailed into sub-subfunctions. These functions are mainly concerning methods and means to acquire analytical data on the amount of NHL-antibody and impurities in *Biotherapeutica's* production process.

The *management functions* are on different levels: the operative management and control of the production plant, the management of analytical data related to production capacity, and the management of quality requirements. These also concern the assignment of objectives in terms of production economy, product quality, and regulatory demands. Obviously, these functions are all interconnected to the information functions and the technical functions responsible for generating data in a timely manner and with sufficient resolution. These functions concern the operational management of the production plant and compliance with regulatory issues.

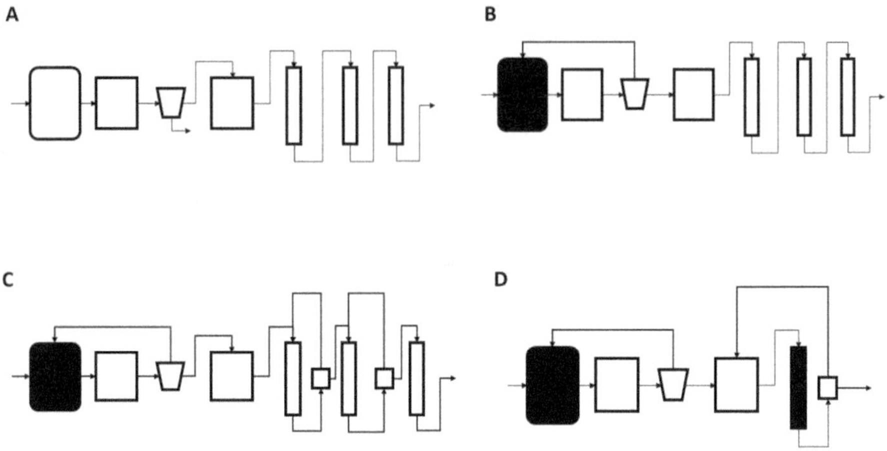

Fig. 7.3 Four conceptual configurations for production of a therapeutic NHL-antibody in continuous or single-use units

The *human functions* concern the ability of operators, technicians, and managers to handle the transformation process adequately, the capacity of support personnel to carry out maintenance of the process, and the function of supporting customers in issues related to the product and quality. This will result in training routines and procedures for these human resources. In relation to the assignment, new process techniques related to continuous processing and single-use equipment are part of this. A new advanced biotherapeutic product also requires special knowledge.

The purpose of conceptual analysis is to facilitate the designers to envisage process configurations for producing the monoclonal antibody within the frame of the assignment prerequisites. Four configurations appear to satisfy the objectives in the assignment (Fig. 7.3).

A first configuration, close to a conventional process with limited continuous operations but where single-use units can be included, is useful for comparison (Fig. 7.3a).

A configuration for continuous bioprocessing can be limited to the bioreaction stage by recycling and reprocessing of the effluent from the bioreaction (Fig. 7.3b). This is close to a conventional perfusion process. It is followed by a train of unit operations for recovery and separation of the antibody product and impurities. This allows for the introduction of single-use units where feasible. These may be the bioreactor units, small-scale or larger, the chromatographic columns, and the ultrafiltration cassettes. Depending on the extent of the exchange of units, the configuration will accordingly, with an effect not only on mainly investment cost but also on operational cost. A detailed process flow diagram will be easy to work out due to the repetitive character in the design and to calculate investments in equipment cost.

A more elaborate configuration is to add a recycling and reprocessing loop in downstream separation steps (Fig. 7.3c). This approach is a completely integrated process. Such a design requires a slitter function between the chromatographic columns. Already at this conceptual stage, it is apparent that it is a more technically advanced and cost-demanding process but could potentially reduce operational costs. Thus, it will be within the frames of the objectives and functionality mentioned above.

Another configurative arrangement is the number of downstream steps reduced by using more efficient separation (Fig. 7.3d). This relies on applying novel separation methods to be available from vendors. The recycling loops are needed. If it could be realized, the use of only two recycling loops should be attractive. With lesser number of steps, the recovery, yield, and process time should be favored, and operational cost and total investment costs reduced.

These four configurations are likely to cope with the ambition of *Biotherapeutica* to implement a continuous and integrated operation, use of single-use technology, and efficient separation. The configuration in Fig. 7.3a appears close to many existing plant bioprocesses, while the Fig. 7.3d configuration is the most integrated design but also the most demanding.

These three configurations seem justified to consider for further detailed design and are in the following referred to as a *non-recycled design*, a *triple-recycled design,* and a *double-recycled design.*

7.3.3 Detailed Design of the Selected Conceptual Configurations

Detailed designs and flow sheeting of the three prioritized conceptual configurations will integrate conventional unit operation equipment in combination with novel biotechnical equipment (Heinzle et al. 2006; Petrides 2015; Pollock et al. 2017; O'Brian 2019). Of special interests to investigate are:

- How to design recycling loops in the upstream and downstream steps.
- Whether stainless-steel bioreactors can be replaced with single-use bioreactors in volumes up to 2000 L, where the size depends on the production target.
- The use of prepacked chromatographic columns with separation materials containing biologically active ligands.
- The potential for scaling up the designs.

These options are investigated in the following detailed design alternatives:

A *non-recycled design* uses a continuous bioreactor (chemostat) for culturing CHO cells that express the NHL-antibody. The antibody is expressed directly into the culture medium. The effluent from the bioreactor with CHO cells and NHL-antibodies is passed to a continuous centrifuge that removes the cells and recovers the antibody in a storage tank. This is subsequently followed by three chromatographic steps for purifying the NHL-antibody (ion exchange, size exclusion, and protein A chromatography). These steps use established chromatographic methods, with the ion exchange separation materials to remove remaining culture media constituents, size exclusion chromatography to remove multimeric IgG forms, and protein A chromatography to remove adverse antibody forms and increase monomeric NHL-antibody purity. This is subsequently followed by virus inactivation, diafiltration, and freeze-drying (Fig. 7.4a).

Already in this non-recycled design process design it would be possible to consider single-use equipment and new separation materials. However, in the example, it is limited to conventional equipment items.

This non-recycled alternative is included to compare the recycled alternatives for showing the effects on investment and operational costs.

A scaling up of the process will mainly follow linear dependencies on equipment size and consumables.

In a *double-recycled process,* the CHO cells are attached to microcarriers where they express the NHL-antibody to the culture medium. The culture medium with CHO cells is recycled by a continuous ultrafilter unit (recycle I). The CHO cells and microcarriers are recycled to the perfusion bioreactor for continued expression of antibody. The ultrafilter (cutoff 500 kD) separates the CHO-expressed NHL-antibody. The recovered NHL-antibody is collected in a storage tank.

The antibody is then first purified by an ion exchange chromatography column. The eluted pool is reprocessed (recycle II), resulting in a higher separation. The collected pool is further purified by a protein A chromatography column (with no reprocessing) for removing remaining adverse forms of the antibody. This is followed by diafiltration, virus inactivation, and freeze-drying (Fig. 7.4b).

The recycling of the bioreactor has the advantage of reusing the culture media, being one of the expansive consumables. It also reduces waste from the process. The recycled bioreactor uses single-use equipment (culture bags) up to a reactor volume of 2000 L.

The recycling of the first chromatography step increases the purity of the antibody but with some loss of yield.

In the *triple-recycled design,* the first recycling is the same as in the double-recycled design, consequently with the same benefits of reuse of cells and microcarriers (recycle I). The recovered NHL-antibody pool is, in this process design, first purified in a chromatography column using a new ion exchange separation material with a higher separation factor. The eluted pool is also here reprocessed (recycle II).

The collected pool is further purified by an exclusive affinity chromatography column with reprocessing (recycle III) that removes all adverse forms of the antibody and other impurities. This reprocessing allows use of a lower amount and volume of separation material. This is again followed by diafiltration, virus inactivation, and freeze-drying (Fig. 7.4c).

The process has been provided with a recycling loop from a centrifuge back to the bioreactor as well as with recycling from the first chromatographic step (Fig. 7.4c). Thus, the alternative has a clear ambition of continuity both in the upstream and downstream processing. It presupposes efficient control of the system in setting recycling ratios. This requires advancement of online monitoring of involved operational units. The alternative is adaptable for using single-use equipment units,

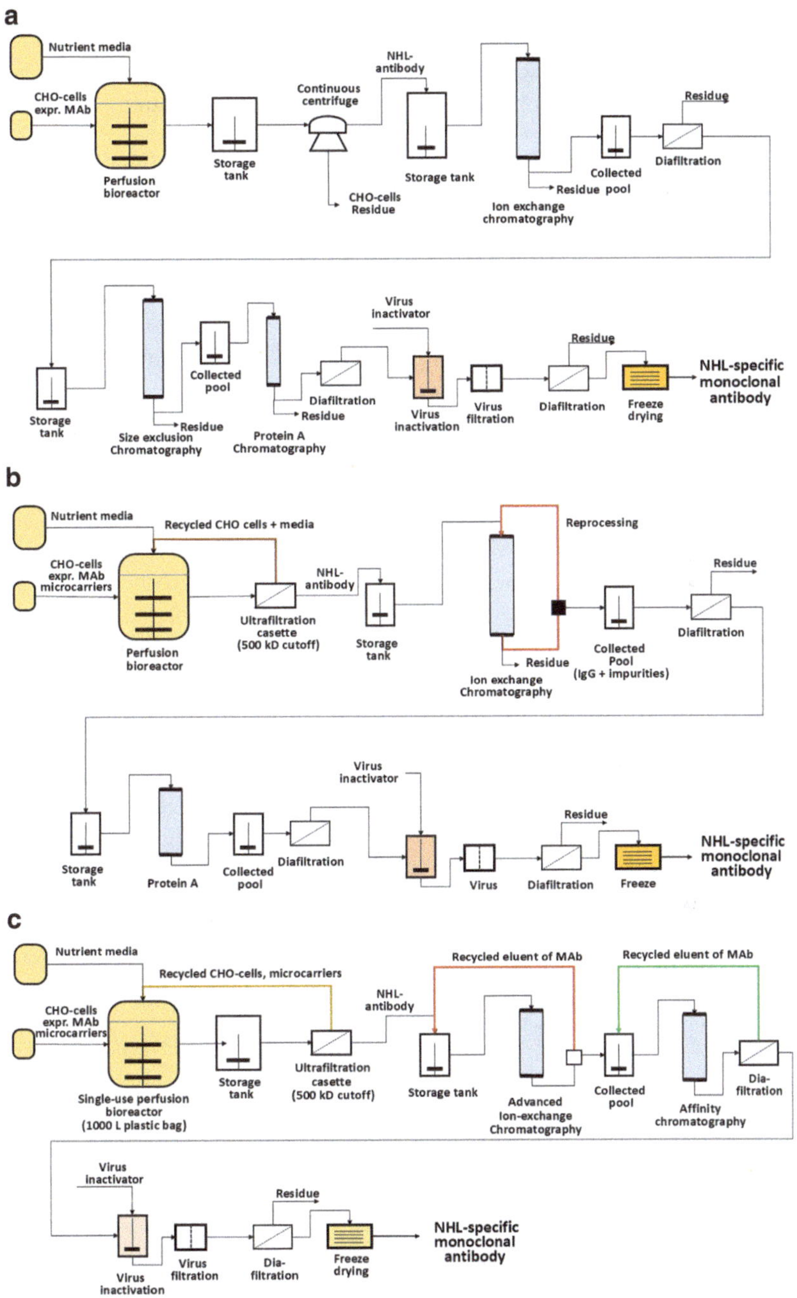

Fig. 7.4 Three design alternatives for production of the NHL-antibody. (**a**) A non-recycled semicontinuous process with CHO cells in suspension culture. (**b**) A double-recycled process where CHO cells, bound to microcarriers, are recycled in a perfused bioreactor and one of the chromatographic columns is recycled. (**c**) A triple-recycled process where CHO cells, bound to microcarriers, are recycled in a perfused bioreactor, and two of the chromatographic columns are recycled

which is also assumed in the economic evaluation below. The alternative is expected to strongly enhance the possibility of reaching the annual production target even in a smaller plant size.

In these three designs, the need for monitoring and control will increase, resulting in additional measurement devices and flow control equipment. Also, trained technicians and engineers for operations and qualified support are needed. With one operation step less, investments in equipment are also reduced and quality controlled simplified. Demands for maintenance of a larger process are reduced as well. A more compact and spacious plant that reduces personnel costs can therefore be anticipated. The designs also call for more control and automation that consequently leads to additional investments, installation, and validations.

The end-to-end double-recycled design seems to best comply with the ambition of *Biotherapeutica*. It could easily be assessed economically.

Scaling up the alternatives could be an issue of larger sizes of equipment, higher yields, and closer to 100% continuous processing. Also, the improvement of the cell line's productivity by optimization could increase production capacity. *Biotherapeutica*'s ambition to increase from 200 to 600 kg per year could be attained with such development, while keeping the size of equipment and facility unchanged, and with only marginal restraint in personnel time. This will be done at the cost of additional production R&D.

It is necessary to ensure that the design alternatives can comply with legal IPR procedures, and that existing patents or patent applications do not infringe on the design priorities.

Several IPR applications that have a potentially infringing impact on the bioprocess design of continuous systems need to be considered (Dierckx et al. 2022; Bartake et al. 2019; Broadley and Garrahy 2021). Other IPR applications concerning the combination treatment using monoclonal antibodies for non-Hodgkin's lymphoma should also be considered although they do not directly involve the production methods per se (Wolin et al. 2003; Goldenberg and Wegener 2016; White and Grillo-Lopez 2010; Frendeus and Mattsson 2012; Frendeus and Hansson 2014; Sims and Bartlett 2021).

7.3.4 Production Economic Evaluation for Three Detailed Designs

The objective of the economic evaluation is to perform a preliminary assessment of the relative economic consequences of the three design alternatives (Peters et al. 2003; Kristiansen 2006; Towler and Sinnott 2012; Stamatis and Farid 2021). The primary aim is to reduce the total production costs through a more cost-efficient design, and to do this without compromising the quality of the NHL-antibody product. The designs must also comply with the assignment objectives of Biotherapeutica and the needs and requirements of users. Three issues that are directly related to the production economy are especially considered:

- How will a scale-up to an annual production of 600 kg NHL-antibody product influence the production costs?
- Which specific cost items dominate the total production costs?
- Are the price levels of specific items (consumables or investments) critical to consider in the design?

The estimated investment costs in the three alternatives can be expected to differ considerably due to the use of equipment for carrying out recycling, the use of single-use equipment, and the utilization of microcarriers for cultivation. These technological features also require considerable process development, which will become a part of the investments. These investments must then be covered, resulting in high annual payoff costs.

In the economic evaluation in Table 7.2, the most influential cost items are presented. The differences in costs are related to the appreciated costs for heavy equipment (reactors, hold tanks, centrifuges, filtration equipment, recycling pumps, chromatography columns, freezer, and control equipment), expensive consumables (culture media, separation media, filters), and additional expenditures (installations, labor, buildings, etc.). Standard factors are used to estimate typical standard costs. Cell line rights and IPR costs are included as separate items.

In the non-recycled process, conventional process equipment is used, including bioreactors, chromatography, centrifuge, storage tanks, filtration equipment, and a freeze-drying unit. The most expensive operational costs are consumables: culture and separation media, microcarriers, and chromatographic separation materials. The consumption of culture and separation media is higher because non-media is reused by recycling.

In the triple-recycled process, the continuous centrifuge is replaced by a continuous ultrafiltration unit; perfusion is used with recycling. The main bioreactor is replaced by a single-use reactor, which consumes culture bags. The number of chromatography units is less but has more advanced technology and expensive separation materials (expanded-bed chromatography, affinity-based separation). A high cost is the investment in equipment for the three recycling loops (pumps, vents, flow controllers).

In the double-recycled process, the continuous centrifuge is used in the cultivation step. Several of the other cost items reappear as in the two previous designs. The equipment for recycling is limited to two recycling loops (the bioreactor and the first chromatographic separation step). The double-recycled process uses, as the triple-recycled process, more advanced chromatographic techniques.

As can be seen in the economic evaluation, most production costs are almost the same despite the rather fundamental redesigning of the production of the NHL-antibody. Upfront basic production R&D, patent filing (IPR), cost for acquisition of cell line, virus inactivation, quality control, cost for buildings and laboratories, and management costs are almost the same. Still, there is a significant investment in new equipment, that requirement production development (upfront) and pre-validation. These costs must be covered by the sale of the NHL-antibody product.

Table 7.2 Economic evaluation of three designs for NHL-specific antibody production

Type of costs	Non-recycled process (kEUR)	Triple-recycled process (kEUR)	Double-recycled process (kEUR)
Investment costs			
Upfront production R&D			
Process R&D	100	900	1500
IPR filing	100	500	700
Cell line licensing	100	100	100
Total upfront production R&D	*300*	*1500*	*2300*
Equipment and instrumentation			
Bioreactors	1000	1000	1000
Recycling equipment	–	200	400
Separation equipment units	80	80	80
Virus inactivation	70	70	70
Quality control instrumentation	50	50	50
Total equipment and instrumentation	*1200*	*1400*	*1600*
Additional expenditures for production			
Installation of equipment (×0.5)	600	1150	1400
Project planning (×0.3)	360	690	840
Taxation (×0.1)	120	230	280
Buildings (×0.3)	360	690	840
Total additional expenditures	*1440*	*1680*	*1920*
Total investment costs	**2940**	**4580**	**5820**
Operational costs (200 kg MAb/year)			
Consumables for production			
Consumables and raw materials	180	80	80
Chromatography media	100	100	100
QC consumables	50	50	50
Single-use units	–	–	100
Formulation materials	20	20	20
Total consumables for production	*350*	*250*	*350*
Additional operational expenditures			
Labor in production facility	1900	1000	300
Renting of buildings	100	100	100
Taxation	30	30	30
Annual IPR expenditure/ licenses	150	150	150
Management	50	50	50

(continued)

Table 7.2 (continued)

Type of costs	Non-recycled process (kEUR)	Triple-recycled process (kEUR)	Double-recycled process (kEUR)
Total additional operational expenditures	*2230*	*1330*	*630*
Total operational costs	**2580**	**1580**	**980**
Annual payoff (5 years)	*588*	*916*	*1164*
Total annual production costs	**3168**	**2496**	**2144**
Production cost 1 g NHL-antibody (EUR)	15.84	12.48	10.72

The distribution of costs is compared in circle diagrams (Fig. 7.5). The payoff is considerable in all the alternatives and growing for the recycling alternatives. Still, the total production cost is decreased in the assessment. As seen from the figures in Table 7.2, this is mainly due to lower labor cost and the continuous production (day-and-night operation, size of the plant size for the annual production target of 200 kg product).

Scaling up to an annual production of 600 kg product will most likely be possible in the new designs: (i) by tighter production scheduling or (ii) by increasing the downsized equipment.

In the mono-recycled alternative, the CHO cells are retained in the bioreactor by returning the centrifugate from the continuous centrifuge to the bioreactor. The top fraction is consequently a cell-free flow with the same antibody concentration as in the bioreactor. This flow with antibodies is purified in three chromatographic steps (see Fig. 7.4b). The bioreactor is a conventional steel bioreactor with equipment for sterilization and reuse. Thus, the investment costs for equipment will be relatively high.

In the triple-recycled design alternative, CHO cells on microcarriers are retained in the bioreactor by recycling from a microfilter unit. The filtered antibody-containing broth is separated by chromatography. This is carried out in two chromatographic columns, each recycled once using a splitter (Fig. 7.4c). The bioreactor CHO culture is carried out in single-use bags, and chromatographic stations use prepacked chromatographic columns. The recycling ratios are possible to be optimized by modelling. The investment in the triple-recycled alternatives is expected to be higher than in the non- and mono-recycled designs, but the operational costs are likely to be considerably reduced due to a higher degree of automation.

The cost structure of two interesting alternatives, the triple- and double-recycled processes, is compared with the non-recycled alternative (Table 7.3).

Table 7.2 provides an overview of the costs. As could be expected, the recycled designs have higher investment costs than the non-recycled design due to their less

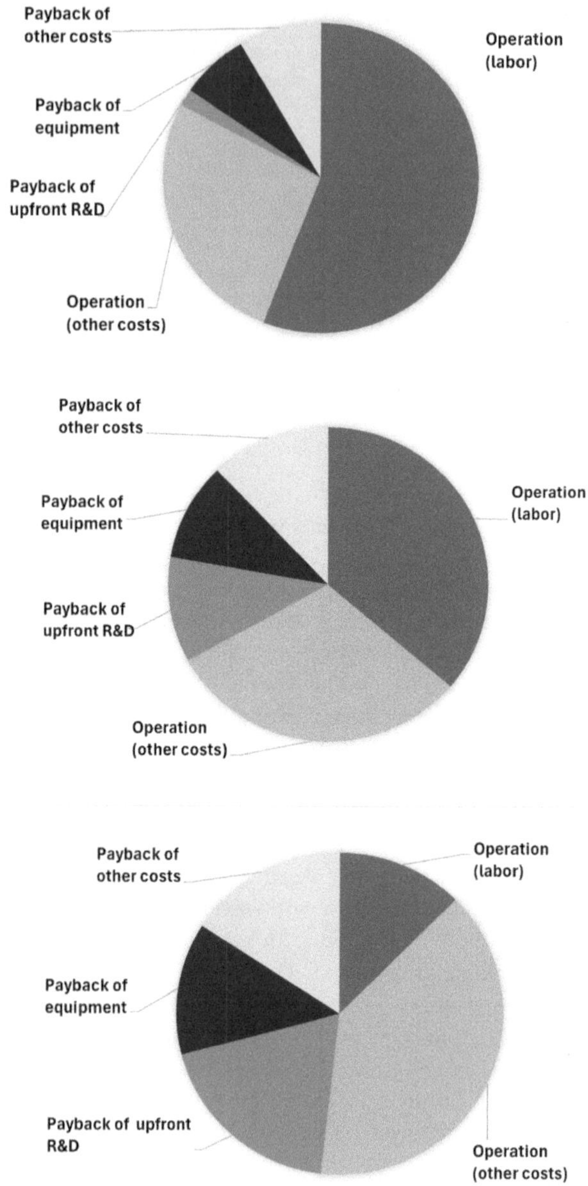

Fig. 7.5 Distribution of costs in the three design alternatives. (**a**) Non-recycled process. (**b**) Triple-recycled process. (**c**) Double-recycled process

modern or exclusive equipment. However, the recycled alternatives have lower labor costs, lower volumes, and other costs for consumables for single-use disposables and media qualities. Some of these costs will become more apparent if the production volume increases.

Table 7.3 Objects of optimization using factorial design or mechanistic modelling

Object of optimization	Expected outcome	Applicable optimization technique
Expression system antibody in the applied cell line	Increase in specific production rate of NHL-antibody	Factorial design of experimentally available parameters (factors)
Cultivation parameters in perfusion bioreactor	Increased growth rate of cells leading to higher rate of NHL-antibody	Factorial design of selected bioreactor parameters
Cultivation media composition	A favorable media composition for production under controlled media cost	Factorial design of selected components and concentrations
Chromatographic operation parameters	Improved separation performance affecting purity and yield	Factorial design of critical separation parameters
Chromatography media composition	Favorable media compositions of separation media	Factorial design of components in media
Effects of recycling rates on productivity	Improved productivity, downsizing and process time	Mechanistic bioreactor modelling
Reactor dilution and recycling rates related to kinetic parameters	Improvement of production, scheduling of process	Mechanistic bioreactor modelling

Importantly, the additional R&D costs for the recycled alternatives will be higher, as will the testing and validation of a plant design with novel technology.

The outcome of the mechanistic modelling is anticipated, and it is assumed that there is a loss of volumetric productivity due to the process integration in the configurations in double- and triple-recycled alternatives. This is estimated to be 85% and 75%, respectively. These values need to be experimentally confirmed but could, at this stage, contribute to grasping the effects and indicate the trend of cost change.

Under all circumstances, the scale needs to be increased to a degree corresponding to the reduced productivity. The trade-off is to find when the set annual production can be reached by the shorter integrated processes.

The second question to determine is how much the scale-up must go for attaining the primary annual production goal and the long-term threefold annual production goal.

The precision at this stage, given the details of the items in the calculations, is limited. A collection of accurate procurement costs should be made to adjust values. However, the principal way of carrying out the assessment remains unchanged. Thus, the relative economic benefit of integration of the process may vary depending on actual price levels and purchase agreements. The noted trends should remain.

To reach the high annual product level, parallel production lines may be considered as an alternative to a larger single-unit plant. The access to larger single-use equipment and its cost may motivate this. As this is simply a multiplicative effect, there is no difference between alternatives, whereas reduced cost and profit are achieved.

The circular charts illuminate that a threefold scale-up will change the distribution of costs of the investment costs as well as the operational cost per unit, resulting in a lower total production cost (Fig. 7.5). In conclusion, the gradually increasing integration of the plant requires higher initial investments that may be returned over time. But they are also at risk, as this return is not guaranteed.

7.3.5 Optimization of the Selected Recycled Designs

Once a decision has been made on how to prioritize the designs, a further optimization of these is motivated (Sioshansi and Conejo 2017; Martins and Ning 2021). It is likely that there are some differences in aptitude for optimization because of the degree of integration. The more compact recycled processes may have less opportunities for optimization. Still, several optimization opportunities are at hand that may result in better performances of the recycled processes (Table 7.3). The goals and expected outcomes are to improve productivity, increase yields, reduce use of resources, and decrease process time, all having a positive impact on production economy.

Optimization of Perfusion Cultivation by Design of Experiments The performance of the recycled design alternatives is possible to optimize by using design of experiments (DoE) methodology (Brereton 2003; Montgomery 2020; Mandenius and Brundin 2008). Primarily, three kinds of optimization objectives should be considered: (1) the medium composition of the culture media, (2) the operative conditions of the cultivation, and (3) the expression kinetics of the NHL-antibody. At this stage of design development, it is worthwhile to identify factors that seem likely to improve kinetics and yields in the process.

Examples of experimental factors associated with kinetics and yields are mentioned in Table 7.4. Glucose, galactose, essential and nonessential amino acids,

Table 7.4 Factors and responses for optimization by DoE

Objects for optimization	Factors in DoE plan	Responses to measured
Culture media composition	Glucose Galactose Nonessential amino acids Essential amino acids Selenium Lipids	Growth rate of CHO cells Yield of cells per medium components Rate of antibody expression Yield of antibody per cell Side-product formation Formation of adverse antibody structures
Cultivation conditions	pH Temperature Agitation rate Dissolved oxygen Ratio of microcarriers	
Expression conditions of the cell line	Plasmid copy number Induction time	

selenium, and lipids are such factors worthwhile to test. To find out how factors such as pH, temperature, stirrer speed, and starting concentration during seeding procedures could positively improve cell growth and antibody productivity, it is recommended to apply a DoE plan available on established DoE software programs (e.g., Modde, MiniTab) and perform reduced experiments by measuring growth rates and expression rates of NHL-antibody.

Several other factor-response combinations can be considered. The parameters in the downstream processing steps could certainly be optimized by DoE methodology. Their effect on process performance can be profound.

Optimization of NHL-Antibody Production by Mechanistic Modelling Mechanistic modelling provides the opportunity to optimize the continuous process conditions (Nielsen et al. 2011; Doran 2013). This could concern the upstream phase of the process as well as the downstream antibody separation phase (Jain and Kumar 2008). Within the process flow diagrams, critical parameters can be identified (Fig. 7.6). Of most interest are those parameters that can be controlled or influenced either by direct actions, e.g., by tuning flows and by process control, or by preemptive actions, e.g., by improvements of cell lines and expression systems. Both these conditions are objects for model studies. Due to the design configurations outlined above, it is possible to identify the parameters and possibly also rank their potential value for the performance of the production process and their proneness to being influenced or controlled. This could ensure an optimal recycling of cells and nutrient media, depending on the configurations in the alternative designs. Basically, it becomes a matter of volumetric effects of expression and growth of cells, yields and rates, and how these parameters reflect on productivity and, consequently, on production economy.

The operation of the process influences the production outcome. This can be evaluated in a structured mechanistic model. Key operational parameters to investigate would be:

- The perfusion rate of culture media through the continuously operated bioreactor, whether the perfused effluent is recycled or not

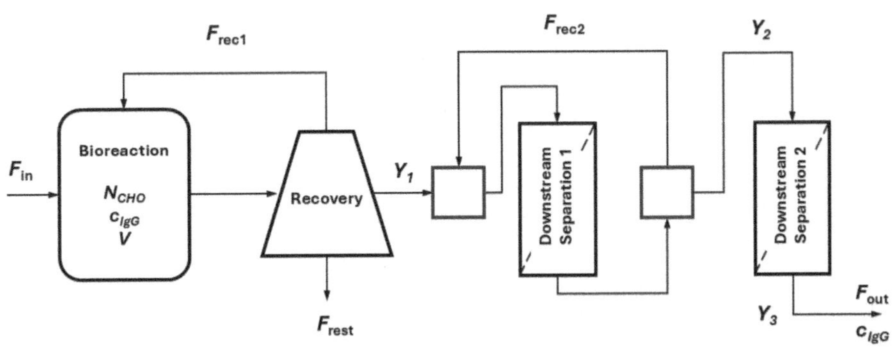

Fig. 7.6 Structure of a mechanistic model for semicontinuous integrated bioprocess

- If the cells are recycled to the bioreactor, how do the recycling rates or ratios influence the performance
- The influence of the specific rates of expression and growth of the CHO cell line
- The dependence of the yield in the process, including relations between culture media, death of CHO cells, and IgG stability and denaturation
- Chromatographic materials capacity, volumetric throughput, and yields
- Centrifuge or ultrafilter performances

Some of these operational parameters are amendable to DoE studies as mentioned above. Undoubtedly, it can also be an interactive combination of optimization methods.

The mechanistic modelling has the obvious advantage of not requiring time-consuming experiments, if reasonable kinetic parameters are available, e.g., from literature data.

Here, three examples are shown to illustrate the potential of the mechanistic modelling:

- The influence of perfusion rate in the bioreactor on total antibody production, cell concentration and cell line properties.
- If the cells produced in the bioreactor are recycled by using a centrifuge or ultrafilter while the antibodies dissolved in the media are recovered for further purification.
- If the perfusing rate and recycling ratio are adjusted, how will the production of antibodies be influenced.

In the examples, the model is based on the following mass balance-derived differential equations:

Mass balance for the IgG product:

$$dc_{\mathrm{IgG}}/dt = q_{\mathrm{IgG}} \cdot N_{\mathrm{CHO}} - k_e \cdot C_i + k_f \cdot C_i / V_{\mathrm{bioreactor}} \tag{7.1}$$

Mass balance for the CHO cells:

$$dN_{\mathrm{CHO}}/dt = \mu_{\mathrm{CHO}} \cdot C_{\mathrm{media}} - F_{\mathrm{in}} + k_{\mathrm{in}} \cdot C_i / V_{\mathrm{bioreactor}} \tag{7.2}$$

Mass balance for the limiting culture media component(s):

$$dC_{\mathrm{media}}/dt = k \cdot C_{\mathrm{media}} - k_e \cdot C_i + k_e \cdot C_i / V_{\mathrm{bioreactor}} \tag{7.3}$$

Relevant perfusion and recycling rates, or ratios, should be included in the modelling. This can be done as dilution rate (*D*), or through flow rates (F_{in}, F_{rec}) and bioreactor volume (*V*), where $F/V = D$. The model structure easily allows testing of the impact of specific growth rate of CHO cells (μ) and specific expression rate of monoclonal antibody (q_{IgG}), as well as uptake of the limiting media component (c_{media}).

These model frames are used in the modelling examples in Fig. 7.7.

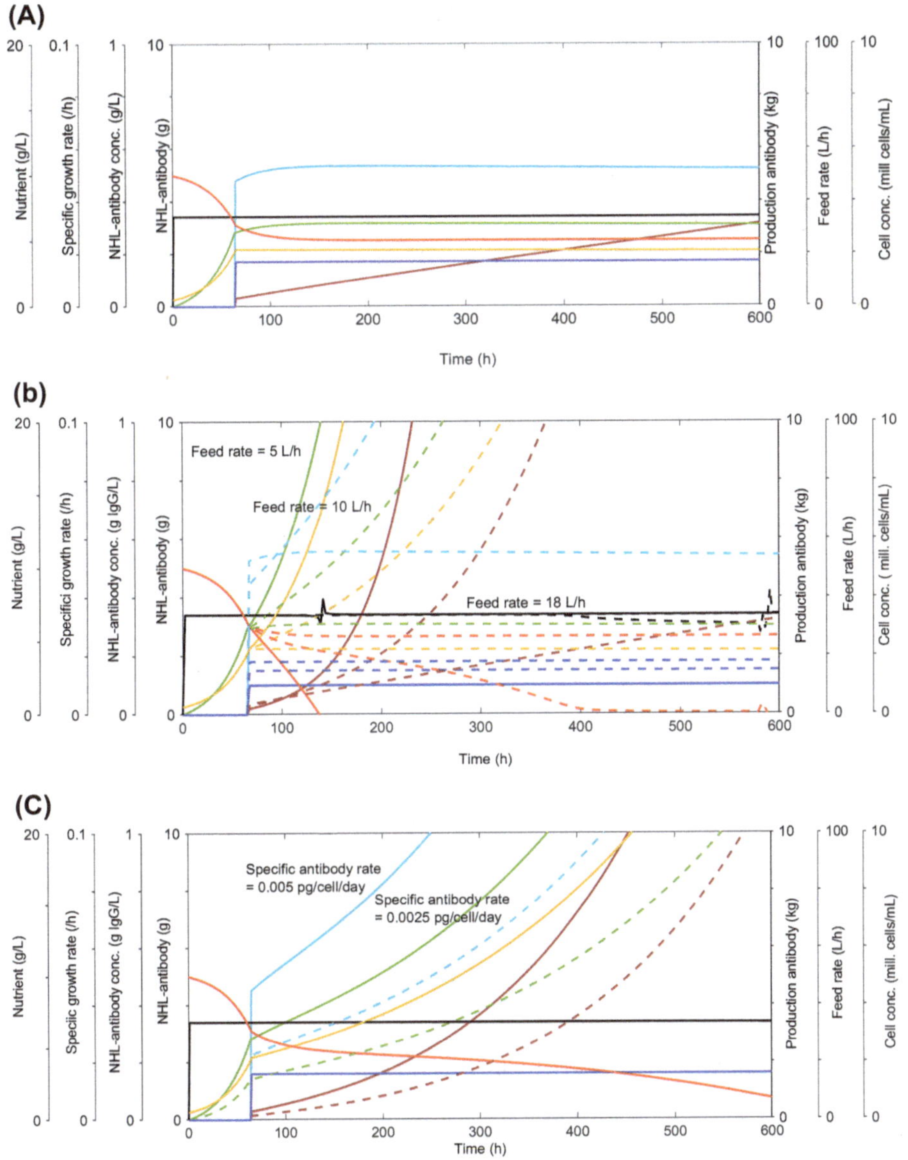

Fig. 7.7 (**a**) Continuous perfusion in bioreactor with CHO cells expressing the NHL-specific MAb without recycling. The feed concentration to the bioreactor is 20 g/L (red line) and 10 g/L (dotted red) at the same dilution rate (0.34 h^{-1}). (**b**) Cells are recycled to the bioreactor at three rates, 5, 10, and 18 L/h. (**c**) Cells recycled as in B at antibody expression rates of 0.0050 (line) and 0.0025 (dashed) pg/cell/day

The *first example* investigates different perfusion rates but without recycling, which relates to the design alternative. This interesting issue is here to judge how productivity can be enhanced by a higher perfusion rate without losing IgG in the reactor effluent.

In the *second example*, cells are recycled. This can be done at different recycling ratios, while IgG is recovered in the centrifugation, i.e., the top fraction of the centrifuge.

In the *third example*, different specific rates are added to the second diagram. This shows the potential impact of cell line improvements through cell engineering and media optimization.

In the simulation graphs, concentrations of cells and product and total production of product were plotted versus time. The reactor volume and flow rates were varied, and different assumed specific growth and production rates were used for systematically investigating the influence on the total production of the product.

The complexity of a continuous process becomes very apparent with the three process configurations dealt with in this assignment. The key parameters that decide the outcome of the production process are obvious: the specific rate of the antibody expression, q_{IgG}, and the specific growth of CHO cells, μ_{CHO}. Important for cost assessment is the bioreactor volume, $V_{\text{bioreactor}}$, which should be minimized with remained antibody output. Next is to include in the modelling the amount of antibody per outflowing volume and time (g/h). This is what goes out from the final stage of the process, and that should be lyophilized or concentrated by diafiltration. The relationships between the parameters and what should be expected to be optimized by tuning their dimensions should be clarified (Table 7.5). It ends up in the size and cost of equipment per amount of produced antibody.

The model allows simulations of the design alternatives during 600 h-periods. The continuous bioreactor with a volume of 1000 L, inoculated with a seed of

Table 7.5 Parameters useful in mechanistic modelling for antibody production optimization

Parameter investigated	Model	Expected outcome
Perfusion rate to the continuous perfusion reactor	Kinetic mass balance based on specific growth rate of CHO cells	Productivity timing of operation
Expression rate of Mab	Kinetic balance with specific growth and expression parameters	Mab productivity per reactor volume
Volume of culture system	Culture density reached under various volumetric conditions	Optimization of volume of plant in relation to time
Total Mab output	Balance based on yield factors in the DSP train	Total productivity related to downstream steps
Recycling rate from centrifuge back to continuous reactor	Mass balance with recycling ratio adjustable	Effect of cell number and MAb conc. In bioreactor effluent
Yield in downstream steps based on efficacy	Simple factorial effect of centrifuge or filter and columns	Estimation of effect of total yield on productivity of end-to-end system

10 million CHO cells, can be studied at varying perfusion rates (Fig. 7.7a). These cells are assumed to come from a prepared working cell bank at *Biotherapeutica* that can be provided regularly at no nominal cost. At F_{start}, feeding is commenced with a feed containing an optimized composition of nutrients (here 50 g/L of the limiting substrate is assumed while all other nutritional factors are in excess). The expression of antibodies starts constitutively. Both cells and antibodies reach steady-state concentrations, as apparent in the graphs. The effluent flow from the bioreactor contains both cells and antibodies. There is no recycling while the effluent flow goes to centrifugation for removal of cells and retention of antibodies that are collected in a hold tank.

This non-recycled process serves as a benchmark for comparison with the recycled process using the same parameters, where cells are recycled from the centrifuge to the bioreactor (Fig. 7.7b). It shows the flow rate adjusts to the steady-state level. By increasing the flow rate, a lower steady-state level results while the antibody output (g/L/h) goes up. This results in increased steady-state cell antibody concentration levels. When the recycling rate from the centrifuge is increased, a further elevation of the levels is attained.

This can be followed up, still with the same basic parameters, by investigating different recycling ratios (Fig. 7.7c). The accumulated antibody output is included in the diagram, which allows estimation of the total effect of using the end-to-end continuous process.

In summary, it is obvious that the mechanistic modelling allows a more complete assessment of the productivity of the system. The bioreactor volume that could supply the required amount of antibody can be assessed. This improves the assessment of costs for investment in equipment and of operation with or without a cost structure related to single-use units to a degree as originally suggested by *Biotherapeutica*.

7.4 Conclusive Suggestions for *Biotherapeutica*

It is suggested to use alternative designs based on recycling. The costs associated with these alternatives are analyzed and compared. It is obvious that continuous and integrated end-to-end bioprocess systems have considerable operational advantages. Thus, the most ambitious alternative, the recycled process design, is the preferred choice. By including streams that are realistic for recycling, the unit production price of the monoclonal antibody is considerably reduced. With an increasing production volume through scaling up, the economic gain is amplified. Going from 50% of the production cost to an assumed market price at the estimated dosage schemes of the non-Hodgkin's lymphoma antibody in combination with Rituximab, the production cost is estimated to decrease to 25% at a threefold increase in production volume and to decrease further to 10% at a sevenfold increase.

This will consequently cover *Biotherapeutica's* objectives in the assignment.

However, it should be emphasized that the fully integrated continuous bioprocess requires extensive investment in new advanced equipment. This should be depreciated according to *Biotherapeutica's* business plan, thus within a period of 5 years. A margin of 50% between market price and production cost will be required for paying back the investment in a new plant over a 5-year period.

This estimate presupposes that during this 5-year period, the sale reaches 20% of the estimated market. This cannot be guaranteed.

Three alternatives are at hand to alleviate this effect:

- To extend the payback time, e.g., to 10 years, which means that sales volumes or price levels can be lower. If the investors can cope with that, it is a feasible way.
- Reduce the initial investment in a new plant to change the prerequisites. An alternative with a double-recycled design could offer this.
- A further optimization of the biological system's capacity to produce more antibody per cell and/or increasing the cell density to enhance the volumetric productivity of the plant.

The first and second alternatives are possible with a changed business plan, and the third alternative is possible with additional R&D efforts.

A fourth possibility could be to develop the pharmaceutical conditions by applying a therapeutic antibody with higher efficacy, thereby reducing the dosage per treatment. This would lead to a linear economic effect from a production perspective.

A fifth possibility could be to improve the bioprocess technology further, e.g., by developing an even more integrated and compact plant, finding a cell line with higher productivity and potentially culture density, but probably then also leading to higher R&D and/or investment costs.

It is therefore suggested that *Biotherapeutica* at this stage choose the recycled process. This would be expected to favor *Biotherapeutica's* competitive position on the market and be able to offer the product at the lowest price to the presumptive customers.

7.5 Tutorial Perspectives on the Assignment

The specific challenge in the assignment is to advance the production technology of the monoclonal antibody by process integration and the use of state-of-the-art technology, and to do so in a production-economic fashion without compromising product quality.

The suggested approach accomplishes this by utilizing continuous around-the-clock end-to-end manufacturing processes at a relatively modest scale and implementing single-use equipment in approximately half of the units. This configuration makes it easy to reach the global production goal. It is claimed that this results in a lower cost, mainly due to reduced equipment size as well as lowered personnel and maintenance costs.

The training challenges are related to identifying these techniques and technological solutions. This requires the trainees to understand what to identify and how to capture the state-of-the-art and its availability. This becomes a critical stage in the design work, where conceptualization is especially helpful.

A major hurdle in that workflow is to understand the consequences of the conceptualization and, within the training team, to discuss, negotiate, and agree on potential alternatives. The fact that host-vector systems using genetic engineering platforms are numerous (production cell lines, expression systems, protease influence, and protein stability versus structure in relation to possible production media) and that upstream process equipment alternatives generate many possibilities makes it difficult to come to agreements and to determine on what grounds those agreements should be made. Here, tutorial intervention and assistance in structuring pros and cons in relation to the assignment are probably needed.

Another hurdle is that the lack of experimental data during the initial ranking of alternatives hampers decision-making substantially. Iterative design in the first training phase can, for inexperienced trainees, be partly confounding. The introduction of experimental reasoning (factorial design) can, in the short term, facilitate this process on both a factual and psychological level. The structuring of biological and process parameters in the design of experiments (DoE) plan (cf. Mandenius and Brundin 2008) will then simplify and lead to more straightforward decisions.

A few additional hurdles are likely to appear:

- The training can benefit considerably if the trainees do not get trapped in finding precise rates and prices and instead run the evaluation of the alternatives conceived using rough estimates. This will accelerate the workflow and save time.
- It is important to pass the conceptual stage relatively quickly and continue to outline the potential possibilities using available means for continuous processing. The risk is becoming too theoretical. It is better to return and reiterate the conceptualization structure based on reality.
- Trainees may neglect existing designs that are already known. This means they must actively scrutinize the state of filed patent applications as well as technical and scientific publications to see if these are in the process of IPR prosecution.

Thus, tutorial actions must monitor the progress of the trainees in these directions and appropriately push them into design work that allows them to realize these possibilities.

References

Agarwal H, Sharma AK, Kateja N et al (2016) Continuous processing for the production of biopharmaceuticals. BioPharm Int 29:14–19

Al-Rubeai M, Naciri M (eds) (2014) Stem cells and cell therapy. Springer, New York. https://doi.org/10.1007/978-94-007-7196-3

Bartake H, Gadgil H, Banerjee A et al (2019) Automated integrated continuous system and bioprocess for producing therapeutic protein. Enzene Bioscience Ltd, US Patent Application PCT/2019/052654

Brereton RG (2003) Chemometrics, data analysis for laboratory and chemical plants. Wiley, Chichester

Broadley ST, Garrahy RJ (2021) Single-use bioreactor assembly with integrated pump heads. Broadley-James Corp, US Patent Application 17/2015823

Dierckx K, Vandeput J, Farouk A (2022) Integrated continuous bioprocess production platform. Simabs NV, Patent Application WO 2022/248623

Doran PM (2013) Biochemical engineering principles, 2nd edn. Elsevier, Amsterdam. https://doi.org/10.1016/C2009-0-22348-8

Frendeus B, Hansson M (2014) Use of antibodies against ICAM-1 in combination with anti-cancer drug in the treatment of patients. Bioinvent International AB, US Patent Application PCT/2014/050274

Frendeus B, Mattsson J (2012) Screening methods and use thereof. Bioinvent International AB, US Patent PCT/2021/068576

Goldenberg DM, Wegener WA (2016) Combined therapy with anti-CD74 and anti-CD20 antibodies in patients with relapsed and refractory B-cell non-Hodgkin's lymphoma. Immunomedic Inc, Canadian Intellectual Property Office, No 2 970 738

Heinzle E, Biwer A, Cooney C (2006) Chapter: Antibody. In: Development of sustainable bioprocesses. Modelling and assessment. Wiley, Chichester

Jain E, Kumar A (2008) Upstream processes in antibody production, evaluation of critical parameters. Biotechnol Adv 26:46–72. https://doi.org/10.1016/j.biotechadv.2007.09.004

Jungbauer A, Hammerschmidt N (2017) Integrated continuous manufacturing of biopharmaceuticals in continuous manufacturing of pharmaceuticals. Wiley VCH, Weinheim

Karlsson I, Gertsson S, Kilany S et al (2021) Phase 1/2a clinical trial of BI-1206, a monoclonal antibody to Fcγriib, in combination with Rituximab in subjects with indolent B-Cell non-Hodgkin lymphoma that has relapsed or is refractory to Rituximab. Blood 138(Supplement 1):1354. https://doi.org/10.1182/blood-2021-147452

Kristiansen B (2006) Process economics. In: Ratledge C, Kristiansen B (eds) Basic biotechnology, 3rd edn. Cambridge University Press, Cambridge, UK, pp 239–252. ISBN: 9780521549585

Luo J, Craver A, Bahl K et al (2022) Etiology of non-Hodgkin lymphoma: a review from epidemiologic studies. J Natl Cancer Center 2:226–234. https://doi.org/10.1016/j.jncc.2022.08.003

Mandenius CF, Björkman M (2011) Biomechatronic design in biotechnology: a methodology for development of biotechnology products. Wiley, Hoboken. https://doi.org/10.1002/9781118067147

Mandenius CF, Brundin A (2008) Bioprocess optimization using design-of-experiments methodology. Biotechnol Prog 24:1191–1203. https://doi.org/10.1002/btpr.67

Martins JRRA, Ning A (2021) Engineering design optimization. Cambridge University Press, Cambridge, UK. https://doi.org/10.1017/9781108980647

Montgomery DC (2020) Design and analysis of experiments, 9th edn. Wiley, New York. ISBN: 978-1-119-63842-1

Nielsen J, Villadsen J, Lidén G (2011) Bioreaction engineering principles, 3rd edn. Springer-Nature, New York

O'Brian D (2019) Engineer 4.0: Life science handbook for medical devices and biopharmaceuticals. Kindle. ISBN-13: 978-1795753340

Patel A, Gujar S, Savita Pohekar S et al (2021) Non-Hodgkin's lymphoma, a case report. J Pharm Res Intern 33(53B):264–267. https://doi.org/10.9734/jpri/2021/v33i53B33705

Peters MS, Timmerhaus KD, West RE (2003) Plant design and economics for chemical engineers, 5th edn. McGraw-Hill & Co, New York

Petrides D (2015) Bioprocess design and economics. In: Harrison RG, Todd P, Rudge SR et al (eds) Bioseparations science and engineering, 2nd edn. Oxford University Press, New York, pp 441–510. https://doi.org/10.1093/oso/9780195391817.001.0001

Plosker GL, Figgitt DP (2022) Rituximab, a review of its use in non-Hodgkin's lymphoma and chronic lymphocytic leukemia. Drugs 63:803–843. https://doi.org/10.2165/00003495-200363080-00005

Pollock J, Coffman J, Ho AV et al (2017) Integrated continuous bioprocessing: Economic, operational, and environmental feasibility for clinical and commercial antibody manufacture. Biotechnol Prog 33:852–866. https://doi.org/10.1002/btpr.2492

Pörtner R (ed) (2021) Cell culture engineering and technology. Springer Nature, New York. https://doi.org/10.1007/978-3-030-79871-0

Sapkota S, Shaikh H (2025) Non-Hodgkin lymphoma. In: StatPearls. StatPearls Publishing, Treasure Island. Available from: https://www.ncbi.nlm.nih.gov/books/NBK559328/

Sims RB, Bartlett NL (2021) Anti-CD30 antibody drug conjugates and their use for the treatment of non-Hodgkin lymphoma. Seagen Inc., US Patent Application PCT 2021/015685

Singh R, Shaik S, Negi BS, Rajguru JP, Patil PB, Parihar AS, Sharma U (2020) Non-Hodgkin's lymphoma: a review. J Family Med Prim Care 9(4):1834–1840. https://doi.org/10.4103/jfmpc.jfmpc_1037_19. PMID: 32670927; PMCID: PMC7346945

Sioshansi R, Conejo AJ (2017) Optimization in engineering, models and algorithms. Springer International Publishing, Berlin. ISBN 9783319567679

Stamatis C, Farid SS (2021) Process economics evaluation of cell-free synthesis for the commercial manufacture of antibody drug conjugates. Biotechnol J 16:2000238. https://doi.org/10.1002/biot.202000238

Towler G, Sinnott R (2012) Chemical engineering design: principles, practice and economics of plant and process design, 2nd edn. Elsevier, Amsterdam

Ulrich KT, Eppinger SD, Wang MC (2019) Product design and development, 7th edn. McGraw-Hill, New York

White CA, Grillo-Lopez A (2010) Treatment of intermediate and high-grade non-Hodgkin's lymphoma with anti-CD20 antibody. Biogen-Idec Inc, European Patent Application EP 2 264 070 A1

Wolin M, Milan S, Hurst D (2003) Methods of therapy for non-Hodgkin's lymphoma. Chiron Inc, Canadian Intellectual Property Office, No 2 469 045

Yazawa N, Hamaguchi Y, Poe JC et al (2005) Immunotherapy using unconjugated CD19 monoclonal antibodies in animal models for B-lymphocyte malignancies and autoimmune disease. Proc Natl Acad Sci 102(42):15178–15183. https://doi.org/10.1073/pnas.0505539102

Zhang Y, Stobbe P, Orrego Silvander C et al (2015) Very high cell density perfusion of CHO cells anchored in anon-woven matrix-based bioreactor. J Biotechnol 213:28–41. https://doi.org/10.1016/j.jbiotec.2015.07.006

Chapter 8
Case 3: Using a Xenograft Zebrafish Model for Evaluation of Oncogenic Drug Candidates

8.1 Assignment: Background, Description, and Objectives

The aim of this assignment is to design a production system for *Drug Technologies*, a biological testing service company. The company utilizes a zebrafish model to evaluate oncogenic drugs on clinical samples provided by customers. Consequently, the commercial product delivered to clients consists of the knowledge and information generated from this testing (Vijaykumar et al. 2011). The assignment focuses on designing a production system specifically for biological information, with the primary training objective of applying design principles tailored to a knowledge product (cf. Sect. 4.3.1).

Drug Technologies provides drug evaluation and prediction studies to advanced customers, including big pharma, hospitals, and medical academic institutes. Typically, these customers send tumor biopsies collected from patients, which the company then tests within its zebrafish model. To conduct these evaluations, the company utilizes its own protected zebrafish xenograft platform and proprietary testing protocols (Patton et al. 2021).

Drug Technologies has been in operation for 5 years. Its primary aim is to establish the company as a reliable provider of a qualified and unique testing service. Investors have provided *Drug Technologies* with startup capital support but expect improved rentability of investments and more business-oriented management. They have 15 employees with medical and cell biology competence. It is located close to a research park and in the vicinity of a medical university.

Drug Technologies has previously developed its testing platform based on the zebrafish tumor xenograft (ZTX) platform for several applications, including the prediction of immune-therapeutic drug candidates (Ruggeri et al. 2014; Kowald et al. 2023; Ali et al. 2022; Wu et al. 2017). The ZTX platform model uses mainly tumor-reactive T-lymphocytes for therapeutic drug treatment of various cancer forms (White et al. 2013).

C.-F. Mandenius, *Bioengineering Design Methodology*,
https://doi.org/10.1007/978-3-032-33940-9_8

Drug Technologies wants to streamline its analytical testing services, which evaluate drug effects on patients for oncogenic clinics and pharmaceutical companies developing new oncogenic drugs using its zebrafish xenograft platform. Supported by its investors, the company has approached an engineering consultancy company with an assignment to improve and streamline its service operations. The main objective is to reduce production costs and turnaround times for the service without compromising the present market position of *Drug Technologies*.

Several criteria and objectives must be met in the design of *Drug Technologies'* analytical service:

- Redesign the ZTX platform by exploiting automation and AI technology to increase testing capacity and reduce operational costs.
- Achieve this ambition through the extensive automation of testing procedures, the integration of robotics, and the deployment of other digital methods throughout the testing workflow.
- Deliver two design alternatives for the testing service based on the ZTX platform. These alternatives must increase *Drug Technologies'* testing capacity from the current 250 tests per year to 2500 tests per year, while allowing for future scalability up to 10,000 tests per year.
- Include the testing of immunotherapeutic drug candidates within the design alternatives, ensuring independence regarding injection procedures, T-lymphocyte sources, yields, and cost structures. The alternatives must also secure a permanent, in-house supply of zebrafish embryos, which require specialized fish culture facilities.
- Adhere to strict financial constraints, accepting a maximum investment of 2 MEUR in new equipment and a maximum increase in annual labor costs of 0.25 MEUR.

Drug Technologies has added a few additional caveats:

- Comply with current certification standards (International Organization for Standardization 2016, 2022) across all proposed designs.
- Accept subcontracting of parts of the testing service, provided that it is proven to be economically feasible.
- Manage intellectual property rights (IPR) under a strict budget, noting that while the company holds or has filed patents for the ZTX-platform, automated redesigns will require new filings; total preparation and filing costs must not exceed 100 kEUR.
- Limit the payback period for all investments in the redesigned testing procedures to a maximum of 5 years.

8.2 Training Scenario for the Assignment

The training scenario is based on the following prerequisites:

- The trainees act as consultants within an established firm hired by *Drug Technologies* (cf. Chap. 4, Fig. 4.3b). Trainees are assumed to be either Master of Engineering students or practicing engineers undergoing continuing professional development. The consultancy firm has access to standard engineering design tools, including software for computer-aided design (CAD), modelling, and system optimization.
- Trainees maintain close contact with relevant expertise from *Drug Technologies,* represented in this scenario by industrial tutorial experts. These experts are prepared to share operational data and discuss the company's current testing service conditions and procedures. Specifically, they will provide the trainees with information regarding (i) the zebrafish model, (ii) analytical protocols, (iii) operational and analytical instrument pricing, and (iv) patents and other intellectual property rights assumed to be controlled by Drug Technologies.
- Progress and final results must be delivered to the *Drug Technologies* management through both oral presentations and written reports. The typical timeframe for this assignment ranges from 3 to 4 months, though this schedule can be compressed if reporting requirements are reduced. All reports must be concise and adhere strictly to typical company standards (see also Sect. 4.4.7).

8.3 A Recommended Design Approach

8.3.1 Structuring the Assignment and Establishing User Requirements

In the description of the assignment, its objectives and the background of *Drug Technologies'* business concept and structure of operation are given (Fig. 8.1). The company has developed the ZTX platform into a methodology for evaluating effects on tumors. The platform allows *Drug Technologies* to provide testing services to pharmaceutical companies, hospitals, and academic research establishments. They must secure a net income to cover their investments in upfront R&D and in production facilities, operational costs, and dividends to investors. This includes all expenditure for their testing service, consumables, provision of zebrafish embryos, instrumentation for testing, facilities labor, and payoff of investments.

Drug Technologies has identified oncogenic drugs as a potentially profitable business opportunity for testing services. They believe that the ZTX platform provides a unique opportunity to detect malignant cells using immunoanalytical screening techniques. For this, the company must ensure quality-assured delivery of testing results to potential customers.

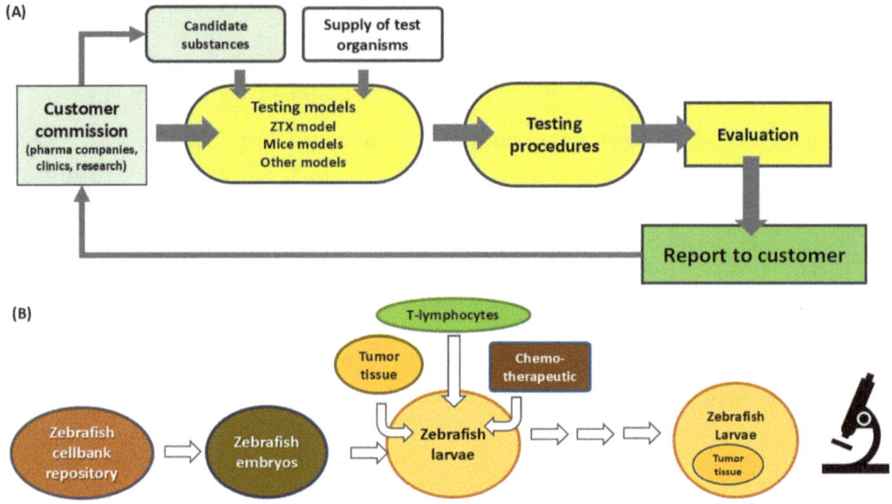

Fig. 8.1 (**a**) The overall structure of the assignment, highlighting key operational conditions, critical parameters, and essential system factors. (**b**) Zebrafish embryonic growth progressing to the larval stage. Cells are exposed to candidate drug substances to observe and monitor their longitudinal effects on metastatic development

Drug Technologies also must correctly assess the size of the market and what a competitive price is for the testing service.

Drug Technologies believes that it is necessary to improve the efficiency of testing and believes automation would be best.

Thus, the focus of the assignment from *Drug Technologies* can be summarized as follows:

- To assess the effect on production costs for the testing by replacing today's hands-on procedures with automated procedures
- To ensure that the redesigned testing service has at least the same quality of performance and meets the customers' expectations
- To perform the scale-up from today's testing service to levels in the assignment objectives without compromising the zebrafish model and its performance to evaluate T-lymphocyte stimulated response from potential potent drug candidates

The ZTX platform makes it possible to design several alternative configurations for a more successful implementation of the testing service. However, functionality and stability are critical aspects in the testing procedure. Thus, several known biological conditions must guide the design work including:

- That 70% of the genome is the same as the human genome, and 80% of the disease-related genes are the same in zebrafish and humans.

- The embryos are transparent, and tumor development or regression can be microscopically observed with fluorescence technique. Small molecules and drug substances can easily be taken up in the embryonic cytoplasm of the zebrafish.
- Transformation is significantly shorter in the zebrafish than in humans.

These advantages together create favorable conditions for drug evaluation studies in terms of precision, time, and costs. It is obvious that these conditions are also critical factors for *Drug Therapeutics'* customers, whether they are pharmaceutical companies developing new drugs, clinicians using drugs for the treatment of patients, or researchers investigating scientific issues.

As in previous design cases, the starting point of the design work is to interrogate the potential users about their requirements on the testing service product (Table 8.1).

Table 8.1 Requirements and specifications with priorities provided in the perspective of Drug Technologies and their customers

Requirement	Target specification	Priority
Customer requirement on the *testing with the ZTX platform*		
Testing of oncogenic drugs on tumors using the ZTX platform shall provide reliable responses in a majority of tested compound	Success rate should be >95%	Very high
The method shall be able to predict responses for additional cancers and chemotherapeutics This is of value for expanding the product platform to other therapeutic applications in cancer therapy by the customer	Within 10 years, the method shall predict urinary cancer and adequate immunotherapeutic drugs for the disease	At present low
Drug Technologies requirements for improving their testing service		
The investment shall be paid back before next product testing. The company must show profitability relatively early given the investors' expectations	Payoff of investment less than 5 years	Very high
The laboratory procedure shall be highly automated, resulting in lower production costs for the testing, mainly due to higher throughput and less labor	Continuous steps shall be carried out by robots	Very high
The method must comply with ISO-13485[a] and ISO-15189[b], as required for in vitro diagnostic products and for clinical laboratory service	All regulatory requirements shall be met	Very high
The method must be used on the global market. The relatively small size of the product requires a global market	European clients shall be the market target	High

[a]International Organization for Standardization (2016)
[b]International Organization for Standardization (2022)

As important is to interview the personnel at *Drug Technologies* about their requirements in the operative testing work.

The requirements on the design are naturally of highest relevance to consider at the early design work. As highlighted in the table, statistical confidence is a very high priority. Also of top priority is the capacity of the testing to show stability, reproducibility and representativity of patient samples.

The fidelity of the zebrafish embryos to develop after transformation under phenotypic conditions is a key issue in the design of the production line.

The pharma customers expect accurate data that can be used to verify other parameters in their drug development, in the preclinical and in the forthcoming clinical phases.

These requirements, with accompanying target metrics, do all connect to the customer's confidence and acceptance of the service product and the price for the product per unit.

8.3.2 *Conceptualization of the Assignment*

Based on the prerequisites of *Drug Technologies'* testing platform, the assignment objectives and the expressed user requirements, a conceptual mapping should be developed (Fig. 8.2). The map should provide a conceptual overview of the transformation process describing the testing and all functions involved in the entire transformation process for delivering test results and drug evaluation (Pahl et al. 2007; Ulrich et al. 2019; Mandenius and Björkman 2011).

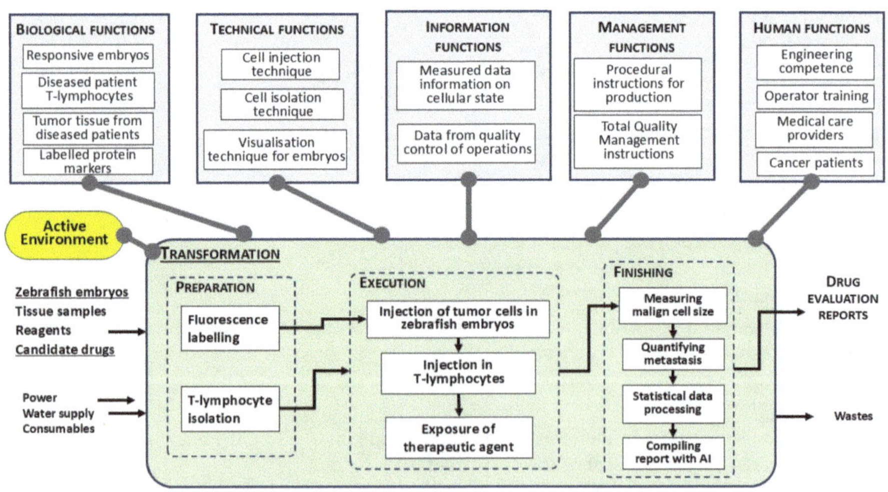

Fig. 8.2 Functional diagram for the procedures at Drug Technologies for testing of drugs and cell samples related to patients on their zebrafish xenograft platform

The transformation process has three phases shown in the map: (i) preparation of zebrafish embryos, lymphocytes, and other testing materials, (ii) exposure of drugs to the prepared embryos and observing effects, and (iii) analyzing and compiling the observed effects and reporting the resulting data and conclusions to the customers.

The procedures in the transformation phases interact with conceptual functions.

The biological functions are the most complex part of the conceptualization, comprising the zebrafish biology, the biology of the tumor, the action of the T-lymphocytes, and biopharmacological actions of the biotherapeutic drug candidates. These biological systems involve subfunctions, such as selective biomarkers for bioanalysis, nutrients for zebrafish, and stimulating factors related to the ZTX platform. These functions and biosystems are interconnected and interplayed with other functions in the operation of the testing service.

The *technical functions* for transforming the biological entities in the testing also have a high degree of complexity because of the biological systems' complexity. The technical functions for culturing the zebrafishes under conditions that favor their proliferation, as well as functions that uphold other conditions for the ZTX model requirements, such as (i) safe containment of the zebrafish culture, (ii) control of the environment of the containment, and (iii) the provision of components required for proliferation. These comprise several technical sub-systems. The functions required for transforming the zebrafish larvae and transferring tumor tissue and T-lymphocytes are integral parts of the functionality of the procedures. The functions of maintaining or preserving tumor tissues and lymphocytes and to collect of provide these are typically separate functions. Special treatment is required prior to the testing procedures. The testing of the assembled biological platform on a technical device over time demands additional technical functional solutions. The bioanalytical techniques for monitoring cells and analyzing biomarkers are several and are also dependent on each other.

The *information functions*, which are the actual delivery of the testing service, have a decisive role in the design. The information functions should (i) deliver the ZTX model result for drug effects on tumors based on observations and analysis of the embryos, (ii) provide the technicians and management of *Drug Technologies* with information on the operative performance of instrumentation used in the testing. This also includes the conditions for the zebrafish culture. Thus, the information comprises a variety of biological and technical data dependent on technical analytical and measurement systems.

The *management functions* include the negotiation of commissions from customers and the presentation of results from the customers' testing orders. The management should guard the intellectual property rights (IPR) of the company and secure additional protection of their technology. The assurance of regulatory and certification demands on the testing service is another important management function.

The *human functions* include (i) the patients for which the drugs are intended, (ii) the developers at the commissioning customers, (iii) the management and technical personnel at *Drug Technologies*, their training and education, and (iv) other collaborative partners involved in the production flow.

There is an *active environment* that the design must consider as well. This could be that (i) new, maybe better, animal models developed by other testing service companies and (ii) new technical methodology and instrumentation are likely to appear. The legislation that regulates drug development and drug products may change. The bioanalytical methods may undergo improvements with better performances. An environmental pressure exerted on the biological system, the embryos, will also change in an unpredictable way. These changing factors in an active environment must be considered in the design for achieving sustainable design solutions.

Given these conditions, several configurations of the testing service can be conceived that comply with the conceptual description and constraints. Four of these configurations are here identified as realistic alternatives (Fig. 8.3). These configurations all comply with the assignment objectives and the prioritized requirements (Table 8.1).

In one of the configurations, the operation of the testing procedures is fully manual, and the supply of zebrafishes is subcontracted (Fig. 8.3a).

In another configuration, automization of some procedures is introduced in the operation of the testing with the potential implication of reducing labor costs and streamlining the flow of testing (Fig. 8.3b).

In a third configuration, the degree of automation is extended to almost all of the procedures that are possible to automize with robots, while the supply of zebrafish embryos is carried out in-house (Fig. 8.3c).

In a fourth configuration, machine learning and AI are applied when it is convenient for interpreting data from imaging and for reporting to customers (Fig. 8.3d).

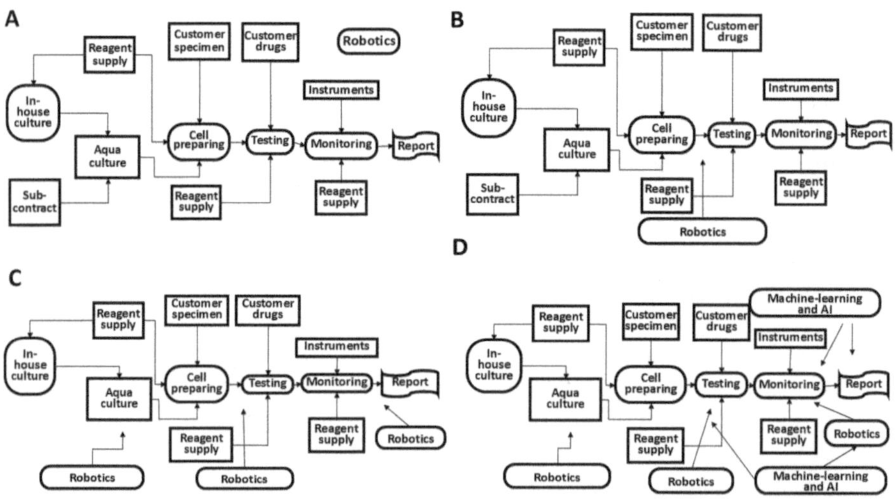

Fig. 8.3 Configurations based on the conceptual analysis. (**a**) Configuration with subcontracting is exploited. (**b**) Configuration where automation with robots is employed to a limited degree. (**c**) Configuration fully automized with robots. (**d**) Configuration utilizing machine learning and artificial intelligence methods in the testing service

8.3.3 Detailed Design of Selected Conceptual Configurations

Two of the conceptual configurations presented in Fig. 8.3 are selected for further detailed design due to their potential to improve testing throughput and ensure the efficient use of labor and other resources. These configurations are considered to fully comply with the assignment objectives and the specified user requirements.

In the first design alternative, which is based on the configuration in Fig. 8.3b, a tenfold upscaling of the testing volume to 2500 tests per year is proposed (Fig. 8.4a). This throughput is achieved by introducing a few strategically placed robotic systems. This configuration leaves operational room for the ongoing development of bioanalytical procedures, such as refining the methodologies for injecting or co-injecting T-lymphocytes, tumors, and candidate drugs. The zebrafish embryos in this design are supplied entirely by in-house aquaculture facilities. Consequently, this design alternative will require capital investment in robotic devices, alongside a focused development effort to adapt current testing methods and technical protocols to automated systems.

In the *second design alternative,* the configuration outlined in Fig. 8.3d is developed. A 40-fold upscaling to 10,000 tests/year is considered (Fig. 8.4b). At this scale, the advantage of automation is assumed to be profound. Therefore, all procedures are automatized by robotic procedures, and machine learning and artificial intelligence (AI) methods are introduced to replace manual operations. This will require substantial investment in robotic equipment and software for ML and AI. It will require substantial development work to adapt all testing procedures to robotic routines. Development of software for AI applications adapted to the procedures for data analysis and reporting to customers. The zebrafish embryos are supplied in this alternative by an external partner by subcontracting. It is considered to be a demanding activity to supply that number of embryos in-house, and the efficiency of supply is worth the costs for subcontracting. The second alternative will allow better time scheduling and use of personnel. The throughput in the second alternative (10,000 tests per year) automation is even more advantageous and will benefit day-and-night operation, less staff for surveillance per test, less spill-offs, and better reproducibility.

Today's testing with a throughput capacity of 250 tests per year is detailed to allow comparison with the new design alternatives (Fig. 8.4c). The operation of the testing is shown with in-house supply of zebrafish embryos.

For the detailed design work, commercial digital design tools can be useful, even if supplied with generic computational units. The software can facilitate the sizing of equipment and consumables based on assumed production volume.

Although the flow diagrams do not include all units and procedures, the designs will suffice to allow the evaluation of economic differences between design alternatives. It will tell the investors about potential and opportunity as well as further investment requirements.

The two new designs are not infringing on any previous intellectual property rights (IPR). Only a few IPR exist in the patent literature that need consideration (de Figueiredo et al. 2022; De Willians and Woon 2014; Wang and Guo 2021). Thus, the objective in the assignment for IPR of a new design is met.

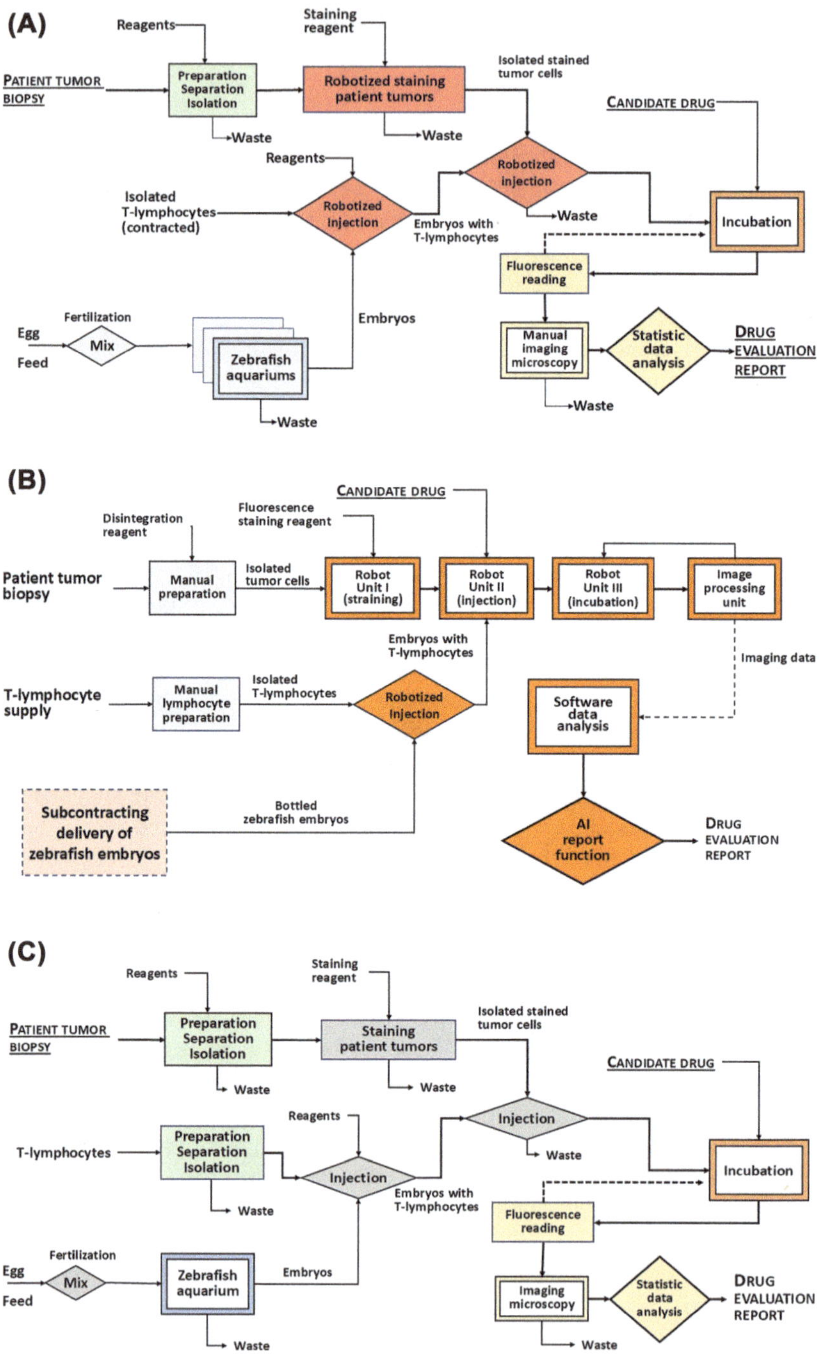

Fig. 8.4 Detailed designs of conceptual configurations that are considered for the testing production. (**a**) A scaled-up and partly automized testing production for 2500 tests/year (robots in red). (**b**) A fully robotized and AI-supported production for 10,000 tests/year (robots in red). (**c**) Today's testing production at Drug Technologies with testing of 250 tests/year

8.3.4 Evaluation of Economics of the Testing Service

In the economic evaluation, it is of interest to investigate how capital investment and operational costs are influenced when scaling up the annual volume of tests. Two questions are of particular interest to evaluate:

- To what level must the annual number of ordered tests be increased to compensate for significant investments in robotics and digitalization?
- What price must Drug Technologies charge its customers to pay back the investments under the assumed conditions?

The investment and operational costs for the two robotized and upscaled alternatives (tenfold and 40-fold upscaling) are compared with today's testing baseline using established economic evaluation methods (Kristiansen 2006; Peters et al. 2003; Ray et al. 2022).

The investments are distinguished into upfront R&D investments, equipment, and other investments for implementation of the robotized testing (Table 8.2). In the upfront R&D costs are included development of procedures required for automation of testing procedures, use of machine learning (ML) and artificial intelligence (AI) for imaging and data analysis and reporting to customers, and costs associated with filing of new IPR (e.g., patent applications). In equipment investments are included costs for purchase of robots and instruments for preparation and analysis of embryos. In other investment costs are included costs for installation of new equipment, and costs for building and certification of the testing facilities.

The operational costs are distinguished into consumables for the testing, supply of embryos either by in-house production or by purchase from subcontractors, labor costs, annual fees for IPRs, public fees, and renting costs for the building.

The consumable costs are comparatively low in relation to investments and personnel costs. Of course, a scaled-up production consumes more consumables, but these costs are quite low compared to the other costs.

The total estimated production cost is within the targeted values for both alternatives. The critical trade-off is to decide about further expensive investments in robotics, digital methods, and higher labor costs for less automated testing work or higher labor costs for technicians. Automation may have some effect on costs for consumables but marginally. Investments are long-term and fixed, while staff costs are more flexible (Table 8.2).

The circle diagrams illuminate how the cost structure is shifted from today's test capacity to a tenfold or 40-fold scale-up (Fig. 8.5). The proportion of costs seems to convincingly support the introduction of robots due to a lower unit cost. It is seen in the diagrams that the scale-up of robotics requires more investment. The win is lower for labor costs. Thus, mainly costly larger production volumes favor costly investments. However, a few caveats should be mentioned:

- Investments in equipment are a long-term risk-taking. Here, a 5-year payoff time is assumed. Thus, the larger production must remain over at least this period. If not, economic loss can be considerable. Investors are aware of that risk.

Table 8.2 Evaluation of production costs for today and scaled-up robotized testing

Type of costs	Today's testing (kEUR)	Tenfold scaled-up robotized testing (kEUR)	40-fold scaled-up robotized testing (kEUR)
Investment costs			
Upfront testing R&D			
Testing development	300	300	1100
IPR filing	–	100	100
Total upfront testing R&D	*300*	*400*	*1200*
Equipment and instrumentation			
Standard laboratory equipment	70	140	200
Advanced robotics	–	300	800
Fluorescence microscopes	50	50	100
Cryopreservation/ freezers units	40	70	200
Micromanipulators	20	20	40
Software (incl. AI)	20	20	60
Total equipment and instrumentation	*200*	*600*	*1400*
Additional expenditures for testing			
Installation of equipment (×0.5)	90	300	700
Project planning (×0.3)	60	180	420
Taxation (×0.1)	20	60	140
Buildings (×0.3)	60	180	420
Total additional expenditure for testing	*230*	*1120*	*1680*
Total investment costs	*730*	*2120*	*4280*
Operational costs (testing/year)			
Consumables for testing service			
Consumables for laboratory work	30	300	1200
Consumables for quality control	10	100	400
Salaries in production	700	400	200
Customer reporting	100	100	100
Total consumables and laboratory work	*840*	*900*	*1900*

(continued)

Table 8.2 (continued)

Type of costs	Today's testing (kEUR)	Tenfold scaled-up robotized testing (kEUR)	40-fold scaled-up robotized testing (kEUR)
Additional operational expenditures:			
Zebrafish supply (subcontracted)	10	30	60
External maintenance of equipment	20	20	20
Renting of buildings	80	100	150
Taxation	50	50	50
Annual IPR expenditures and licenses	10	10	10
Management	100	100	100
Total additional operational expenditures	*270*	*310*	*390*
Total operational costs	*1110*	*1210*	*2290*
Annual payoff (5 years)	*146*	*424*	*716*
Total annual production cost	**1256**	**1634**	**3006**
Production cost per testing (EUR)	*5.02*	*0.65*	*0.30*

- Salary costs seem to be possible to reduce by increasing automation. The caveat is here that robotics requires specially trained technicians. This will increase costs. Qualified staff is attractive for employment by competitors. A confidentiality agreement can reduce risk for knowledge transfer.
- Competitors will certainly show up. IPR gives time-limited protection. High technology is a sales argument, but IPR tends to give away too much intrinsic know-how.
- *Drug Technologies* needs to have a next commercial step in mind, either new testing methods, disease targets, or therapy forms. A wise automation strategy should therefore have flexibility for the next step to reduce start-up time and costs.

In the economic assessment, a 5-year payoff time is assumed. This can be shortened or prolonged, thereby changing the margin for net income. Automation will allow a lower price given an increase in testing orders can be made. A 10-year payoff will allow for a further price reduction.

The production economics can potentially be further improved by optimization of media, productivity, and yields in the testing steps, with direct consequence on the size of the testing procedures. At this stage of production, however, it is realistic to assume that such effort may be in the order of not more than 10 to 30%. At this stage, it is not directly possible to see if optimization favors one design more than another.

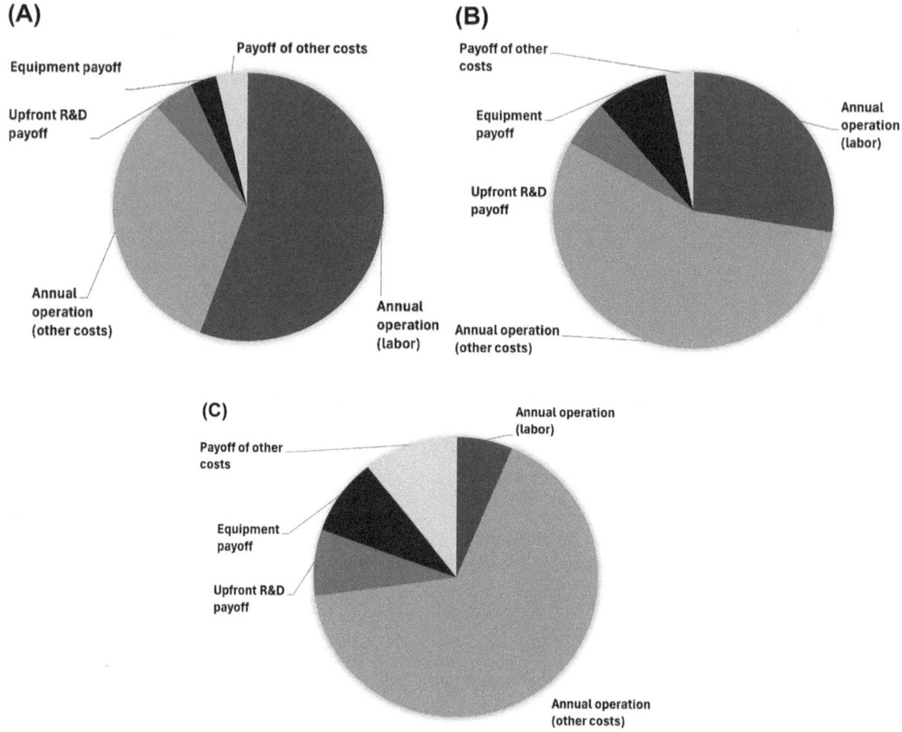

Fig. 8.5 Distribution of costs for the testing service. (**a**) At today's level of testing with 250 tests/year. (**b**) Scaled-up with robotic testing to 2500 tests/year. (**c**) Scaled-up with robotized testing and digital evaluation to 10,000 tests/year. The payoff time is 5 years

8.3.5 Optimization of the Design of the Testing Service

This assignment offers various actionable opportunities for trainees to systematically optimize both turnaround times and operational costs within the biological testing service framework (Sioshansi and Conejo 2017; Martins and Ning 2021). Because the company's final deliverable is inherently service-based, maintaining strict data quality and testing accuracy remains a critical, non-negotiable optimization constraint throughout the process. Applying established engineering and operational optimization techniques to each individual step will have a cumulative impact across the entire testing value chain, particularly regarding bottleneck elimination, workforce scheduling, and labor efficiency. Several specialized modelling techniques and analytical approaches should be actively considered by the trainees (Table 8.3); however, because executing these comprehensive methods can be exceptionally time-consuming, they must be carefully prioritized in direct alignment with the assignment's core objectives and financial boundaries.

Table 8.3 Objects for optimization of the testing service that can be enhanced by various techniques

Object for optimization	Intended outcome	Potential optimization technique
The zebrafish culturing time	Short delivery time for zebrafish larvae, less culture media and labor cost	Factorial design of experimentally available parameters and culture media components
Shortening time and improving accuracy for imaging evaluation	Shorter delivery time to customers with better accuracy	Factorial design using different software and sampling parameters
Reducing consumption of consumables	Optimizing consumption in operational steps	Factorial design of critical parameters
Reducing runtime in robotized units	Better adaptation of operational steps to robotized procedures	Factorial design
Reducing lags in production	Shorter total production time, higher throughput and productivity	Mechanistic modelling and factorial design, scheduling techniques in CAD software

Design of Experiments for Optimizing the Testing Service The testing service line of testing procedures can most probably be improved by optimizing many of the conditions in the procedural steps from the preparation of embryos, analytical procedures in analyzing the responses during exposures of drug candidates, or in the interpretation of imaging data (Montgomery 2013; Mandenius and Brundin 2008). A collection of potentially relevant parameters to optimize by DoE can easily be identified (Table 8.4). The table focuses on parameters that can be optimized by applying reduced factor experiments in design of experiments (see Chap. 3 and other cases in Chap. 5). The factorial parameters are, as recommended, investigated by screening at two or three levels. Some are subsequently selected for further optimization.

Also, other statistical optimization methods related to reporting results, imaging, comparison between robot procedures, and use of personnel time may be of interest to investigate with DoE and relate to critical costs, as evident in the table of investment and operational costs.

Optimization of the Testing Service by Mechanistic Modelling Using mechanistic modelling in this design case is different from other presented cases, but still has the objective to improve testing procedures, leading to better performance in service and economy. To turn this into models could be to study the impact of changes on productivity. Here, this can be related to:

- Production cost per testing order (e.g., assay number; time per assay; instrumental occupation of instrumentation)
- Performing testing by robotic procedure or labor-demanding manual procedures

Example of parameters that are of particular interest to model in relation to the objectives of the design assignment could be the following:

Table 8.4 Objects for optimization by design of experiments in zebrafish xenograft model

Object for optimization	Factors in DoE plan	Responses to measure
Culturing conditions for producing the zebrafish	Composition of culture media with additives. Physical culturing parameters in aquarium tanks. Procedures for recovering the zebrafish	Cell density and yields. Rate of growth. Quality properties of the grown organism
Performance of the testing procedures	Time instances and periods of applying test substances, and T cell. Amount of substance	Visual observation of cell morphology and size. Assays of characteristic biomarkers
Performance of assay procedures used in the testing	Assay procedure parameters expected to influence the analytical performance	Verified sensitivity, limit of detection, and reproducibility
Quality and precision of the predictions of the testing	Factors that affect predictions may include number of tests, materials, size of assays, diversification of test materials in terms of T cells and tested substances	Statistics of observed responses of cells and tumor development in assays

Number of tests, average production cost per order, average income per order, use of investments per test, time per test, and average labor cost. These parameters are of interest to investigate due to their influence on efficiency and cost between the design alternatives.

Assuming that the operation costs for testing are reduced with higher quantities of tests due to lower cost of consumables per test and other auxiliary costs that are not influenced by quantity. Thus, linear relationships are not expected. Instead, there is a stepwise gradual decrease of cost/test. In the model, this can be shown by cost factors.

A simple way to model this is to use differential equations:

$$d(\text{cost})/d(\text{tests}) = (\text{labor}) \cdot (\text{tests}) + (\text{consumables}) \cdot (\text{tests}) + (\text{robots}) + (\text{equipment}) + (\text{overhead}) \tag{8.1}$$

where *cost* is the total production cost of tests; *tests,* the number of tests carried out; *consumables* the cost of consumables per test; *robots*, the cost for installation of robots; *equipment*, the cost for other equipment used in the testing independent of number of tests carried out; and *overhead*, other costs associated with the testing that are independent of testing volume, such as facilities and management.

If assuming an inverse relation between robotic capacity and labor needs, the Eq. (8.1) can be extended to:

$$d(\text{cost})/d(\text{test}) = (\text{labor}/n) \cdot (\text{tests}) + (\text{consumables}) \cdot (\text{tests}) + (\text{robots} \cdot n) + (\text{equipment}) + (\text{overhead}) \tag{8.2}$$

where n is the number of robotic functions, either parallel or other robotic capacity measure.

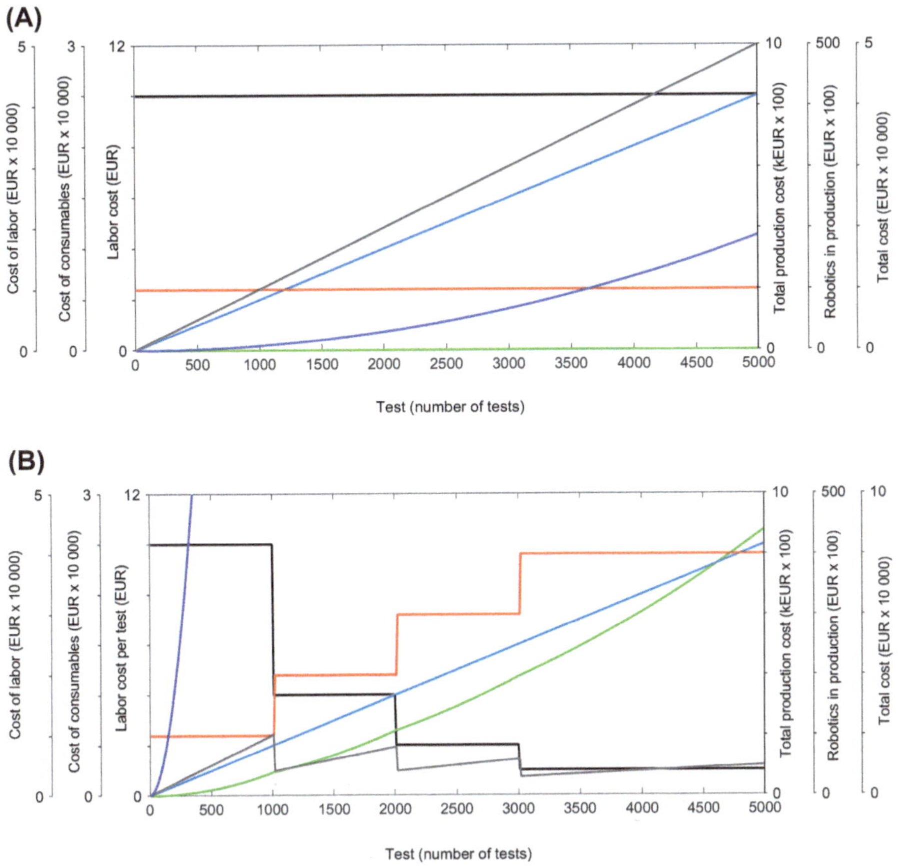

Fig. 8.6 (**a**) The effect of increasing the number of tests on labor cost and robotic cost, price setting per order, and net income. (**a**) At constant degree of automation and labor expenditure. (**b**) At increasing automation with saving of labor

These equations can be used to simulate the changing costs with the volume of tests performed. The changing cost with volume at costs/test is constrained to cost reduction results in a favorable total cost with increasing number of tests (Fig. 8.6a). The simulation is carried out in steps where there is a cost reduction for larger quantities of consumables while labor is unaffected. It is also assumed that the labor cost goes down with test volumes.

The changing cost with testing capacity at higher implementation of robotics, while labor per test is reduced, can also be simulated (Fig. 8.6b). Here, the implementation of robotic functions can involve image processing and other functionalities that offload labor but at a high investment in automation.

8.3.6 SWOT Analysis for the Scaled-Up Testing Alternatives

A SWOT analysis is especially appropriate and highly valuable to carry out for this specific kind of engineering design mission (Shinno et al. 2006). Strategic decisions regarding the ultimate choice between competing production system configurations are often less quantitative and instead more heavily reliant on evaluating qualitative pros and cons related directly to the initial operational requirements of the testing service.

The SWOT analysis should be carefully focused on systematically comparing the tenfold and 40-fold scaled-up production alternatives (Table 8.5), placing a strong emphasis on those critical issues that at this stage seem most relevant to consider for their direct impact on company economics and their long-term importance for product marketing.

Furthermore, other strategic subjects for the SWOT analysis can and should be actively considered by the trainees, such as factors related to the long-term flexibility of producing highly specialized testing services, the ease of access to qualified human resources for future employment, and potential organizational risks.

Table 8.5 A SWOT analysis comparing the upscaled production alternatives

Critical aspects	Scale-up of testing × 10	Scale-up of testing × 40
Reproducibility of testing results	*Strength*: Robotic procedures enhance reproducibility *Weakness*: Surveillance by technicians lower *Opportunity*: Technology ascents	*Strength*: Robotic procedures enhance reproducibility *Weakness*: Surveillance by technicians lower *Opportunity*: Technology ascents
Scalability of testing	*Strength*: Excellent *Weakness*: Equipment cost high *Opportunity*: Market not yet saturated	*Strength*: Excellent *Weakness*: Higher equipment cost *Opportunity*: Market not yet saturated
Sensitivity of tests	*Strength*: Better control by automation *Weakness*: Cells sensitive *Opportunity*: Better technology *Threats*: Regulatory demands Technological challenges	*Strength*: Better control by automation *Weakness*: Cells sensitive *Opportunity*: Better technology *Threats*: Regulatory demands Technological challenges
IPR situation for the testing technique	*Strength:* Methods are protected for at least 20 years *Threats:* Competitors IPRs	*Strength:* Methods are protected for at least 20 years *Threats:* Competitors IPRs
Environmental footprints	*Strength:* Insignificant for a small production *Threats:* New legislative rules	*Strength:* Insignificant for a small production *Threats:* New legislative rules
Economics of testing	*Strength:* Expensive *Weakness:* Access to spare parts *Opportunity:* Flexibility to production volume. Can be adapted to other cells.	*Strength:* More expensive *Weakness:* Access to spare parts *Opportunity:* Flexibility to production volume. Can be adapted to other cells

8.4 Conclusive Suggestions for *Drug Technologies*

Based on the discussion above, *Drug Technologies* is suggested to develop their testing service based on the zebrafish model by:

- Robotizing the procedural steps and methods to save labor, use operational time better, and scale up the service capacity. The robots should be controlled by regulatory-approved functions.
- Utilizing pattern recognition should be used to replace evaluations by technicians for image analysis.
- Utilizing digital techniques to speed up reporting routines to customers.
- Carrying out extensive training in applying new techniques. This will include operation of robots, pattern recognition for microscopic imaging of cell structures, and use of AI-supported reporting formats.

The preliminary economic assessment shows that a scale-up from 150 to 1500 tests per year (tenfold) reduces the effect of investment and operational costs. The cost per commission decreases linearly with the number of commissions. The chosen method seems to be independent of whether drained glands or tumor T-lymphocytes are used.

The use of statistical optimization techniques has the potential to lower the costs for *Drug Technologies*. This may also improve both quality and time for analysis.

Typically, in service-related production, labor costs dominate. Here, these costs are decreased at the price of investments in automation and robotics. This will result in a longer payback time and initially a higher price for service. This is partly a business decision.

- Risk assessment of suggested streamlining of the service production by robots and digitalization shows dependency on too many suppliers of equipment and instrumentation with service agreements for exclusive and sensitive technical systems. Replacements must be at hand on short notice, not to risk delivery to customers. Software companies have occasionally a short lifespan. *Drug Technologies* should therefore consider building up the software and programming competence in-house.
- Another severe risk factor is that the zebrafish model may fail or require more test samples to provide reliable statistical assurance.
- Another risk is the competition situation. The ZTX platform may be challenged by newer and more precise models. A further development of methods and techniques is a wise strategy and does not expect today's methodology to survive more than a 5–10-year period.

A strength in *Drug Technologies* service production is the generality of the zebrafish platform. It is applicable to other disease model systems after some adaptations. This may include adjustments of stepwise procedures, sample volumes in robotized assays, and the ease of reprogramming robotic and instrumental software.

8.5 Tutorial Perspectives on the Assignment

The core of the training in this assignment is about the design of an exclusive testing service in a small company, *Drug Technologies*, with unique competence. The company exploits a zebrafish model's likeness with the human genome to support the development and use of oncogenic drugs. The focus for the trainees is to analyze how this testing service can be carried out more efficiently and result in better business conditions.

Several challenges in the assignment require the tutors' attention:

- *Drug Technologies has* a unique competence in using zebrafish embryos for investigating pharmacological effects of cancer therapeutics. This is for most trainees a new kind of bioproduct production they are not accustomed to. This requires guidance from the tutors.
- Still, the same approach for analyzing design is applicable for service production, where knowledge and information are the actual products. This will initially be confusing for the trainees. To understand, this is facilitated by using conceptual mapping and applying the functionality concept. Probably this needs to be pedagogically explained to ensure a good start to the scenario.
- It is important to understand how the responsibility is shared between the pharma company and *Drug Technologies*. The trainees should not be misled into trying to solve the pharmacology issue. The industrial experts should be helpful in explaining this.
- One of the main challenges is to configure and dimension the operational testing cost per drug, throughput test time, and confidence in the result, as well as patient status.
- These parameters are demanding to rank. The first challenge is to overview the parameters and grasp what factors are most influential. The trainees should be encouraged to focus on these and carefully list the parameters, their characteristics, and criticalities for the outcome. The trainees should realize that this might need the collection of information from several sources and expertise.
- A challenge for the trainees is to establish a cost structure and connect this structure to configuration alternatives, where the cost distribution is different than in a biopharmaceutical process and shows different sensitivities.

For these challenges, the trainees occasionally need much active support from the industrial expert tutors in (i) how to apply divergent thinking, (ii) ensuring the design work is not confounded into details of procedure or optimization of production but held at a structured level, and (iii) ensuring the concept of the knowledge service.

References

Ali Z, Vildevall M, Rodriguez GV et al (2022) Zebrafish patient-derived xenograft models predict lymph node involvement and treatment outcome in non-small cell lung cancer. J Exp Clin Cancer Res 41:58. https://doi.org/10.1186/s13046-022-02280-x

Alvares Cabral de Figueiredo, Cabral de Figueiredo, RL, Barroso Povoa VC (2022) Methods for analyzing tumor innate immune interactions using the zebrafish xenograft model as a living biomarker. US2022265866 (A1)

De Willians DE, Woon DJ (2014) Methods for anti-cancer drug screening using zebrafish human tumor xenograft model. KR20140131754 (A)

International Organization for Standardization (2016) Medical devices. Quality management systems. Requirements for regulatory purposes. ISO 13485:2016. International Organization for Standardization

International Organization for Standardization (2022) Medical laboratories. Requirements for quality and competence. ISO 15189:2022. International Organization for Standardization

Kowald S, Huge Y, Tandiono D et al (2023) Novel zebrafish patient-derived tumor xenograft methodology for evaluating efficacy of Immune-stimulating BCG therapy in urinary bladder cancer. Cells 12:508. https://doi.org/10.3390/cells12030508

Kristiansen B (2006) Process economics. In: Ratledge C, Kristiansen B (eds) Basic Biotechnology, 3rd edn. Cambridge University Press, Cambridge, UK, pp 239–252

Mandenius CF, Björkman M (2011) Biomechatronic design in biotechnology: a methodology for development of biotechnology products. Wiley, Hoboken. https://doi.org/10.1002/9781118067147

Mandenius CF, Brundin A (2008) Bioprocess optimization using design-of-experiments methodology. Biotechnol Prog 24:1191–1203. https://doi.org/10.1002/biot.201100463

Martins JRRA, Ning A (2021) Engineering design optimization. Cambridge University Press, Cambridge, UK. https://doi.org/10.1017/9781108980647

Montgomery DC (2013) Design and analysis of experiments, 8th edn. Wiley, New York

Pahl G, Beitz W, Feldhusen J et al (2007) Engineering design, a systematic approach, 3rd edn. Springer Verlag, Berlin

Patton E, Zon LI, Laneuau DM (2021) Zebrafish disease models in drug discovery, from preclinical modelling to clinical trials. Nat Rev Drug Discov 20:611–628. https://doi.org/10.1038/s41573-021-00210-8

Peters MS, Timmerhaus KD, West RE (2003) Plant design and economics for chemical engineers, 5th edn. McGraw-Hill, New York

Ray SC, Chambers RG, Kumbhakar SC (2022) Handbook of production economics. Springer Nature, New York

Ruggeri BA, Camp F, Miknyoczki S (2014) Animal models of disease: pre-clinical animal models of cancer and their applications and utility in drug discovery. Biochem Pharmacol 87:150–161. https://doi.org/10.1016/j.bcp.2013.06.020

Shinno H, Yoshioka H, Marpaung S et al (2006) Quantitative SWOT analysis on global competitiveness of machine tool industry. J Eng Des 17(3):251–258. https://doi.org/10.1080/09544820500275180

Sioshansi R, Conejo AJ (2017) Optimization in engineering, models and algorithms. Springer International Publishing, Berlin. ISBN 9783319567679

Ulrich KT, Eppinger SD, Wang MC (2019) Product design and development, 7th edn. McGraw-Hill, New York

Vijaykumar G, Vasantha GVA, Roy R et al (2011) A review of product–service systems design methodologies. J Eng Des 23(9):635–659. https://doi.org/10.1080/09544828.2011.639712

Wang M, Guo H (2021) Cancer cell xenograft zebrafish model and construction method and application thereof. CN113767879 (A)

White R, Rose K, Zon L (2013) Zebrafish cancer: the state of the art and the path forward. Nat Rev Cancer 13:624. https://doi.org/10.1038/nrc3589

Wu JQ, Zhai J, Li CY et al (2017) Patient-derived xenograft in zebrafish embryos: a new platform for translational research in gastric cancer. J Exp Clin Cancer Res 36:160. https://doi.org/10.1186/s13046-017-0631-0

Chapter 9
Case 4: Microfluidic Chip for Pharmacological Studies of Organotypic Teeth and Liver Cells

9.1 Assignment: Background, Description, and Objectives

The aim of the training in this assignment is to develop the production of a novel microphysiological chip for advanced pharmacological studies (Volponi et al. 2010; Maschmeyer et al. 2015; Marx et al. 2019).

The assigner is a small biotechnology company, *Biochip Engineering*, which is well-established in developing and marketing microphysiological devices. The company operates excellent research and production facilities located within an industrial park environment close to an international research university. They employ a staff of 40 highly qualified researchers, technical specialists, and a market-oriented management team. The company has historically been successful with its previous generations of organotypic microphysiological products.

The core technology exploited by *Biochip Engineering* is based on perfectly controlled microfluidic circuitries embedded within multichamber chips (Wagner et al. 2013; Sanka et al. 2019; Gao et al. 2022). The required organotypic cells are carefully grafted into these microfluidic chambers before the final devices are delivered to customers, who typically represent the R&D departments of pharmaceutical companies devoted to oral medicines. *Biochip Engineering's* production lines operate in strict compliance with Good Manufacturing Practice (GMP) and Clinical Laboratory Practice (CLP), ensuring highly reliable safety, stability, and cost conditions that allow the products to be presented to the market at a highly competitive price.

Biochip Engineering has decided to expand its portfolio of multi-organ chip products with a combined chip for the study of tooth cells and liver cells. The company intends to market this chip directly to researchers and drug-developing companies. Recently, they have established cell culture protocols for tooth pulpal cells on various supports, and they have previously developed similar protocols for liver cells.

C.-F. Mandenius, *Bioengineering Design Methodology*,
https://doi.org/10.1007/978-3-032-33940-9_9

Biochip Engineering has therefore now assigned its development research group to design an efficient production process for their new microphysiological product. The following objectives must be met in the design:

- Develop two alternative designs for the production of the organotypic tooth and liver microphysiological chip within the company's own manufacturing facilities.
- Establish a competitive design based on robotized production to ensure low labor costs per produced unit. Concurrently, ensure that the total volume of the manufacturing plant is minimized, leading to lower upfront investment costs and a low environmental burden.
- Ensure operational efficiency by verifying (i) that the number of operational units and steps in the plant remains low and comparable to similar products on the market, (ii) that the lowest possible consumption of construction units and raw materials is maintained across all steps of production, and (iii) that a short production time is achieved for this complex manufacturing process.
- Dimension the design for a projected sales volume of 5,000 chips per year for various customers. Designers should assume that these customers are predominantly pharmaceutical companies in the start-up phase of developing a new drug candidate, though the design must accommodate both smaller biotech firms and large pharmaceutical corporations.

Three caveats are added by *Biochip Engineering* to the assignment:

- Integrate the external monitoring instrument, which monitors and controls the flows within the microphysiological chips. This instrument is manufactured and provided by a subcontractor with a 3-week delivery lead time at an internal price of 150,000 EUR per master device. The instrument is pre-equipped with sensors for oxygen, temperature, and pH, alongside flow rate controls. The design of this instrument will be handled by Biochip Engineering separately and is not a part of this assignment; however, the subcontractor requires exact specifications for the chip size.
- Secure necessary regulatory compliance, ensuring that both the final product and the chosen production methods are fully approved and certified by relevant international organizations and regulatory bodies.
- Evaluate the intellectual property rights (IPR) landscape as part of the production system design.

In addition, *Biochip Engineering's* upfront costs for research and development (R&D) for the new design, licensing fees for utilizing external IPR in manufacturing, and the internal cost of goods and services (COGS) for plant production—such as growth media, specialized labor, and facility housing—must be factored into the final analysis. The existing production process baseline is described in internal documents provided by *Biochip Engineering*.

9.2 Training Scenario for the Assignment

For design training of students or other trainees, a scenario should preferably be based on the following prerequisites:

- The trainees are assumed to be a product development team within *Biochip Engineering's* own R&D organization. The trainee team has five to six members with backgrounds in mechanical engineering, measurement technology, biochemical engineering, electrical engineering, and computer programming. They should be familiar with bioanalytical methods using enzymes and antibodies. If not, experts in training management should support the trainees with advice.
- The trainees access all in-house information and documentation about cost issues, marketing conditions, upfront costs, and internal purchase agreements. Cell line specifications are to some extent known but need verification and assessments, especially for alternatives. They have access to laboratory documentations from *Biochip Engineering* for testing culturing induced pluripotent stem cells (iPSC) and other tissue cells. The assignees have access to software for computer-aided design (CAD) adapted to bioprocessing, 3D printing, and manufacturing. They also have access to simulation and modelling tools for design and calculations, as well as software for design of experiments (DoE) and process economic calculations (see also Sect. 4.4.4).
- The trainees are in close contact with expertise from *Biochip Engineering* and can request information from other companies to a limited extent. Drawings of the present process are available showing volumetric capacities and preliminary cost estimations for slightly modified production routines.
- The trainees have access to *Biochip Engineering's* intellectual property rights (IPR) portfolio for the design of microchips. They can also obtain limited specifications from subcontracting agreements for assessment of the subcontracting costs. For procurement of cell materials, for example, liver cells and tooth cell materials, suggestion of purchase costs related to annual quantities is provided. The R&D unit has several test benches for investigating prototypes and performing analytical experimentation of plasma samples.
- The R&D unit of *Biochip Engineering* has previously collaborated with subcontractors for sensor device fabrication and small-scale manufacturing, and experienced expertise is available for the trainees through tutorial experts.
- The trainees should report to *Biochip Engineering* with progress and final reports. The results should be delivered orally and in written form. The typical time frame for the assignment is in the range of 3–4 months. This can be shortened if lower demand for reporting is expected. Deliverables should be concise and follow typical company standards (see also Sect. 4.4.7).

9.3 A Recommended Design Approach

9.3.1 Structuring the Assignment and User Requirements

From the description of the assignment and background of *Biochip Engineering,* the general conditions of the assignment can be structured (Fig. 9.1). Several upfront subcontracting is assumed where preconditions are settled.

Attention should be given to those parts applicable to stem cell derivation and fabrication of microfluidic devices, and a collection of design alternatives complying with the assigner's requirements should be identified. The original idea of the product is partly published (Marx et al. 2016, 2021; Wagner et al. 2013) (Fig. 9.1). The alternatives should be prioritized according to these and after conceptual functional analysis.

The following design challenges for performing the assignment need to be focused on the following:

- To ensure a low-cost production of cells for testing and physiology study
- To ascertain delivery of hardware instrumentation to customers for control of microfluidic systems from external suppliers
- To assemble the microfluidic platform according to the customers' requirements
- To assess and compare the economic outcomes of configurations and compare these with *Biochip Engineering's* demands of production volumes, production costs, and net income
- To ensure that the designs comply with regulatory requirements
- To carry out a risk analysis for the product and competition strength from a longer perspective

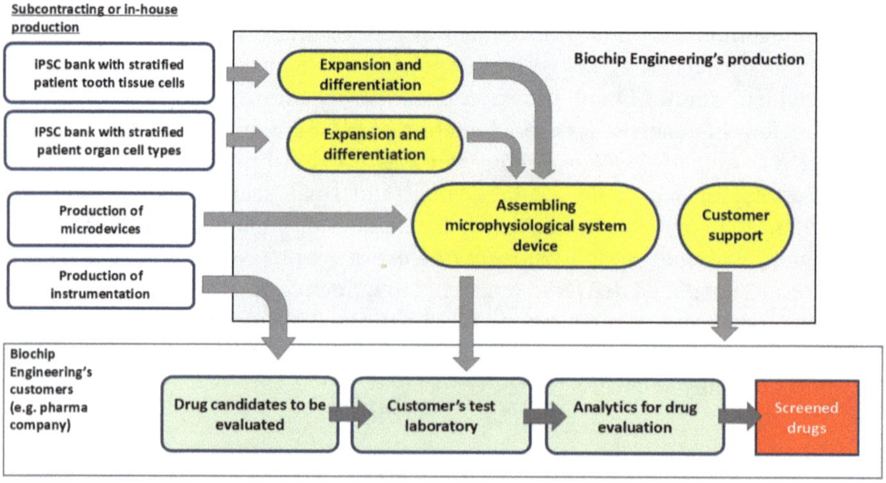

Fig. 9.1 The overall structure of the assignment in relation to Biochip Engineering development of microphysiological systems (white) and production (yellow) to customers (green/red)

The requirements should be seen from viewpoints about the critical parameters and their metrics for product stability and longevity, expected consumption of chips and supply, volumetric conditions, purity needs, market volume, and estimated size of the production plant. Two configuration alternatives that should be considered for reaching the target values need to be considered. These alternatives can then be configured with suitable equipment units.

Different stem cell systems could be compared in relation to biological parameters, accessibility of cell systems, requirements and criteria for R&D efforts, and auxiliary facilities for quality control (QC). Different chip fabrication and assembling methods are compared in relation to coping with the derived stem cell components' biological parameters, accessibility of raw materials, requirements and criteria for processing R&D efforts, and auxiliary facilities for control and QC.

The cost of the configurations is based on standard cost estimates for consumables and needed investments known to the purchase and procurement department of the company and used in the company. The risk of fault in cost assessments is to be considered, as well as its potential impact on total costs. The conceptual mapping provides great help in covering the diversity of these costs. Especially time and personnel needs are to be carefully examined for the alternatives.

A thoughtful strengths-weaknesses-opportunities-threats (SWOT) analysis to increase the precision of the ranking order is recommended. The two top-ranked alternatives could then be further studied, and the estimated costs refined.

The first action to be taken is to analyze the requirements expressed in the assignment. This could be done by discussing eye-to-eye with the assigners from the company, primarily to repeat and confirm the goals and constraints of the assignment and transform this where possible to metrics or other defined specifications. It is recommended to distinguish between the company's requirements and metrics and the potential customers' needs. *Biochip Engineering's* economy and production people could easily quantify their requirements in terms of economic figures such as production costs and investments, quality criteria, product shelf-life, and market price conditions. These are all possible to either express desirable values or even critical values for reaching criteria for profitability or affordability of product dissemination. Also, legal aspects could easily be mentioned and more precisely defined.

The needs in a pharmaceutical R&D unit are well known for pharma companies, where many are general, such as efficacy and safety of drugs. Experienced medical experts or pharmacologists should be interrogated and targeted.

Some of these requirements and needs coincide with company production conditions and customer expectations.

Prioritized requirements are expressed by *Biochip Engineering* and their users (Table 9.1). The tables also provide target metrics for each requirement and a first assessment of priorities on four levels.

Those needs that the design must fulfill are, of course, of the highest relevance to identifying at this early stage. These need to be verified with the assigner through dialog.

Table 9.1 Requirements and target specifications with priorities from the perspective of Biochip Engineering's production and customers

Requirement	Target specification	Priority
Customer requirements (e.g., pharmaceutical companies)		
Precision and reliability of using the microphysiological chip with different cell types should be very high and in compliance with regulatory agencies' expectations	< 5% accuracy; 95% repeatability of results	Very high
Equipment should be easy to handle for R&D personnel	Training in using the equipment should take less than 1 week	Very high
The price should be competitive versus alternatives	50–90 % of competitors	High
Biochip Engineering shall provide online support and troubleshooting	Troubleshooting time < 1 day	
Laboratory space requirement for the microphysiological system should be low	< 10 m^2	High
Storage stability of the microphysiological chips should be high	Up to 6 months	High
Requirements on production at Biochip Engineering (production management/operation)		
Cost of production should be much lower than the planned market price	< 30% at an annual production of 10000 chip units at a market price of 900 EUR/unit	Very high
A tenfold increase in production volume should be possible in the same plant with minor reinvestment	From 10000 units/year to 30000 units/year. Reinvestment < 25% of original investment	Very high
Day-and-night production should be possible by automation to minimize labor costs	Two operators working in three shifts should operate	Very high
The chips' shelf-life at customers should minimize supply logistics	Shelf-life of chips > 4 months	High
Plant size at lowest production volume (10000 units/year) shall be reduced	Chip fabrication < 2 m^3	High

As the tables highlight, purity and stability of the protein product have top priority. This connects to protein biology and the relationship with environmental conditions during the production stages and storage of the products.

Also of top priority is the capacity of the biological production system, i.e., the cell's capacity to express the product protein in a correctly folded form.

The choice of host-vector system is therefore a critical design condition that *Biochip Engineering* has already devoted much effort to under the restriction of their Intellectual Property Rights that they access or could acquire.

The capacity of the host cells to grow after transformation with the gene for the product protein is a matter of design optimization where culture media design plays a decisive role.

These requirements with accompanying target metrics do all connect to production economy and price for product per unit. The better performance of all these metrics, the better production economy and market price could be attained.

The customer's role is obvious but can be distinguished from the economic incitements.

The safety of the delivered product has very direct implications for the design of the production process, especially on the purification steps. The higher the demands, the more elaborate processing is required, which results in a surge in production costs, both in investments and in consumables.

The customer uses the delivered product as long as possible and under conditions not requiring freezing or refrigeration. It should be convenient to administer where oral dosage is desired, but for this product not realistically carried out.

9.3.2 Conceptualization of the Assignment

Once the analysis of needs and specifications is ready, the functionality of the product must be realistically discussed and understood (Ulrich and Eppinger 2011; Pahl et al. 2007; Mandenius and Björkman 2011; O'Brian 2019). Mapping of the functions required for a transformation process based on cell systems for physiological studies, the protein established, and the typical categories of functional systems that should be combined for achieving a production process that could copy with all the requirements that Table 9.1 highlighted. A general outline of functional systems for production and use of the multi-microphysiology device should be drawn (Fig. 9.2). Already, this overall depiction of the production process and use procedure elucidates the complexity of the task and how diverse competences must be merged into a functional production and user system.

The transformation process is close to a conventional flowchart diagram with inputs and outputs that include biological materials, construction materials and components, consumables, analytes to be investigated, and analytical and computed results. Secondly, inputs and outputs are added to this, such as power and waste. The transformation steps in the map show more than most engineering flowcharts, as it also brings in sub-steps for preparation, execution, and finishing phases, while a typical flowchart has a focus on the main process box where conversions and separations occur. A particular reason for taking this wider scope is that many of the cost-intensive parts of the process are included in the preprocessing and after-processing steps on the production train. If these are not involved when creating and analyzing the design alternatives, cost estimation will suffer markedly. In this case, preparation of media and handling of cell banks for tissue derivations are time-consuming, as are testing of the final product with all quality control and related analytics for allowing release of devices and auxiliary supply reagents and media. Efficiency in these may determine and impact production cost decisively.

The conceptual map differentiates between the biological and technical functions. It is obvious that the biological systems require biology competence to adequately understand and engineer the design efforts. The technical systems involve, to a large degree, materials science, biophysics, hydrodynamics, and biochemical engineering. These systems, and subsystems, need to be efficiently and economically designed.

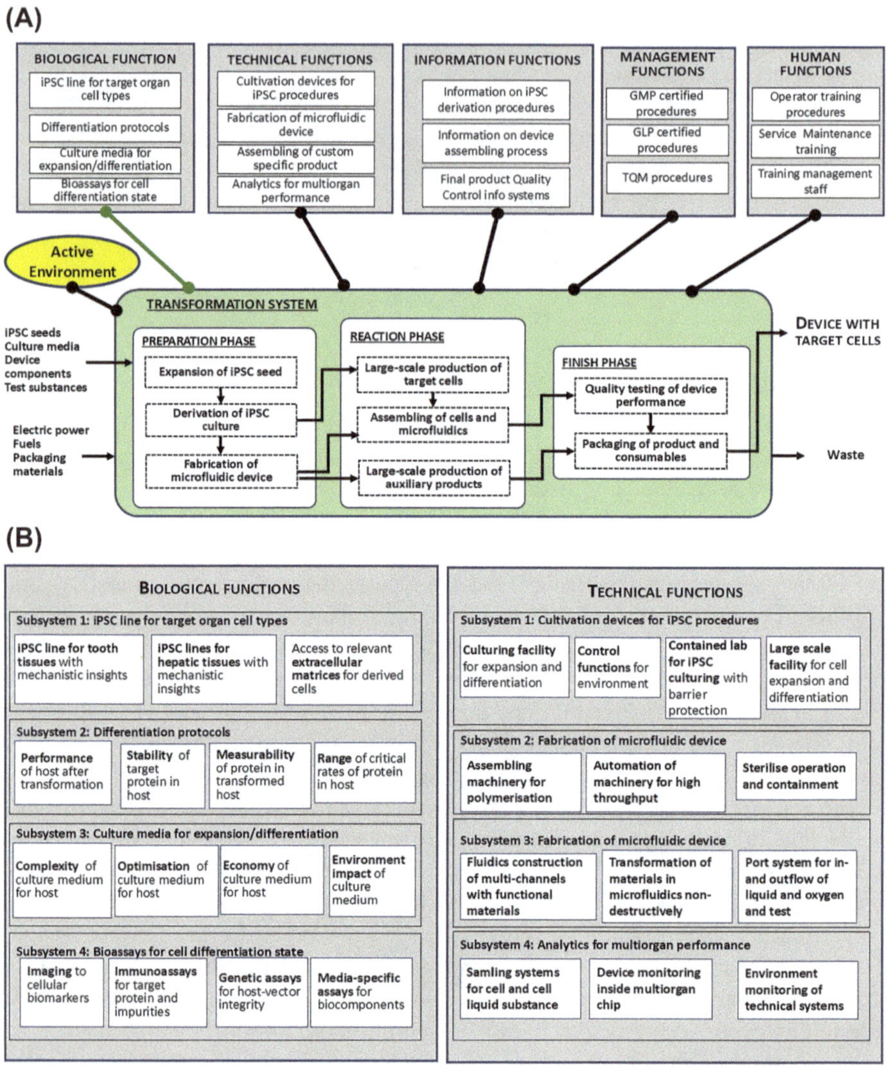

Fig. 9.2 Conceptual diagram of the functions and transformations for the product in the assignment from Biochip Engineering. The biological and technical functions are detailed into subsystems

This must also be the case between the conditions of biology and the technology as intertwined in the design. This will lead to several decisions between alternative technical and biological choices. These two systems are the most complex (Fig. 9.1b), and the interactions between the systems and the transformation process are intricate. Anticipating all possibilities of interactions that may occur and interaction matrix is recommended.

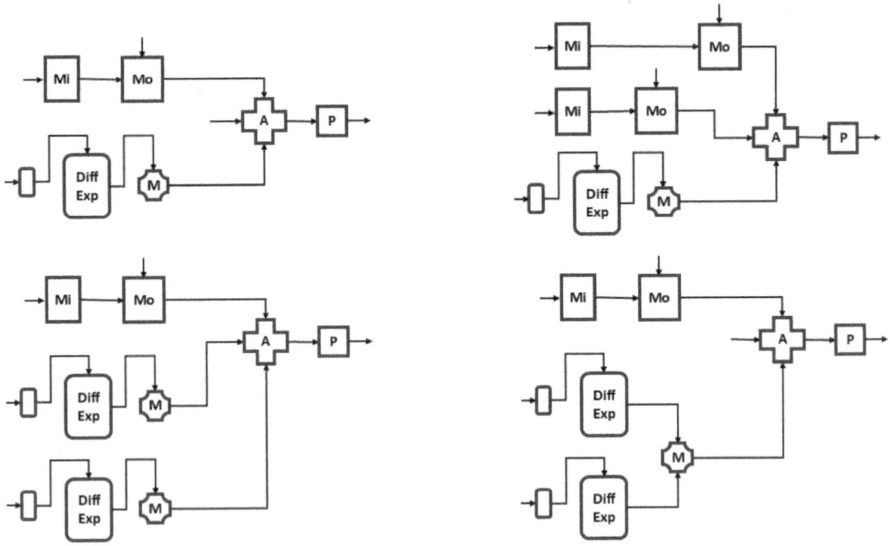

Fig. 9.3 Four alternative configurations. The upper two schemes (**a, b**) are configurations with one cell type derived from iPSC and with one or two types of microfluidic chips; the lower two schemes (**c, d**) show configurations where two types of cells derived from iPSC are infused into the same microfluidic chip

The conceptual map includes information functions, systems, management functions as well as human functions. Certainly, these can be detailed in several subfunctions with interaction nodes. The impact may also be considerable here, where, for example, a high complexity of technical systems will require more education and training for involved technicians.

Management systems in the biotech industry are known for their demanding documentation and inspection routines from authorities when it concerns pharmaceutical products, and supply to be used in conjunction with that. Management of quality, both overall and at a lower level, are other concerns affect design and choice of biological and technical systems. Economic consequences of these factors are sometimes neglected in design work. Here, e.g., the Food and Drug Administration (FDA) and corresponding authorities will surely scrutinize quality and do consequence assessments, especially when the microchip product is intended for verification of preclinical and clinical data in the R&D work in drug development. This will certainly favor design solutions that are able to comply with such demands.

In general, the educational level in biotech production of supplies is high. A large company can be expected to have established in-house and probably departmental structures for training operators and process engineers. Smaller companies' organizations may need to rely on external support and consultancy services for this in combination with their own expertise.

When the conceptual map of the production process for the assignment is developed, alternatives of process configurations can be conceived (Fig. 9.3).

Four configurations are established around an assembling unit. The first configuration has one process line for fabricating the microfluidic chip unit and one line for cell culture and introducing cells into the microfluidic chip (Fig. 9.3a). The second configuration includes either a single-line processing setup or parallel lines for chip fabrication (Fig. 9.3b). In a third configuration, different cell types are cultured in separate lines and introduced into the microfluidic chip consecutively (Fig. 9.3c). In a fourth configuration, the cells are cultured in separate lines but mixed together before they are introduced into the microfluidic chip (Fig. 9.3d).

The final architecture of the fabricated chips could, due to the layout, differ considerably. But could also its finished cell-filled product be the same. It is obvious that already at this basal representation of the configuration, investment and production cost will be influenced by which alternative is chosen. Consequently, it is important at this stage to compare how the requirements from Table 8.1 are fulfilled.

From this initially rather simple, but logical, reasoning, it is obvious that the alternatives C and D may provide the customer with the most flexible device. This is a desire distinctly expressed in the user requirements, to increase the versatility for the user. Certainly, this also strengthens the potential of the product for *Biochip Engineering*. This is most relevant if it can be achieved in a cost-effective way in the fabrication and supply chain. A relevant question will be whether the same fabrication machines and lines can produce more than one type of chip over periods.

It seems that the overall assignment conditions can be accomplished with all the alternatives or with a combination of them. Of course, much remains to be further designed, but already at this point the priorities in Table 10.1 can be evaluated. At this stage, it seems that the preliminary assessment above supports the order of priorities in concordance with the overall objectives of the assignment from *Biochip Engineering*.

Note that technical fabrication units are not yet scrutinized. Thus, the kind of machines, materials, mechanics, and automation, and possibly robotics, remain to be considered in their details. Should it be continuous fabrication, a combination of manual and automated procedures, as automated as possible. Will it require day-and-night production, or are the production cycles limited in time and can be campaigned? Should the supply of cell cultures be an in-house business, should it be subcontracted, or should the customers themselves take pre-cultivation steps to be structured differently?

These kinds of questions require much more consideration in the design studio work. CAD, market investigation, and optimization possibilities play a valuable resource in determining the space and conditions for different design alternatives. The relation to market needs over time, cost of production and dissemination of products, and the after-sales and customer support are issues not entirely design engineering judgments. Design engineering may primarily focus on the constraints and input design conditions and analyze these with the key engineering tools that can exploit the biology and technology of relevance. Other paths of *Biochip Engineering* have the responsibility and insights for managing the subsequent decision-making.

9.3.3 Detailed Designs of Selected Configurations

Of the four configurations considered for device fabrication, the two configurations that involved two cell types (C and D) seem favorable to be selected for detailed development with real objects (Fig. 9.4). The rationales for the selection are the following:

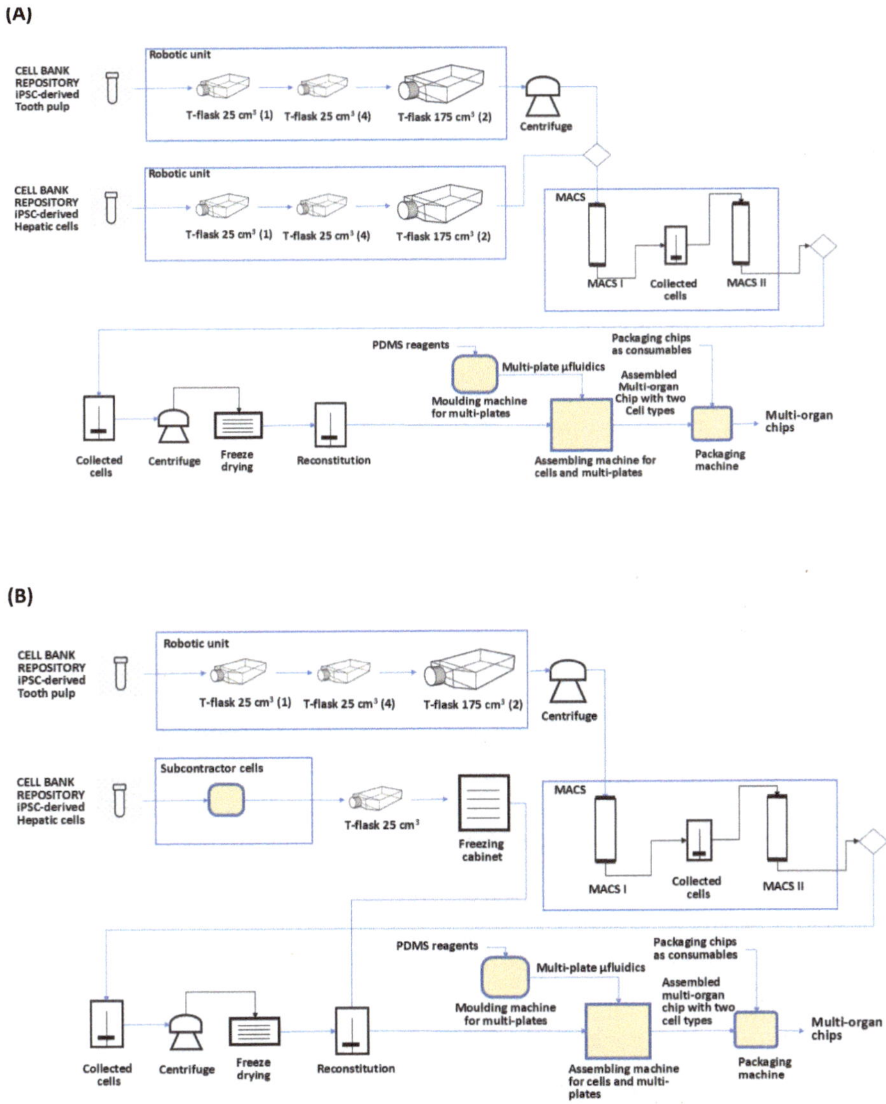

Fig. 9.4. Detailed design of the two selected configurations. (**a**) Production in-house within the company. (**b**) Production that is partly supported by subcontractors

- The microphysiological system should be able to mimic the fluidic and spacious dimensions of the in vivo situation, in terms of perfusion rates, diffusion distances, and gaseous levels and gradients.
- The microphysiological system should be able to be infused and to accommodate relevant tissue cultures.
- The microphysiological system must be controlled with sensors and other technical means to sustain conditions long enough to permit meaningful physiological and pharmacological studies.

Thus, configurations where cells are infused into the microfluidics separately or as a co-culture. This is mainly a critical biological choice. Could a mixed culture mimicking a tissue be an adequate representation of the in vivo system? This would depend on cellular biology. It opens up extracellular matrix reasoning of the in vitro model. The possibility to add biopolymers into the microfluidic system. On the other hand, the best representation of in vivo conditions is to separate the tissue-representing mimics and let them cross-talk between flown microunits through the microfluidic transfer in the device.

The main purpose of the digital tools is to establish a process layout including real and realistic unit operations for all steps. Thus, a digitalized flow sheet will include tubing, channels, pumps and syringes, micro-vents, micro-supply containers for media and other culture factors, as detailed inflow and outflow streams. Commercial digital software is recommended for speeding up this work (e.g., SuperPro Designer). The software is tailored for the case, as the necessary units are not standard. Thus, dimensions, volumes, sequential procedures for inflows and outflows, flow rates, and air supply can be added in tailored boxes. This required some technical work for the designers but could, after that, be reused in the forthcoming design work. It also paved the way for continuing optimization by Experiment-of-Design and mechanistic modelling.

The software allows it to set price levels on parts of the components used, although that could more efficiently be done in economic calculations.

Scaling equipment, either in number of units or each unit, could be done. Either scaling is a matter of adjusting size to a realistic physiological unit, or, to render the platform the desired capacity and multiplicity.

The obvious conclusion from the detailed design is that alternative D has less investment needs. Cell cultures are expanded in-house from commercial, proprietary induced pluripotent stem cell (iPSC) banks within the two design configurations shown in the detailed layouts (Fig. 9.4). Before immersion into the microfluidic devices, the derived pulp tissue and hepatic cells are reconstituted and carefully transferred into the microfluidic chambers of the device. The baseline cell bank materials originate from tooth pulp cells and hepatic cells developed by commercial laboratories. In Alternative A (Fig. 9.4a), *Biochip Engineering* differentiates and expands both the tooth and liver iPSCs in-house using standardized protocols and robotic units. Cell separation in this alternative is carried out via the magnetic-activated cell sorting (MACS) technique. In Alternative B (Fig. 9.4b), a subcontractor differentiates and expands the hepatic cells instead. These expanded cells are then freeze-dried for subsequent integration into the microchips by *Biochip Engineering*. In the assembly stage, empty plastic microplates are filled with cell cultures using an automated machine, which is directly followed by packaging in an automated packing system. The finished devices from the packaging machine are stored at low temperatures before being subsequently distributed to customers.

The Alternative B layout, where expanded hepatic cells are sourced directly from a subcontracted biotechnology company, is motivated by the fact that expanded hepatic cell culture batches have been commercially available for over 10 years; consequently, market price pressure has become favorable enough to justify direct purchasing. Furthermore, the reliable delivery track record of the primary subcontractor, along with the availability of alternative subcontractors, ensures a stable and secure provision of hepatic cells. These subcontractors fulfill all regulatory quality criteria from authorities and perform rigorous quality control (QC) and product testing. Within *Biochip Engineering's* facility, the final QC of the production process is carried out manually both before and after assembly, representing a highly personnel-demanding phase of the production line.

9.3.4 Production Economics for the Two Selected Design Alternatives

The capital investment and operational production costs for the two selected alternatives are compiled, structured, and analyzed using established economic evaluation methodologies (Kristiansen 2006; Peters et al. 2003; Towler and Sinnott 2012). As mentioned in the preceding section, specific pieces of equipment represent heavy capital expenditures that heavily influence the overall production economics.

The evaluation therefore must especially clarify the following economic issues:

- Analyze investment differences between the design alternatives and determine how alternative operational setups influence the overall cost structure.
- Investigate how subcontracting influences the final unit production cost, evaluating both positive and negative financial impacts.
- Analyze how a scale-up of production volume influences the economies of scale and the resulting unit costs for manufacturing.

The major distinction between the alternatives centers on the extent of subcontracting and the strategic advantage of securing the supply of key product components from external partners. For instance, the microfluidic unit can be fabricated externally and then assembled and populated with cells in-house at Biochip Engineering. Similarly, the control instrument unit can be manufactured externally based on blueprints provided by Biochip Engineering. Ultimately, the chosen investment and operational strategy for logistics is decisive for the total production cost.

At this stage, an approximate estimate of production costs is possible to make for the subcontract and in-house production alternatives (Table 9.2). The cost structure is divided into investments to establish the production and annual operational costs for the two alternatives. These costs are distinguished into cell production, cell separation, microfluidic fabrication, and quality control to detail as given in the flowcharts in the previous section.

Several of the costs in the assignment are provided by *Biochip Engineering*. Costs for procured materials and consumables from external vendors or subcontractors include human cell lines from repositories (e.g., United States National Institute for Medical Research 2023), plastic microfluidic units, and assembling machines for microfluidic fabrication. Such technically advanced machines should mold chips with microfluidic channel structures in plastic materials, have viable designs for filling, connecting these functions, and preparing them for a control instrument device with pumps or syringes and valves. *Biochip Engineering* already has technical systems on the market for similar products adaptable to microphysiological chip designs using computer-aided design and manufacturing (CAD-CAM) and 3-D-printing.

It may seem risky for *Biochip Engineering* to rely on the production line of subcontractors. Still, from a production economics perspective, it will be a typical subcontracting procurement of the assembling machine; the expense will be a dominating part of the production costs (in the range of 0.8–1.2 MEUR).

Standard multiplication factors have been applied in the table for typical cost items such as buildings, installations, piping, and construction and project planning (see Sect. 4.4.4, Table 4.4). These cost factors include labor costs. which are therefore not accounted for separately.

Operational costs are reported separately and divided into the biological section, mechanical section, and QC. Raw materials and consumables are substantial, as are labor costs. Additional costs with energy and support functions that are scale-dependent are shown. Some of the user fees also depend on the scale of production.

As stated in the assignment, R&D costs and the annual payoff of 5 years are added. This payback time can be shortened or prolonged.

Due to these approximations, the precision of total production cost is at the level of ± 25 %.

The total estimated production cost is for both alternatives within the targeted values. The most favorable alternative is the in-house production, mainly due to the smaller size of equipment which also is mirrored in the lower operational costs.

Investments and operational costs are added to R&D, license costs, other fees and taxes, funding from public sources and other costs that may be relevant to include. Which of these costs that in the end should be considered as costs to be paid back from the revenue from the new product, is only partly obvious and a matter of judgement and strategy from *Biochip Engineering*. For *Biochip Engineering*, which has around 5 to 10 products in its pipeline, it will be possible to share some of the payoff costs between products. That are multi-purpose machines and other equipment, procurement of raw materials that can be used in several production lines, personnel that can work with related products in parallel, marketing units responsible

Table 9.2 Evaluation of production costs for in-house and subcontracted alternatives

Type of costs	In-house production (kEUR)	Combined subcontracting (kEUR)
Investment costs		
Upfront production R&D		
Upfront production development	200	200
Subcontracted production development	150	100
Total upfront production R&D	*350*	*300*
Equipment and instrumentation		
Robotic units for cell culture	900	450
Separators for cell selection (MACS)	200	450
Cell storage/preservation (freezers, lyophilizers, tanks)	100	100
Chip fabrication machines (assembling, grafting)	500	500
Automatic packaging machine	200	200
Quality control instruments	200	200
Total equipment and instrumentation	*2100*	*1900*
Additional expenditure on investments		
Installation of equipment (x 0.5)	1050	950
Project planning (x 0.3)	630	570
Taxation (x 0.1)	210	190
Buildings (x 0.3)	630	570
Total additional expenditure on investments	*2520*	*2280*
Total investment costs	**4620**	**4180**
Operational costs (50 000 chips/year)		
Consumables for production		
Consumables cell production (media, factors)	70	40
Consumables chip fabrication (polymer, chip, reagent)	10	10
Consumables quality control (reagents, materials)	10	10
Total consumables for production	*90*	*60*
Additional operational expenditures		
Subcontracting fee of cells from iPSC bank	100	200
Subcontracting microfluidic chips	100	100
External maintenance of equipment in facility	10	10
Labor in production facility (incl QC)	110	80
Renting of buildings	100	100
Taxation	20	20
Annual IPR expenditure and licenses (cell lines)	50	40

(continued)

Table 9.2 (continued)

Type of costs	In-house production (kEUR)	Combined subcontracting (kEUR)
Management	20	20
Total additional expenditure for operation	*490*	*370*
Total operational costs	**580**	**630**
Annual payoff of investment (5 years)	924	126
Total annual production cost (50 000 chips/year)	**1504**	**756**
Production cost per chip (EUR)	30,1	15,1

for sales activities and customer support. Therefore, the costs associated with such activities could, in the calculation of one new product, be relatively modest and adapted to actual conditions at *Biochip Engineering*.

The cost for the control instrument unit is a one-time payment for the customer in the range 50–70 kEUR per instrument. The marketing strategy could be to supply the station at the actual manufacturing cost without any net income, assuming that the total number of stations is low and not a lucrative market while the microfluidic chips will lead to a high net income.

The distribution of types of expenses shows the sensitivity of the investments and potential for upscaling production (Fig. 9.5).

9.3.5 Status of Intellectual Property Rights for Microphysiological Systems

The new production process for the microphysiological chips is dependent on strong intellectual property rights (IPR) that protects the production from infringement (Farnley et al. 2004; Demir and Stamhuis 2023). Therefore, it is important to have a detailed knowledge about existing patents and patent applications that describe similar production systems that are based on identical or similar techniques. Companies like *Biochip Engineering*, as well as other competing companies in the marketing of microfluidic products for the same customer purposes, have most probably filed several patents and applications of relevance. Table 9.3 lists a collection of patent applications that are closely related to *Biochip Engineering's* microphysiological concept. These patents do especially challenge the following design aspects:

- Creation of fluidic conditions appropriate for cells and tissues that mimic the in vivo environment (Trietsch et al. 2023; Bishard et al. 2022)
- Creation of intra-fluidic networks that mimic multi-organ systems in the body (Vulto et al. 2022)
- Creation of conditions allowing differentiation of cells (Marx et al. 2019)

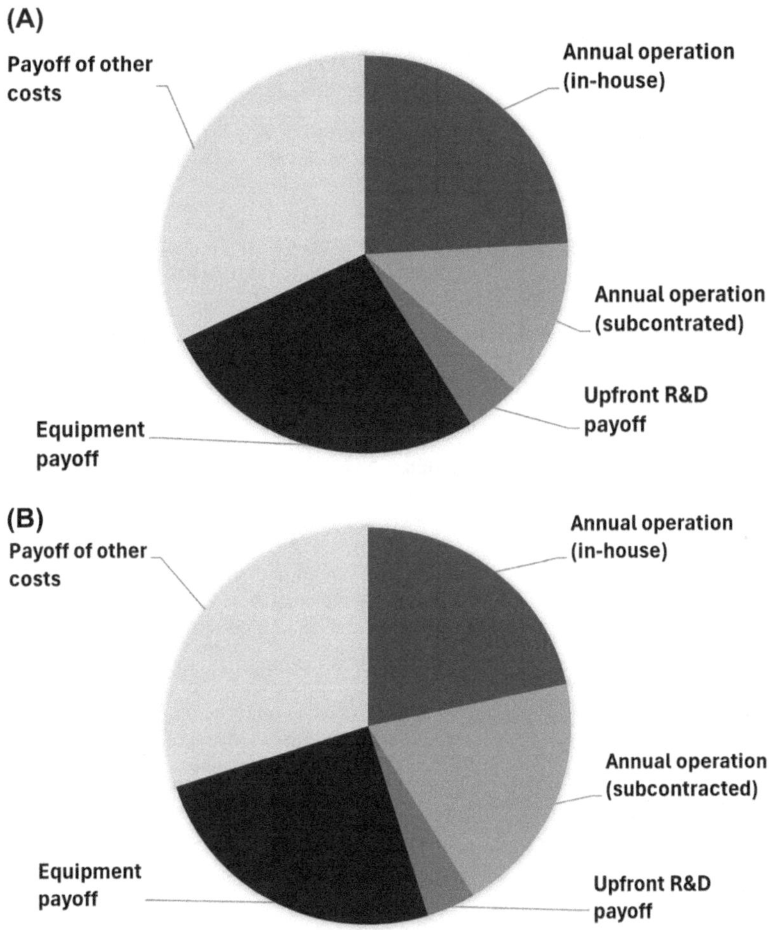

Fig. 9.5 Distribution of costs in the two alternatives. (**a**) In-house. (**b**) Subcontracting

- Allowing testing of drug candidates to circumvent animal studies (Fatehi-Varkani et al. 2012)
- Allowing testing of mechanical stress in the in vivo system (Vulto et al. 2022)

Biochip Engineering must ensure that they fully control the intellectual property rights (IPR) landscape, utilizing either proprietary-owned rights or appropriately secured licensed rights. Concurrently, they must conduct a comprehensive risk analysis regarding potential new, competing IPR filings within the same technology domain. Importantly, the evaluation should address whether there is potential to patent a specific function or structural feature within the new microphysiology design. Furthermore, it must consider how external ownership of related IPR

Table 9.3 Patents that may treat the microphysiological system alternatives

Patent or patent application	Protection	Patent number, reference and owner
Microfluidic cell culture device	Methods for creating a fluid-fluid interface and for investigating a cellular response to a stimulant	US2023/250377 Trietsch et al. (2023) Mimetas, Leiden
Microfluidic cell culture system	Microfluidic structures are in fluid communication with each other via a communication channel	US2022/395833 Bishard et al. (2022) Mimetas, Ledien
Novel multi-organ chips establishing differentiation of iPSC-derived cells into organ equivalents	Multi-organ-chips establishing the differentiation of iPSC into organ equivalents	WO2019/122291 Marx et al (2018) TissUse, Berlin
Microfluidic devices implementing blood and urine circuit formulating homeostatic microphysiological system	For pharmacokinetic-pharmacodynamic analysis in the context of administration, distribution, metabolism, and toxicology (ADMET) profiling. Comprising a first "blood" circuit with one or more cell culture compartments, and a second "urine" circuit comprising a renal filtration	WO2019/122349 Marx et al. (2019) TissUse, Berlin
Device for assessing mechanical strain induced in or by cells	The device comprises a base, a microfluidic channel and a cover, and the base comprises a diaphragm forming at least part of an inner surface of the microfluidic channel. The device finds use in methods for assessing mechanical strain induced in or by cells, such methods also being described.	US2022/017846 Vulto et al. (2022) Mimetas, Leiden
3D in vitro biphasic cartilage-bone construct	A 3D in vitro biphasic cartilage-bone organoid comprising (a) a layer of artificial cartilage tissue and (b) a layer of artificial bone tissue, wherein the artificial bone tissue comprises a structure-giving scaffold and a bone marrow structure	ES2739201 Fatehi-Varkani et al. (2012) TissUse, Berlin

might change the company's competitive situation and determine whether there is viable space for further design improvements and patentable innovation.

It is important from a design perspective to know when implementing a new design that the process is robust to infringements or other potential threats to protect their product production and marketing. The ten patents listed in the table are those which are considered to have the highest actuality in these respects.

Given these conditions, the suggested subcontracted design alternative is still a robust choice for the system and its large-scale production of chips.

9.3.6 *Optimization of the Microphysiological System Alternatives*

Once a decision has been made on how to prioritize the designs, a further optimization of these is motivated (Sioshansi and Conejo 2017; Martins and Ning 2021; Cortez 2021). Due to the differences in the design, the likelihood of improving the performance of the microphysiological chip could be expected to vary significantly. The more compact design may have less opportunities for optimization. Several optimization methods are at hand. Several design aspects are possible to optimize by various optimization techniques, and with potential benefits and outcomes (Table 9.4). Basically, the goal is to improve the productivity of chips, increase yields of cells and other materials, reduce use of labor resources, and decrease process time, all having a positive impact on production economy.

Design of Experiments for Optimizing Microphysiological Chip Performance The overall design of a system can, in most cases, be significantly improved by systematically altering operational conditions within the structural design of the product itself, as well as during its fabrication and production stages (Brereton 2003; Mandenius and Brundin 2008; Montgomery 2013). Several distinct options are readily available for optimizing the entire manufacturing and fabrication procedure of microphysiological chips through the application of design of experiments (DoE) methodology.

Optimization of the geometry of the chip versus the performance is one example. This may concern the dimensions and geometric ratios of the design. This spans across the design of the flow chamber, the flow conditions, the attachment of cells in the flow chamber of the chip, the supply of oxygen, and the choice of construction

Table 9.4 Optimization methods of the microphysiological product's performance

Object of optimization	Expected outcome	Applicable optimization technique
Production of target cells for the microphysiological chips (pulp and liver cells)	Increase in specific production rate of cells	Factorial design of experimentally available parameters
Proliferation parameters in the perfusion microphysiological chip	Increased growth rate of cells	Factorial design of selected parameters
Dimensions (or aspect ratios) of the microphysiological chip	A favorable media composition for production and media cost	Factorial design of components
Production conditions in the assembling machine of the microphysiological chip	Improved performance of the assembly of the chips resulting in faster production	Factorial design of critical production parameters Mechanistic modelling for production
Assembling time of the microphysiological chips	Shorter assembling time with impact on productivity, size of fabrication plant	Mechanistic modelling for production

materials of the chip. In the chip fabrication step, again qualitative and quantitative parameters are possible to identify. Choice of materials in the chip, its geometry, the precision in the molded channels, and the air permeability are examples of parameters that can be determined and investigated. The response converges to productivity and quality. Sometimes these go in opposite directions, sometimes they do not. That is, a higher speed of flow-through in the assembling machine may result in larger variability in channel dimensions, in applied cell amounts, etc.

If also the supply of cells, pulp cells, and liver cells, this may include stem cell differentiation and expansion steps which are appropriate targets for optimization where productivity related outputs of the optimization are of interest. This could also include the composition of culture media, stimulating factors added to the media, time schedule in the culture protocols, supply of air, agitation, surface in culture vessels, and others.

The DoE will allow time-saving experimental plans, but it is also obvious that the number of parameters as quoted above may easily rise to 50 or more. Experienced designers may initially reduce this number to 10–20 parameters (as factors in DoE).

Then it should also be realistic to observe the responses without too complicated and time-consuming and cost-intensive resource allocations. *Biochip Engineering* is not interested in doing so fully but will accept some efforts if it is certified that it will pay off. The design team is detrimental to this activity.

It is therefore suggested to prioritize those factors that have the highest likelihood of paying back with an improved production economy and a competitive edge in the quality of the product (Table 9.5). The DoE procedures should follow the methodology described in Chap. 4 using reduced factor analysis at two or three levels. Analytics for response assessments could follow standard bioanalytical procedures.

Optimization of Chip Production Using Mechanistic Modelling By studying growth and maturation of iPSC using mechanistic modelling critical conditions can be investigated and favorable procedures identified for reaching the objectives of the assignment (Doran 2013; O'Brian 2019). Using mass balances and kinetic equations and simulating these with time under a variety of assumptions such as seed concentration, plate and flask volumes and growth conditions, better conditions can be established (Nielsen et al. 2011).

One of the focuses in the modelling should be the kinetics of the differentiation and expansion of the iPSC cells and tissue cells derived from these. Thus, the properties of cell biology, i.e., how cells differentiate from the iPSC and how differentiated cells expand at optimal rates and yield and at scales appropriate for the production target. This is best carried out after the DoE optimization as parameters of high relevance become clearer there.

The following model equations (Eqs. 9.1, 9.2, and 9.3) predict the dynamics of the differentiating and expanding cells before being seeded into the microphysiological chip:

Table 9.5 Optimization of microphysiology system by DoE plan

Optimization object	Factors in DoE plan	Responses to measure
Composition of the expansion media for tooth tissues	Basal media. Commercial media. Trace elements and vitamins. Cell differentiation factors	Density of viable cells. Cell purity. Microscopic verification
Composition of the expansion media for hepatic cells	Basal media. Commercial media. Trace elements and vitamins. Cell differentiation factors	Density of viable cells. Cell purity. Microscopic verification
Composition of the differentiation media for tooth tissues	Basal media. Commercial media. Trace elements and vitamins. Cell differentiation factors	Density of viable cells. Cell purity. Microscopic verification
Composition of the differentiation media for hepatic cells	Basal media. Commercial media. Trace elements and vitamins. Cell differentiation factors	Density of viable cells. Cell purity. Microscopic verification
Physical and chemical conditions in the above cultures	Environmental conditions in the cultures (pH, temperature, dissolved oxygen, ionic strength)	Growth rates and yields
Centrifugal separation of expanded tissue cells	Centrifuge rate and diameter. Density of culture media.	Cell yields in centrifuge outflows
Environment of the microphysiology chip	Oxygenation flows. Surface treatment of cells. Heat transfer. Flow dynamics	Microanalysis in the device
Assembling machine operation for molding unfilled microphysiological chips	Reagents and polymers for molding. Composition. Reaction time	Channel precision. Flow cell precision
Filling pulp and liver cells in the assembling machine	Amounts of tissue cells. Rate of filling. Sterility. Temperature	Cell viability. Cell survival

$$dN/dt = k_{cell} \cdot N \tag{9.1}$$

$$dS_{media}/dt = k_{cell} \cdot Y_{S/N} \tag{9.2}$$

$$k_{cell} = k_{max} \cdot S_{media}/(S_{media} - K_{sat}) \tag{9.3}$$

where N is the cell concentration of the tested cell type, S_{media} is the concentration of the limiting nutrient, and V is the volume or area of the flask/plate where the cells are cultured. Constraints that can be introduced in the equations are the number of multilayers of cells and the confluence limit of cells. $Y_{S/N}$, K_{sat}, k_{max}, and k_{cell} are values for describing the kinetic and yield constants of the cells.

The microphysiological chip can initially be modelled using three equations (Eqs. 5.5.4, 5.5.5, and 5.5.6) to capture the cell growth in the continuously perfused chamber of the chip (Fig. 9.6):

$$dN_{\mu F}/dt = k_{tox} \cdot N_{\mu F} + k_{\mu} \cdot N_{\mu F} – N_{\mu F} \cdot F_{filter}/V_{\mu F} \tag{9.4}$$

$$dDrug/dt = -N_{\mu F} \cdot k_{drug} – Drug \cdot F_{chamber}/V_{\mu F} \tag{9.5}$$

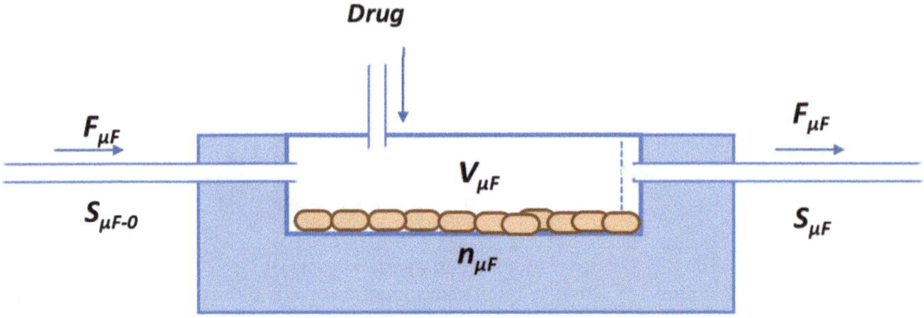

Fig. 9.6 Model for microphysiological chip chamber perfused with a nutrient medium, seeded with cells (pulp or liver cells) and exposed to a candidate drug (or toxicant). The outlet of the chamber has a filter that allows the drug to pass while the cells, to a large extent, are retained

$$if\ Drug < 0; dN_{\mu F}/dt = 0 \tag{9.6}$$

where $N_{\mu F}$ is the tested cell's concentration in the microfluidic unit, $F_{chamber}$ is the flowrate through the microphysiological chip, $V_{\mu F}$ is the volume of the chamber of the chip, S_{media0} is the concentration of the limiting nutrient S at the inlet to the chamber, and S_{media} is the concentration at the outlet. The constant k_{μ} is the specific growth of the test cells; k_{tox} is the rate of degradation of test cells due to the toxicity of the drug. Drug is the concentration of the drug, $V_{\mu F}$ is the volume of the chamber, and F_{filter} is the nominal flow rate of test cells escaping the chamber. The constant k_{drug} is the uptake of drug by the test cells, which is not equivalent to k_{tox}, as drug uptake does not per se is degrading the cells.

The externally cultured test cells are infused into the chamber and are assumed to immediately adhere to the inner surfaces of the *chamber.*

Three sets of simulations show the outcome of the model where the conditions are varied and constrained as described (Fig. 9.7).

The *first example* shows differentiation and expansion of iPSC-derived liver cells over a period of 170 h at stepwise increased concentration of culture media (Fig. 9.7a) (Eqs. 9.1, 9.2 and 9.3). The media concentration is increased by 0.10 mg/mL in each plot, allowing the culture to grow to higher concentration. The specific growth rate is unchanged while surface concentration on the plate increased stepwise. This may go on until the plate surface has reached confluence. After that, growth sizes, as multilayer growth is not permitted (which is conditioned in the model equations). This can experimentally be changed by using a flask with a larger surface area. The simulation can easily be adapted to cell expansion with other cell types and other specific growth rates (not shown). The information on actual specific growth rate can be collected from literature.

In the *second example,* the differentiated cells from the plate are transferred into the microphysiological chamber of the chip, where the test cells directly adhere to the chamber surface (Fig. 9.5b). The media composition is assumed to be optimized by DoE. A potentially toxic drugs are infused. The plots show a nontoxic drug, a medium toxic drug, and a highly toxic drug. Their effects are seen in the number of test cells in the microphysiology device.

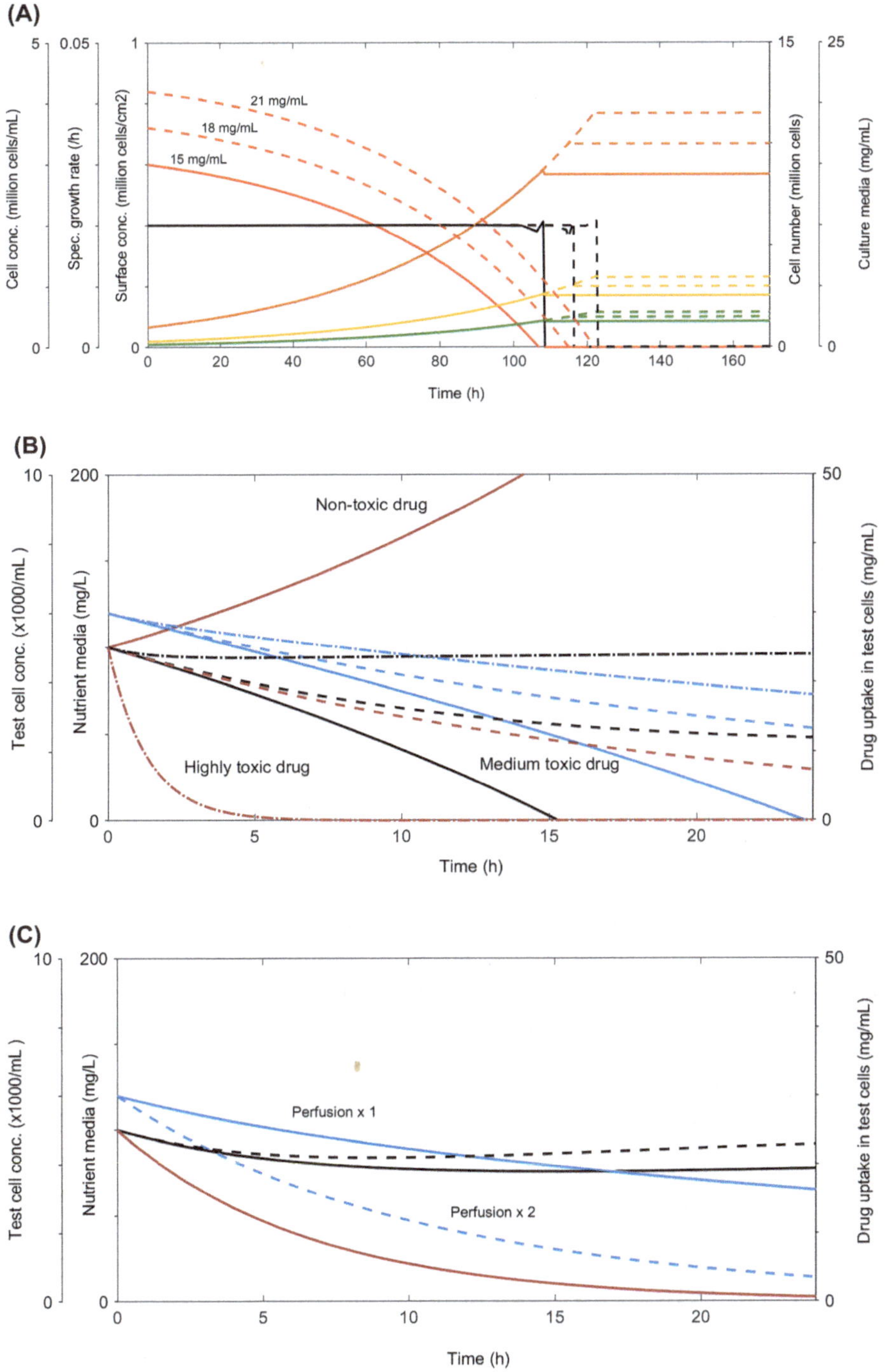

Fig. 9.7 (**a**) Propagation of tooth or liver tissue test cells in a culture plate. Culture media concentration is increased in steps (red plots). Growth rate and area of the culture plate are unchanged. (**b**) The cultured test cells are transferred to a chamber in a microphysiology chip and exposed to a drug candidate. The amount of drug is increased (blue plots). (**c**) The perfusion rate through the chamber is increased (gray)

In the *third example*, the simulations above are repeated at different perfusion rates through the microphysiological chamber (Fig. 9.5c), for example, the effects on the test cells for the drug with medium toxicity. Obviously, the flow rate influences the test cells.

Other parameters are possible to investigate with the models, for example, the volume of the chamber, the seeding of each test cells, and the effect of the nutrient medium.

9.3.7 SWOT Analysis of the In-House and Subcontracted Alternatives

It is advised to perform an evaluation of pros and cons for the prioritized design alternatives by using analysis of strengths, weaknesses, opportunities, and threats (SWOT) (Shinno et al. 2006). This should be carried out with regard to the priorities in Table 9.1. The SWOT analysis provides a broader analysis than a simple pros and cons list, as it also anticipates future opportunities and threats. The SWOT analysis compares those issues that at this stage seem relevant to consider and that are assumed to have strong impact on economics and marketing of the microphysiological product (Table 9.6). The analysis is purely qualitative and to a minor degree based on concrete performance values. Still, it serves the purpose of notifying which issues are worth spending more time on in the design work and needs further attention. The table below highlights a few things in that respect.

Many of the critical conditions are favorably appraised in the SWOT table. The fact that an additional cell type (matured hepatic cells) is provided through subcontracting has not so severe impact of the production platform. The economic benefits are relatively modest, and it if the arrangement with subcontracting approach can be questioned. The cost for setting up of small-scale in-house production can be considered. Given the fact that many customers still prefer the provision of cells through their own resources or agreements this may be of minor importance.

Eight aspects are analyzed in the SWOT scheme. Additional aspects can be included. However, these eight aspects encircle the most sensitive issues that design engineering can negate or promote by smarter design solutions. From a design engineering perspective, it is possible to reconsider the design alternatives at this point and with relative minor adjustments strengthen the performance of the design of microphysiological product.

Here, it should especially be mentioned:

- New cell types with better in ex vivo mimicking ability through cell engineering.
- Other technological structures using, e.g., nanotechnology.
- The development toward personalized medicine
- Severe cost reduction for production by artificial intelligence methodology

Finally, the pharma industry's future role will determine the market forces and the societal economy's potential for exclusive technology in pharmacy.

Table 9.6 SWOT analysis of the in-house and subcontracted alternatives

Priority criteria	In-house production	Subcontracted production
Scalability of multichip plant	*Strength:* Technology is scale independent *Weakness:* Exclusive machines limit upscaling *Opportunity:* Adaptable to other cell types with SME company *Threats:* All depends on one type of machine	*Strength:* Exploit time of subcontractor's development *Weakness:* Dependable on that expertise *Opportunity:* Speeding up time to market. *Threats:* Dependable on one external cell supplier
Microphysiology environment in the device	*Strength:* The alternative development of in vivo drug testing is multiple times higher *Weakness:* The microfluid design is not in proportion to physiological dimensions *Opportunity:* Nanotechnology is in steady development *Threats:* Improved mimicking by nanotechnology seems likely	*Strength:* A substantial reduction in production costs can be achieved. *Weakness:* This may not be enough in comparison to technical solutions. *Opportunity:* The use of already existing cell systems gains time in competition. *Threats:* The real competition is other biological systems with better mimicking properties
Design of fabrication method	*Strength:* Small with low cost *Weakness: Too complex* *Opportunity: Can be optimized* *Threats: Competitors better*	*Strength:* Smaller with lower cost *Weakness: Too complex* *Opportunity: Can be optimized* *Threats: Competitors better*
Flexibility of fabrication of multichip plant	*Strength:* Very flexible *Weakness:* None *Opportunity:* Very expandable *Threats:* Uncertainty about the outcome of follow-up products	*Strength:* Very flexible but less, when additional procedures *Weakness:* None *Opportunity:* Very expandable *Threats:* Uncertainty about the outcome of follow-up products
IPR situation	*Strength*: Owns unique features of fabrication of chips for both systems *Weakness*: Rather many IPRs are required	*Strength:* IPR process ready and positively solved *Weakness*: Subcontractor own rights for part of product may cause problems
Personnel size	*Strength:* Automation reduced costs. *Weakness:* Surveillance suffers *Threats:* The product quality is endangered	*Strength:* Automation reduced costs *Weakness:* Surveillance suffers *Threats:* The product quality is endangered
Environmental impact	*Strength:* A very controlled and contained procedure *Weakness: None* *Opportunity:* Regulators may become more environmentally related *Threats:* Using disposables not accepted	*Strength:* A very controlled and contained procedure *Weakness: None* *Opportunity:* Regulators may become more environmentally related *Threats:* Using disposables not accepted

(continued)

Table 9.6 (continued)

Priority criteria	In-house production	Subcontracted production
Overall business economics	*Strength:* A cost-effective platform *Weakness:* Too few users *Opportunity:* Regulators may become much more demanding *Threats:* Results obtained too inaccurate for demands	*Strength: A more cost-effective platform* *Weakness:* Too few users *Opportunity:* Regulators may become much more demanding *Threats:* Results obtained too inaccurate for demands

9.4 Conclusive Suggestions for *Biochip Engineering*

It is suggested that *Biochip Engineering* apply a design for the microphysiological chip system where the production platform and the supply of both tooth and liver cells are managed entirely in-house. This recommendation is based on the following reasons and cost-related concerns:

- Production costs are easier to control and minimize within an integrated, in-house operational setting.
- The physical footprint of the plant is modest for the intended production volume, which should make it straightforward to minimize capital investments in expensive equipment and its installation in-house.
- A safer, more secure supply of derived cell materials is established through in-house culturing, especially since the baseline iPSCs accessed from public cell banks or commercial suppliers will be used frequently.
- Culture media and other critical consumables required for iPSC processing are easier to monitor, regulate, and control directly.
- Operational costs can be further reduced by leveraging process and production R&D efforts to systematically optimize cell expansion and differentiation conditions.
- Environmental impacts of production remain marginal due to the small manufacturing scale; however, adequate measures must still be taken to negate any external environmental variations that could affect production stability.

It is suggested that *Biochip Engineering* consider a few risk factors in the assignment:

- The product should also be competitive versus the customers' own alternatives, i.e., to buy the cells from their own supplier or to culture them in-house.
- Although the personnel at the production line will be few, they must have qualified competences and training for their jobs. Access to personnel with multi-capacity is required, which results in higher personnel costs for salaries, training, and recruitment.
- Sustainability of the product should be considered with respect to upcoming new microphysiology organ-on-chip products or reengineering organisms.

- According to the economic evaluation, the product is sensitive to price changes. Although the microphysiology platform is unique, it is likely that a second similar product on the market could radically change the price pressure.

  Some additional concerns are:

- The quality control demands in the pharmaceutical industry are significant. The larger companies are usually well provided with such resources. *Biochip Engineering* should therefore focus on the product quality testing and verification of such attributes that are not regularly assessed by qualified customers.
- It is likely that similar microphysiological products are developed by competitive companies with high or higher functionality.
- The scale-up alternative has been seen as the easiest and most flexible way of handling an unpredictable marker request.
- The need to be close to the users motivates plant movability. The modest size of the production makes that possible.

In summary, small-size production, with the lowest investments, and high flexibility are paramount for a successful commercial development. Obviously, the product design with its production economics is the important enabler for this kind of biotech product.

9.5 Tutorial Perspectives on the Assignment

The pedagogical challenges in the training for this assignment are directly connected to combining two novel bioengineering technologies and delivering the final product to highly qualified end-users. The assignment also highlights the critical strategic decision of how to leverage subcontractors for supplying specialized components in the fabrication of both the microphysiological system and the corresponding tissue cells. The specific challenges that will be particularly difficult for the trainees to manage can be concretized into the following five issues:

- Understand how qualified customers utilize the product to optimize and accelerate the development of pharmaceutical drugs.
- Analyze how the multi-organ microfluidic product delivers value to clients who intend to use it for true, high-fidelity physiological cell research purposes.
- Integrate an advanced multi-organ microfluidic platform seamlessly with cutting-edge stem cell differentiation and expansion technology.
- Realize how critical space and time constraints possess the potential to overcome operational thresholds for reaching acceptable production targets, and learn to apply these factors within basic manufacturing models.
- Compare the alternative costs of subcontracting, capital equipment, consumables, and other auxiliary expenses required to produce the target number of microphysiological chips against the inherent uncertainties of introducing a novel product with unique components and instrumentation.

The tutorial actions of the industrial experts should focus on:

- Filling the gaps in knowledge that most trainees are lacking about drug development needs in industry. It is unlikely that previous education programs for academic students have included this notion. This can be largely done at the customer interviews.
- Helping trainees to see the potential of applying for DoE to non-quantified parameters that the production system is in this assignment characterized by. That would mostly be connected to comparing production units versus key production parameters (responses).
- Consider how to act from a subcontractor perspective to ensure that also different subcontractor priorities become apparent.

References

Bishard K, Grasegger J, Trietsch SJ (2022) Microfluidic cell culture system. US2022/0395833 A1

Brereton RG (2003) Chemometrics, data analysis for laboratory and chemical plants. Wiley, Chichester

Cortez P (2021) Modern optimization with R. Springer, Cham. ISBN 9783030728182

Demir E, Stamhuis E (2023) Patenting human biological materials and data: balancing the reward of innovation with the *ordre public* and morality exception. J Intellect Prop Law Pract 18(7): 546–553. https://doi.org/10.1093/jiplp/jpad052

Doran PM (2013) Biochemical engineering principles, 2nd edn. Elsevier, Amsterdam. https://doi.org/10.1016/C2009-0-22348-8

Farnley S, Morey-Nase P, Sternfeld D (2004) Biotechnology, a challenge to the patent system. Curr Opin Biotechnol 15:254–257. https://doi.org/10.1016/j.copbio.2004.04.004

Fatehi-Varkani S, Lauser R, Marx U (2012) 3D in vitro biphasic cartilage-bone construct. EP 2:634 251 A1

Gao P, Shan L, Wang X et al (2022) Dental applications of induced pluripotent stem cells and their derivatives (review article). Jpn Dent Sci Rev 58:162–171. http://creativecommons.org/licenses/by-nc-nd/4.0/

Kristiansen B (2006) Process economics. In: Ratledge C, Kristiansen B (eds) Basic biotechnology, 3rd edn. Cambridge University Press, Cambridge, pp 239–252

Mandenius CF, Björkman M (2011) Biomechatronic design in biotechnology: a methodology for development of biotechnology products. Wiley, Hoboken

Mandenius CF, Brundin A (2008) Bioprocess optimization using design-of-experiments methodology. Biotechnol Prog 24:1191–1203. https://doi.org/10.1002/btpr.67

Martins JRRA, Ning A (2021) Engineering design optimization. Cambridge University Press, Cambridge. https://doi.org/10.1017/9781108980647

Marx U, Ramme A (2019) Novel multi-organ-chips establishing differentiation of iPSC-derived cells into organ equivalents. WO2019/122291 A1

Marx U, Andersson TB, Bahinski A et al (2016) Biology-inspired microphysiological system approaches to solve the prediction dilemma of substance testing. ALTEX 33(3):272–321. https://doi.org/10.14573/altex.1603161

Marx U, Dehne EM, Hasenberg T (2019) Novel microfluidic devices implementing blood and urine circuit for emulating homeostatic microphysiological system. WO2019/122349 A1

Marx U, Accastelli E, David R (2021) An individual patient's "body" on chips: how organismoid theory can translate into your personal precision therapy approach. Front Med 8:728866. https://doi.org/10.3389/fmed.2021.728866

Maschmeyer I, Lorenz AK, Schimek K et al (2015) A four-organ-chip for interconnected long-term co-culture of human intestine, liver, skin and kidney equivalents. Lab Chip 15:2688–2699. https://doi.org/10.1039/c5lc00392j

Montgomery DC (2013) Design and analysis of experiments, 8 eds. Wiley, New York

Nielsen J, Villadsen J, Lidén G (2011) Bioreaction engineering principles, 3rd edn. Springer-Nature, New York

O'Brian D (2019) Engineer 4.0: Life science handbook for medical devices and biopharmaceuticals. Kindle ISBN-13: 978-1795753340

Pahl G, Beitz W, Feldhusen J et al (2007) Engineering design, a systematic approach, 3rd edn. Springer Verlag, Berlin

Peters MS, Timmerhaus KD, West RE (2003) Plant design and economics for chemical engineers, 5th edn. McGraw-Hill & Co, New York

Sanka R, Lippai J, Samarasekera D et al (2019) 3DµF interactive design environment for continuous flow µF device. Sci Rep 9:9166. https://doi.org/10.1038/s41598-019-45623-z

Shinno H, Yoshioka H, Marpaung S et al (2006) Quantitative SWOT analysis on global competitiveness of machine tool industry. J Eng Design 17(3):251–258. https://doi.org/10.1080/09544820500275180

Sioshansi R, Conejo AJ (2017) Optimization in engineering, models and algorithms. Springer, Germany. ISBN 9783319567679

Towler G, Sinnott R (2012) Chemical engineering design: principles, practice and economics of plant and process design, 2nd edn. Elsevier, Amsterdam

Trietsch SJ, Nicolas AYM, van den Broek LJ et al (2023) Microfluidic cell culture device. US2023/0250377

Ulrich KT, Eppinger SD (2011) Product design and development, 5th edn. McGraw-Hill, New York

United States National Institute for Medical Research (ed) (2023) The Human Genetic Mutant Cell Repository: List of genetic variants, chromosomal aberrations and normal cell cultures submitted to the repository, 4th edn. Camden, United States National Institute for Medical Research,, Legare Street Press. ISBN: 10-102149335X, ISBN-13: 978-1021493354

Volponi AA, Pang Y, Sharpe PT (2010) Stem cell-based biological tooth repair and regeneration. Trends Cell Biol 20:715–722. https://doi.org/10.1016/j.tcb.2010.09.012

Vulto P, Trietsch J, Burton TP (2022) Device for assessing mechanical strain induced in or by cells. US2022/0017846 A1

Wagner I, Materne EM, Brincker S et al (2013) A dynamic multi-organ-chip for long-term cultivation and substance testing proven by 3D human liver and skin tissue co-culture. Lab Chip 13:3538–2547. https://doi.org/10.1093/c3lc50234a

Chapter 10
Case 5: Production of Ventricular Progenitors from Induced Pluripotent Stem Cells

10.1 Assignment: Background, Description, and Objectives

The aim of the training in this assignment is to design a commercial production system for ventricular progenitor cells (VPC) for use in regenerative treatment of cardiac patients (Lin and Pu 2014; Saito et al. 2025).

The assigner, *Global Pharma*, is an established international pharmaceutical company with a portfolio of drugs in most pharmacological areas. The company has extensive experience *in* cardiovascular pharmacology and is confident that it can establish a strong global market position with stem cell-derived products. They have identified cardiac treatment as a priority *for the use of* their own protected stem cell technology. The company has facilities *on* all continents and *the* ability to market the product to hospitals and clinics.

Global Biopharma has established competence in large-scale manufacture of human ventricular progenitor cells (VPC) derived from human pluripotent stem cells (Fig. 10.1) (Park et al. 2025). The cardiac progenitor cells are intended for regenerative therapy of patients at hospitals with heart clinics (Eschenhagen and Weinberger 2024; Bissoli et al. 2023; Chien et al. 2012; Hammond et al. 2019).

The goal is to produce clinically potent cells at a level of 70×10^9 to 100×10^9 functional cells per week using novel production methodology (Manstein et al. 2021). *Global Pharma* has developed such methods in collaboration with a smaller subcontractor. Protocols for the production have been established on a laboratory level (Foo et al. 2018). The resulting progenitor cell product must have high clinical applicability and reliability (Hashima et al. 2025).

Global Biopharma has assigned its development unit to develop new designs for the large-scale production of ventricular progenitor cells for cardiac cell therapy. The following objectives are included in the assignment:

- *Global Pharma* would like to have two production alternatives to consider for large-scale production.

C.-F. Mandenius, *Bioengineering Design Methodology*,
https://doi.org/10.1007/978-3-032-33940-9_10

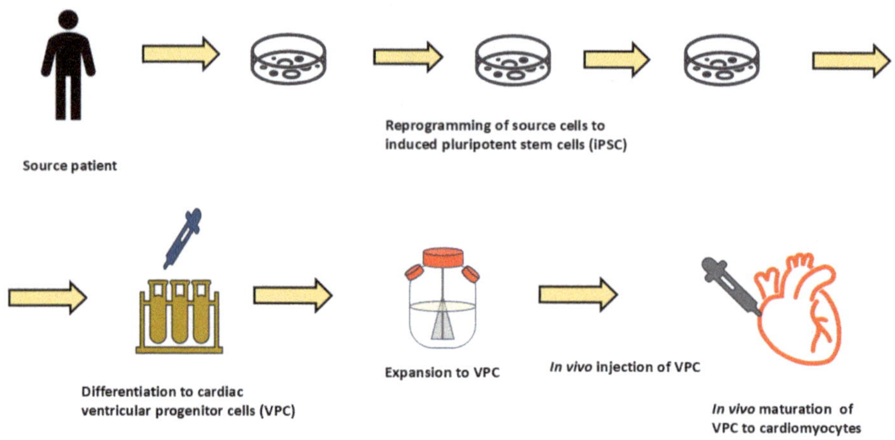

Fig. 10.1 Regenerative cardiac treatment using ventricular progenitor cells (VPC) from induced pluripotent stem cells (iPSC)

- The production alternatives after scaling up shall provide ventricular progenitor cells at low production costs. Both production alternatives should be convincingly evaluated in relation to their quality properties and volume production.
- The production alternatives are not expected to generate profit during the first 5 years. Instead, the objective is to enable *Global Pharma* to successfully enter a new pharma market sector before potential competitors.
- *Global Pharma's* expenditure for upfront R&D in regenerative medicine and stem cell research shall be included in the production costs of the design alternatives.

Global Pharma has assigned its development unit to develop new designs for the large-scale production of ventricular progenitor cells for cardiac cell therapy. The following objectives are included in the assignment:

- *Global Pharma* would like to have two production alternatives to consider for large-scale production.
- The production alternatives after scaling up shall provide ventricular progenitor cells at low production costs. Both production alternatives should be convincingly evaluated in relation to their quality properties and production volume.
- The production alternatives are not expected to generate profit during the first 5 years. Instead, the objective is to enable *Global Pharma* to successfully enter a new pharma market sector before potential competitors.
- *Global Pharma's* expenditure for upfront R&D in regenerative medicine and stem cell research shall be included in the production costs of the design alternatives.

A few caveats are added to the objectives by *Global Pharma*:

- Extended protection of intellectual property rights (IPR) is necessary to establish the proposed production methods. *Global Pharma's* own patent attorneys will carry out the filing of IPR at a cost of approximately 200 kEUR. This cost should be considered when comparing alternative design solutions.
- The production of progenitor cells should be possible to scale up in the suggested design alternatives.
- The cell production should cope with regulatory demands and validation requirements in these countries.
- The trainees may acquire goods such as culture media and factors, single-use equipment, and consumables through Global Pharma's internal procurement.

10.2 Training Scenario for the Assignment

The trainees are supposed to be allocated to an R&D unit of *Global Pharma* with responsibility for the company's R&D in cell and gene therapy and production development. In the training scenario, *Global Pharma* collaborates with external partners that *Global Pharma* subcontracts development of cell lines based on stem cell derivation and protocols, specialized processing equipment for cell culturing, and supply of culture media and other consumables.

- The trainees should preferably be composed of a team of individuals with backgrounds in cell biology, biopharmaceutical technology, process construction, and bioanalytical technology. The trainees should have experience in biochemical engineering through engineering school courses and/or vocational experience from similar industries. During the scenario training, they have access to process design software such as digitalized process design software, programs for economic evaluation, and software for process modelling and experimental design.
- *Global Pharma*'s own manufacturing and quality assurance expertise is made available for inquiries to specify needs and to establish realistic target values for the trainees.
- Internal cost factors for operational costs, including buildings and renting, are provided by *Global Pharma*. Labor costs are to be based on standard employment agreements and added to cost calculations as agreed with *Global Pharma.*
- The trainees' report to the *Drug Technologies* management on the progress and final reports. The results should be delivered orally and in written form. The typical time frame for the assignment is in the range of 3–4 months. This can be shortened if lower demand for reporting is expected. Deliverables should be concise and succinct and follow typical company standards (see also Sect. 4.4.7).

10.3 A Recommended Design Approach

10.3.1 Structuring the Assignment and Establishing User Requirements

Based on the conditions given in the assignment, it is recommended to investigate several conceptual approaches that can fulfill the conditions for establishing alternative production protocols. From the known background, it is conceived that *Global Pharma* wishes to carry out its business activity of the regenerative therapy product for cardiac treatment according to the overviewing scheme in Fig. 10.2. These conditions and constraints form the scenario of the actual training and should guide the design work in a structured manner and should focus on the following considerations:

- The assignment should exploit the potential of using human pluripotent embryonic stem cell systems for differentiation to human ventricular progenitor cells, where these allow further development and maturation into ventricular cardiomyocytes (Cabral et al. 2017; Stacey et al. 2022). The source of cells should be from internal or external cell banks where cell materials have been collected from stratified groups of donors representing the population to which the product is to be offered. Preferentially, this is a limited number of cell lines, assuming that an average cell type can be used for a wider group of patients. This will affect the scale of production substantially.
- The transformation of ventricular progenitor cells to mature cells occurs in the patient's heart tissues during the clinical treatment. Thus, the ex vivo production

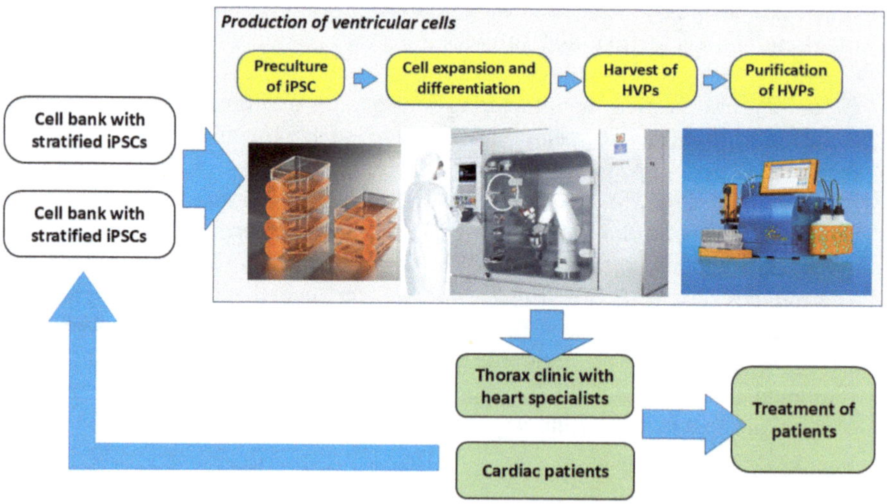

Fig. 10.2 Overview of the scenario of the assignment for Global Pharma's replacement therapy activities. The assignment involves primarily the production of the cell culture product (gray)

of induced pluripotent cells (iPSCs) to ventricular pluripotent cells is the core of the bioprocessing. However, the responsibility of *Global Pharma* primarily stops before that but will certainly be strongly connected to the outcome of the clinical treatment, being directly associated with the quality of the cell product and its potential market success.

- The ventricular progenitor cells to be employed shall be possible to characterize and monitor using current omics methods. This should include critical cell surface antigens (e.g., biomarkers such as TRA-1-60), and physiological parameters for cell growth and nutrient media consumption. These characterization procedures must be integrated into the production protocol.
- All alternative protocols for production developed in the design work should compare personnel intensity, environmental aspects, sustainability, energy demand, degree of automation, and contamination risks to ensure safe production of clinical materials, since these are most likely to be variable and determine total production costs and feasibility for production and scale-up.
- It should be possible to monitor the protocols to control productivity and quality along the production line and to ensure current Good Manufacturing Practice (cGMP). The typical means for this are bioanalytical methods with short delays for delivering results or responses. Imaging and digitalized methods seem like valuable resources for this. Sensor technology applicable online along the production line will be attractive for bioanalytics to use. Bioanalytical methods with high specificity and sensitivity will have a significant impact on monitoring performance.
- The apparent user needs should be compiled and finally compared versus the required functions from a conceptual perspective and, from that, generate alternative protocols.

Prioritized user needs and requirements expected from patients, clinicals and *Global Pharma's* production and marketing units can be identified by interviews with these user groups and stakeholders (Table 10.1). The needs include the medical and patient needs, important to integrate in the development of the design efforts. The needs can, as seen, be very different for patients and production, and there must be a compromise. As concluded in the priorities, the patients' and market needs mostly supersede the production requirements. This means that the designer must be able to find design solutions that can cope with such contradictory situations. Often, this may lead to more expensive production and consequently lower net income *for Global Pharma*. A cost-efficient design must therefore be accomplished.

With these preconditions and with *Global Pharma's* objectives and the established user needs, feasible design solutions can be established.

Initially, several functional requirements should be identified from the conceptual analysis that potentially could be realized with a variety of technical means. These include choice of media components, transcription factors, control methods, culture vessel formats, microcarriers for cells, preservation methods, cell separation and selection methods.

Table 10.1 User requirements and target specifications with priorities for the ventricular progenitor products

Requirement	Target specification	Priority
Patients and clinicians requirements		
Undifferentiated cells in progenitor product must be very low	Due to the sensitivity of some patient groups, a very low limit is set to 0.5%	Very high
Production must comply with regulations for cell therapies	Authority approvals after validation required before regular production	Very high
The sales price must be within ability of the global healthcare systems	The cost/treatment should not exceed 50 kEUR	High
Progenitor product must be preserved at customers	Freezing media and protocols for freezing/thawing provided to users	High
Global Pharma's market requirements		
Production must be considerably lower than sales price	<40% of sales first 5 years	Very high
The progenitor product quality must be able to promote sales	Five cardiac biomarkers (incl. ISL1) shall be in the quality control protocol	High
Production costs must be the lowest on the market to permit a low price	No other production should have a lower cost at the same quality	High
Global Pharma's production requirements		
The plant must have stable production of the progenitor product	The weekly progenitor production should be in the range 5–8 billion cells	Very high
Production plant should be automatized to ensure lower operation cost	>50% of unit operations must be automatized	Very high
Plant shall be a multiproduct plant	Diversified production with 20 different cell types must be done in the plant	Very high
Plant facilities must be safe for contamination	The plant shall have overpressure twice ambient pressure	Very high
The upstream cultivation should be perfectly controlled in terms of operation and cleanliness	Automatic monitoring and control shall be used. The milieu shall be sterile and adapted to room classification B	High
Products must comply with regulations for cell therapies	The plant shall be operated according to good manufacturing practice (GMP) and good laboratory practice (GLP)	High

Important issues for the generation of alternative protocols are to ensure the functional aspects in a conceptual manner. This could direct the therapy concept defined in the assignment, where the scope of the user requirements can be set. Defining the functional technical constraints in relation to the capacity to reach production targets then became decisive for finding the best alternatives. Hereby, the ranges of biological power are established that the stem cell system could endow to derived cardiac cell systems. In parallel, these ranges and constraints should be related to the economic degree of freedom to manufacture and sell the therapeutic cell product. Alternatives generated by this divergent approach should evaluate pros and cons of the alternatives based on priorities and rankings (convergent approach). In this, functionality of elements (cells, devices) becomes fundamental for the comparisons of the methods and protocol alternatives.

Established configurations of the manufacturing protocols should be compared and converged. Two protocols are recommended to be selected for detailed design using a commercial digital design tool such as SuperPro Designer (SPD) (www.intelligen.com; Heinzle et al. 2006; Harrison et al. 2003; Darkins and Mandenius 2014). Here, stem cell-related elements should be transformed into existing technical and biological objects. The digital tool may allow the designers to add estimates of the direct and indirect costs for development and operation of manufacturing. A rough estimation of costs for the two alternatives using inbuilt process economic parameters should be supported by external and updated costs. This evaluation should be used in a first sensitivity analysis, where the impact of price changes of equipment, consumables, and other direct costs was considered.

10.3.2 Conceptualization of the Assignment

Based on the analysis of requirements and target metrics, a conceptual map is developed that identifies the general functions needed for the transformation of iPSC to ventricular progenitors (Mandenius and Björkman 2011; Pahl et al. 2007; Hubka and Eder 1988; Ulrich et al. 2019). Each subsystem could be subdivided further into more specified functions (Fig. 10.3). The transformation process illuminates the basic preparatory, reactive, and finalizing stages required for the transformation of iPSC to progenitors. It opens up many alternative technical systems. The fact that cell culture engineering is going through a continuing development of new techniques makes it wise to be open to many state-of-the-art technologies, such as

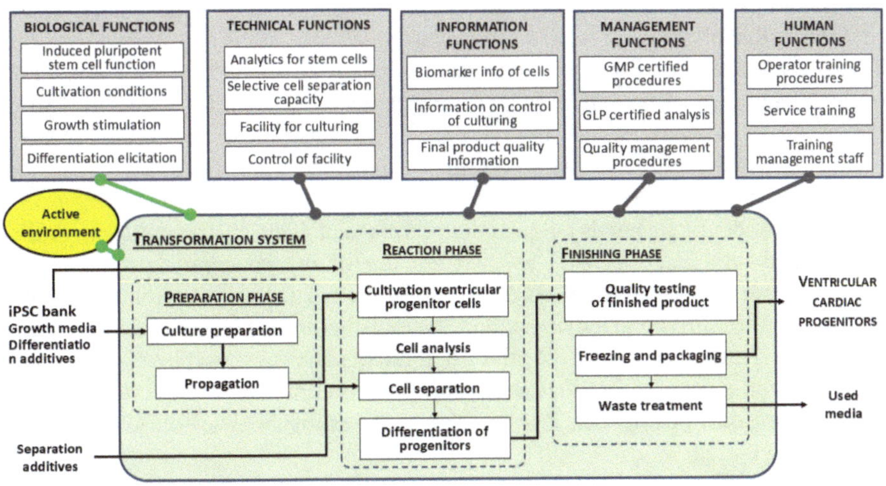

Fig. 10.3 Conceptualization of functions and transformation process for the production of cardiac ventricular cells from iPSC

compact bioreactors, robots for transfer of materials, novel cell separation techniques, and sensitive, cost-efficient analytics.

The map indicates where improvements and optimization possibilities should be sought. Several of the indicated steps in the phases or inputs could be considered, such as the composition of media components, the cultivation parameters in the propagation, differentiation, and expansion phases, and the procedure and additions in the formulation steps and freezing procedure.

The functions for effectuating the transformation are the most critical in the production process. As the figure shows, they concern growth and differentiation qualities, the functionality of the pluripotent cells, the possibility to invoke an effect on these parameters by composition of culture media and growth and differentiation factor compositions, and cell stability and interaction effects.

Once the most promising biological functions are found, a variety of technical functions and systems for realizing these functions should be identified. This includes culture containments, which will pave the way for culture vessels and containers for control functions. Ways to transport and transfer cells and liquids. Instrumentation for analytical methods that can deliver monitoring and quality data in due time for environmental control and quality assessment of cells. Functions for separating functional cells from undifferentiated cells or irrelevant cells and impurities. In the technical systems, robotics and automation technology are also included, specially designed for the purpose of the process.

The information functions are of utmost importance for the transformation process. The main objective must be to evaluate the cells' morphology and cardiac functionality. Here, numerous cell analytical methods are at hand. Here, biomarker information becomes highly important, which then will be connected to what kind of technical systems are required for analyzing these. Information about the cells and the separation conditions in the instrumentation is critical information.

It is obvious that functions for quality control and management have a key role in the production of progenitors for clinical use. Usually, total quality management (TQM) is an important issue for the manufacturing industry and is surely applicable to manufacturing cells, where TQM criteria can be identified and monitored likewise.

Finally, human resources, operators, and technicians' capabilities and their training are of utmost importance to consider.

From the identified needs of *Global Pharma* and their customers (i.e., cardiac patients and clinicians, as well as the structure of the conceptual map), several possible conceptual configurations can be conceived. The configuration can employ traditional cell cultivation practices and state-of-the-art cultivation and separation techniques. Automation and robotics to reduce manpower while also with the intention of improving reproducible handling seem attractive to exploit. If that is a cost-effective design solution, it is well worth investing in. The following alternatives are envisaged:

- Cell culture and cell separation in contained laboratories using conventional methods and equipment based on approved and validated protocols.

- Employing novel techniques, such as magnetic affinity cell separation (MACS), equipment and methods are used to process pluripotent cells downstream. Probably these will be expensive techniques, and labor is still demanding.
- Biomarkers for monitoring production are important to establish. In addition, the culture density and cell morphology also need to be controlled during cultivation. This is most easily done by microscopic analysis. Physical parameters measured in the surrounding medium, such as pH, lactate, and glucose, are required to confirm the cells' metabolism.
- Replacing the first alternative's conventional culture equipment with cultivation vessels or bioreactors that allow higher cell density-based 3D features realized within these devices.
- Combinations with the above options, where as many steps as possible are carried out by robotic machines programmed according to the same protocols and accurately validated. The purpose is obvious: to reduce labor with mechanics, increase capacity, and allow day-and-night production of cells.

The design will most likely include at least one variant of the robotic option. Here, the choice has been to go for conventional culturing but employing microcarrier cultures and the MACS technique and comparing this with a commercial robotic system.

10.3.3 Detailed Designs of Selected Alternatives

From the conceptual analysis, three perspectives should be considered when implementing detailed designs that comply with the assignment, its requirements from customers, and *Global Pharma's* production conditions:

- The quality and precision of the derivation of the ventricular cells.
- The regulatory requirements for this new kind of pharma product.
- The customer requirements when being provided with a personalized product.

A detailed design configuration of manually based production of the ventricular cells is one possible alternative (referred to as the *Manual Alternative*) (Fig. 10.4a). The production starts using iPSCs supplied from a cell bank established and maintained at *Global Pharma*. Cells are manually seeded, expanded, and differentiated in three steps. The procedures use sets of multiple T-flasks at volumes of 25 and 175 cm^3 placed in incubators with controlled gas composition and temperature. In the T-flasks, the cells grow until confluency. The confluent cells are harvested from the T-flasks and transferred to spinner flasks where cells are attached to porous microcarriers. The spinner flasks are also handled manually and maintained in incubators. The spinner flask cultivation proceeds in three steps, at 250 mL spinner-flask volume, which is transferred to 2 L spinner flasks, which subsequently are transferred to 4 L spinner flasks. The production proceeds in three steps in benchtop single-use bioreactors at 50, 100, and 200 L. This allows the process to reach a cell mass of ventricular cells close to the production-specified targeted amount.

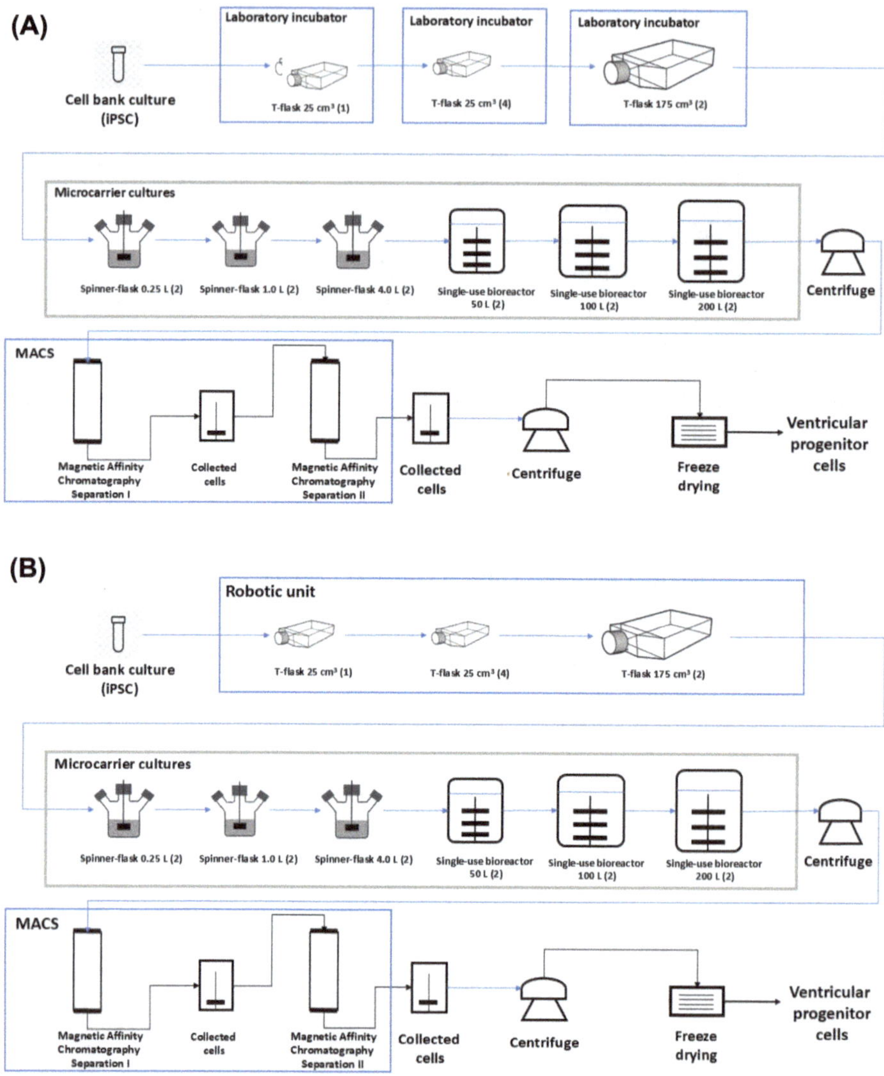

Fig. 10.4 (**a**) The design of pluripotent stem cell-based production of ventricular cardiac progenitor cells using the Manual Alternative. (**b**) The design of the production using robots in the Robotized Alternative

In the separation stage of the *Manual Alternative*, cells are recovered by conventional centrifugation. The effluent flow of the concentrated cells is subsequently transferred to a magnetic activated cell sorter (MACS) unit. The MACS separates the progenitors from non-differentiated cells. This is repeated twice to increase the yield of purified cells. The same MACS unit is reused with little time delay. In the last set of steps, cells are centrifuged and freeze-dried before delivery to the clinic. All the steps and units can be implemented on CAD software with unit procedures created from generic boxes, including influent and effluent flows and sub-procedures (Darkins and Mandenius 2014).

The procedures in each flask encompass (1) thawing of iPSCs, (2) preculture, (3) cell differentiation and expansion, (4) harvesting, and (5) purification and freezing. These procedures are all manually performed by trained technicians according to defined protocols and quality analytics.

In a robotized design, as many as possible of the steps in the manual production should be replaced by robots (in the following referred to as the *Robotized Alternative*) (Fig. 10.4b). The first steps of cultivation take place in T-flasks procedures as in the *Manual Alternative* in terms of size, concentrations, and cell densities. However, in the *Robotized Alternative,* the filling, capsulations, movements, and emptying of the T-flasks are completely robotized using grip tools, controlled pumps, and valves (Fig. 10.2). Examples of convenient robotic systems for cell culturing have recently been developed (Conway et al. 2015; Ochs et al. 2022; Mathew et al. 2022; Melocchi et al. 2024). Robotics also allows operation of desktop bioreactors. As in the manual alternative, the *Robotized Alternative* covers the five phases: (1) thawing of iPSCs, (2) preculture, (3) cell differentiation and expansion, (4) harvesting, and (5) purification and freezing, although implemented with robotic procedures.

The type of robotic systems mentioned for the T-flasks is also possible to consider for the spinner flasks. For the disposable single-use bioreactors, a robotic system is developed where still some manual steps remain, such as exchange of culture bags and harvesting of these bags.

The subsequent production in the *Robotized Alternative* is similar to the steps in the *Manual Alternative*. Thus, cells from the final single-use bioreactor are centrifuged and separated twice in a MACS system. Purified functional ventricular cells are collected and concentrated by centrifugation. The centrifugate is freeze-dried and transferred to storage until delivery to a clinic for treatment of cardiac patients.

10.3.4 Production Economic Evaluation of the Detailed Designs

The aim of the economic evaluation is to elucidate where the highest costs are generated in the design alternatives and if the objectives of the assignment to the development unit are financially sound and compatible with a realistic net income of the product (Peters et al. 2003; Kristiansen 2006; Ray et al. 2022; Petrides 2015; SuperPro Designer 2025). The economic evaluation should provide answers to the following questions:

- Can the substantial investment required for an advanced, robotized production facility be offset by forecasted sales and long-term market share?

- Are there alternative configurations that reduce capital or operational burdens without compromising the biological quality or therapeutic efficacy of the progenitor cells?
- To what extent can bioengineering methodologies (e.g., process intensification or optimized media formulations) maximize yield to improve the net income of the VPC product?

The economic evaluation is based on an annual production of ventricular cardiac stem cells for 5000 cardiac patients.

The production costs for the alternatives differ slightly (Table 10.2). For the *Manual Alternative*, the investment costs for the production equipment are estimated to be 1320 kEUR, while for the *Robotized Alternative* the investment costs rise to 3110 kEUR including installations and other additional costs. The higher investment costs are due to the purchase costs and the installation of the expensive robotic machines (Conway et al. 2015) and the sequential single-use bioreactors for cell expansion. Thus, robotic equipment increases the investment needs more than twice.

Although the single-use bioreactor units have a relatively lower initial investment cost, they generate high expenditures for disposable culture bags.

For the separation of expanded cells, several cost items remain the same in both alternatives. This includes the required process analytics.

The upfront development costs are included in the investments since they are supposed to be one-time costs. In this case, it is assumed that robotic design requires both a high internal R&D effort and externally subcontracted R&D for adapting the culture protocol to the robotic procedure. This is also supposed to increase the initial cost for IPR protection of the unique production process.

Standard cost approximations for installation and building a new plant are added to the investment costs.

It is assumed that the *Robotized Alternative* requires plant area but has higher costs for installation and validation than the *Manual Alternative.*

The operational costs cover a variety of consumables such as culture flasks, culture media, differentiation additives, antibodies for analytics, microcarriers for cell separation (e.g., MACS Microbeads), and other materials and chemicals necessary for culturing ventricular progenitor cells. For the *Manual Alternative*, this amounts to 800 kEUR per year and for the *Robotized Alternative* to 1900 kEUR per year.

The small difference is due to less labor costs for the *Robotized Alternative*, which is supposed to save labor due to the automatic procedures. However, this does not substantially influence the total operational cost as might have been expected. Robotic systems still need continuous surveillance and support. The benefit is instead mainly a quality assurance issue.

In the table are added cost items for renting buildings, maintenance during operation, annual fees for user rights, and local taxes. These costs are set according to standard costs commonly applied in chemical production.

The total annual production costs for the *Manual Alternative* excluding investments are 1340 kEUR. An annual payoff during a 5-year period is added to the total

Table 10.2 Investment and operational costs for the automated production of cardiac cells

Type of costs	Manual alternative (kEUR)	Robotized alternative (kEUR)
Investment costs		
Upfront production R&D		
External R&D (stem cell research)	300	600
External R&D	300	500
Internal R&D	500	600
Total upfront production R&D	*1100*	*1700*
Equipment for production		
Robotic system (centrifuges)	–	1000
Cultivation (bioreactors, tanks)	100	100
Separation (MACS, lyophilizer)	100	100
Standard lab equipment	100	100
Total equipment for production	*800*	*1900*
Other costs for the production plant		
Validation of new robotic plant		300
Installation of equipment (×0.5)	400	950
Taxation (×0.1)	80	190
Buildings for production (×0.3)	240	570
Total additionalproduction costs	720	2010
Total investment costs	**1320**	**5610**
Operational costs (annual per targeted production volume)		
Consumables for production		
Consumables downstream	200	200
Consumables upstream	150	150
Consumables for quality control	80	80
Total consumables for production	*430*	*430*
Additional operational expenditures		
Labor production facilities (incl. Quality control)	300	150
Renting of buildings	70	70
Taxation	10	10
Annual IPR expenditures	60	60
Maintenance of plant	50	70
Management	150	150
Total additional operation expenditure	*640*	*510*
Total operational costs	**1070**	**940**
Annual payoff of investment costs (5 years)	*264*	*1122*
Total annual production cost	1334	2062
Relative difference between alternatives	100%	155%

annual cost of 1604 kEUR. Thus, the payoff cost is, as expected, low due to modest investments.

For the *Robotized Alternative*, the production cost per year is 1210 kEUR, and if a 5-year payoff is added, 1832 kEUR. Thus, although the plant investments are significant in robotic systems, the total annual amount is about the same, with the set payoff time.

From a business perspective, the alternatives are almost equal. What favors robotic design is the quality assurance aspect, being easier to control and validate. Probably the *Robotic Alternative* can be scaled up more easily to accommodate a higher throughput for more patients. And after the payback of the investments, the net income rises in the *Robotic Alternative* due to lower operational costs. A high net income is favored in the *Robotic Alternative*, which will allow *Global Pharma* to set lower pricing and improve competitiveness.

To further illuminate the production cost for the two alternatives, the circular diagram below shows the percentage of the critical costs (Fig. 10.5). The diagrams show that investments have a decisive role in the cost distribution. It highlights that it is important to correctly assess the cost of advanced robotic equipment purchase and MACS and wisely select the appropriate devices for the set production objectives. Certainly, the depreciation time is an important regulator of annual costs, a time that, for a wealthy company, can be extended.

Finally, the net income for the product must be compromised with its competitiveness. A production design that allows a cost-effective upscaling will favor this.

10.3.5 Optimization of Manual or Robotized Production

Following the prioritization of the design alternatives, a focused optimization of critical parameters is necessary to maximize productivity. The susceptibility of these parameters to refinement may vary; for instance, a highly standardized robotic process may offer different optimization margins compared to more flexible manual or semiautomated systems.

To navigate these interdependencies, several established methodologies can be employed (Sioshansi and Conejo 2017; Martins and Ning 2021). Table 10.3 outlines the target objects for optimization, the applicable techniques, and their projected impact on outcomes.

The overarching objective in *Global Pharma's* assignment is to enhance yield and throughput while minimizing resource consumption and processing time, each of which directly strengthens the production economy. Given the company's specific objectives, factorial design or design of experiments (DoE) is particularly well-suited for this scenario due to its ability to evaluate multiple variables and their interactions simultaneously. But, as also mentioned in the table, mechanistic modelling can be very useful for certain optimization tasks.

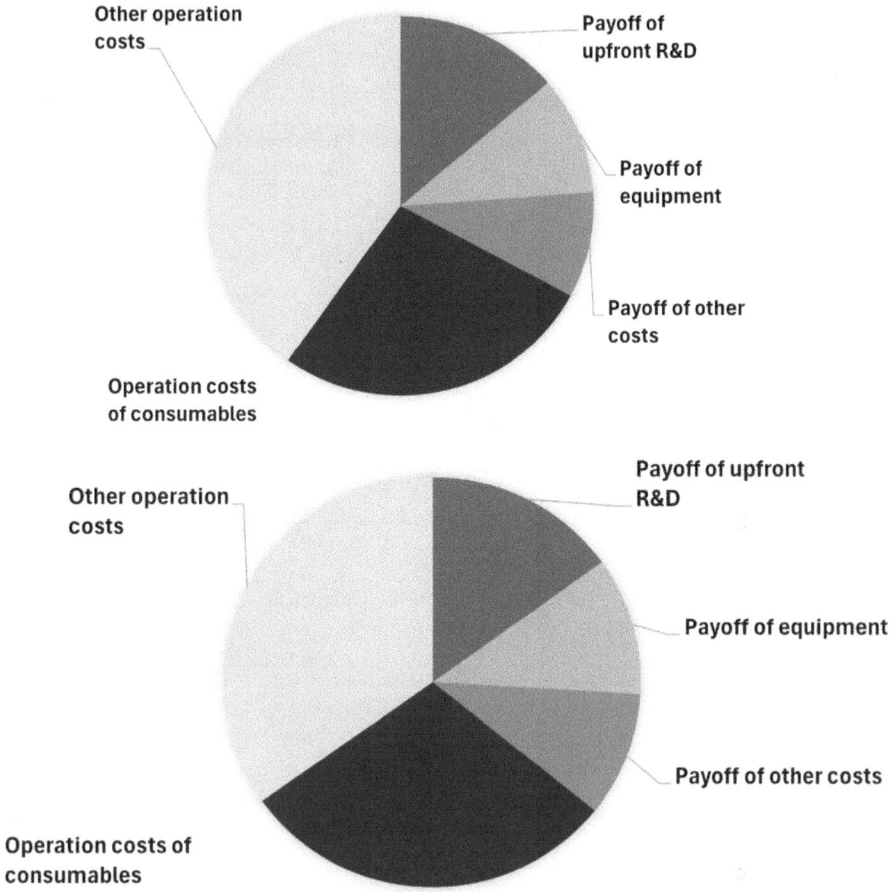

Fig. 10.5 The distribution of investments, operation, upfront R&D, and payback costs for the Manual Alternative and Robotized Alternative

Optimization of the Progenitor Production by Design of Experiments For the manual and robotic alternatives to work optimally, design of experiments (DoE) should be used after investigating which factors affect the final product (Brereton 2003; Montgomery 2020). This is carried out with factor experiments where each individual factor is investigated by experiments at different levels and measuring changes of relevant responses. In cases where two or more factors are examined, a response surface is calculated, where optimal values of the factors appear. In cases with one factor, a diagram is drawn showing the optimal level (cf. Chap. 3). Three levels for each factor with two measurements per level result in representative data that can then be analyzed further.

Several DoE options can be considered (Table 10.4). For example, pre-cultivation is a critical step where it is recommended that the factors (temperature and amount of

Table 10.3 Objects of relevance to investigate for optimizing production of ventricular cells

Object of optimization	Expected outcome	Applicable optimization technique
Media composition in T-flasks and spinner flasks	Increase in specific expansion and differentiation rate	Factorial design of media components and differentiation factors
Culture parameters in the flasks and single-use bioreactors	Increased proliferation rates of cells	Factorial design of controllable parameters such as time, oxygen and temperature
Conditions for differentiation	Improved differentiation and yield for ventricular progenitors	Factorial design of decisive parameters as above
Scheduling of the nine steps	Shorter total time of production of cells	Mechanistic modelling for time to confluency
Centrifugal properties	Separation yield and degradation of expanded cells	Factorial design of speed and flow
Parameters in the MACS procedures	Efficiency of cell separation	Advanced mechanistic modelling

Table 10.4 DoE plan for optimized selected parameters in the production of ventricular cells

Optimization object	Factors in DoE plan	Responses to measure
Proliferation in flasks and spinners	Temperature, pH, media components	Cell density, temperature, pH Ambr, FACS
Bioreactor	Temperature pH, aeration rate	Cell density, temperature, pH Ambr, FACS
Centrifugal recovery	Rotation speed, flow, radius	Yield viability FACS, patch clamp
Cell separation in MACS	Beads, flow rate	Yield FACS
Freezing performance	Freezing medium, temperature, freezing time	Viability, cell number Patch clamp, FACS

nutrients in media) be optimized and where the response (e.g., number of cells) should be increased. As previously mentioned, two observations per level/combination can be conducted, generating a total of 18 different experiments.

Data could be collected with commercial robots (e.g., Ambr™ Microbioreactor, www.sartorius.com) and fluorescence-activated cell sorting (FACS) instruments (e.g., FACS Aria III Cell Sorter, bdbioscence.com). A response surface can be derived from the DoE data. The main difference between the *Manual Alternative* and *Robotized Alternative* is the cell cultivation operation (bioreactor or culture flasks), while other parameters are equivalent. Consequently, only in the bioreactor can the oxygenation flow be modulated.

Mechanistic Modelling for Progenitor Production Mechanistic modelling can help in scheduling the complex multi-stage cell expansion procedures. A mechanistic model that describes the kinetics of the cells should include time, volume, cell concentration, and specific growth rate in time-dependent differential equations (Nielsen et al. 2011). In simulations using the model, starting values and values of various parameters can easily be tested.

The propagation of cells is in the detailed robotic and manual designs carried out from the cell bank vials with iPSC vials transferred to T-flasks, spinner flasks, and single-use bioreactors. The conditions in the vessels can be simulated using the model of Eqs. 10.1–10.5:

$$\mu_{\mathrm{PSC}} = \mu_{\mathrm{PCS\text{-}max}} \cdot S_{\mathrm{media}} \cdot (S_{\mathrm{media}} + K_{\mathrm{S}}) \tag{10.1}$$

$$\mathrm{d}N_{\mathrm{PSC}}/\mathrm{d}t = \mu_{\mathrm{PSC}} \cdot N_{\mathrm{PSC}} \tag{10.2}$$

$$\mathrm{d}S_{\mathrm{media}}/\mathrm{d}t = -\mu_{\mathrm{PSC}}/Y_{\mathrm{NS}} \cdot N_{\mathrm{PSC}} \tag{10.3}$$

$$n_{\mathrm{PSC}} = V_{\mathrm{vessel}} \cdot N_{\mathrm{PSC}} \tag{10.4}$$

$$\text{if } n_{\mathrm{PSC}} > (A \times \text{Confluence}) \text{ then } \mu_{\mathrm{PCS\text{-}max}} = 0 \tag{10.5}$$

where N_{PSC} is the concentration of PSC in the vessel, V_{vessel} the nominal volume of the vessel, μ_{PSC} the varying propagation rate of the PSC, $\mu_{\mathrm{PSC\text{-}max}}$ the maximal propagation rate of the PSC on the support (T-flask surface or microcarrier), S_{media} the concentration of the media based on the limiting components; K_{S}, the saturation constant for the media; Y_{NS}, the yield of PSC from the media; n_{PSC}, the number of PSC in supporting interface of the vessel (plastic surface, microcarrier); *confluence*, the number of cells at confluency in the vessel; and A, the area of surface/interface of the vessel. The values for confluency and surface areas are usually available from suppliers.

For example, PSC in a vial from a cell bank may have a concentration of one million cells/ml, and PSC growth rate can be in the order of 0.018 to 0.022 h^{-1}.

Primarily, the model can be used to estimate the propagation of PSC after transfer of a vial of cells to the T-flask. Of special interest is to estimate the time for the cells to propagate to confluency depending on the number of seeded cells, the T-flask's volume and area for cell attachment, and the cells' propagation rate. Simulations can be divided into different stages in the process, for example from vial to T25-flask (Fig. 10.6a) and for transfer from T25-flask to 175-flask (Fig. 10.6b).

In the propagation stages carried out in spinner flasks with microcarriers, the amount of microcarriers and the bead cell loading limit need to be given in the model. The number of cells transferred from the T-flask to the spinner flask can be compared, and the volume of the spinner flask and the amount of microcarrier in the spinner flask can be investigated in simulations (Fig. 10.6c). There are limits to how many microcarriers can be contained in a vessel, which depends on size and type.

The propagation rate in microcarriers will change depending on the loading of cells. The model equations can be supplied with parameters to compensate for that and reduce the rate when confluence or high cell density is close.

Finally, the propagation of PSC on microcarriers in the single-use bioreactor can be investigated (Fig. 10.6d). The same model equations are useful where the vessel

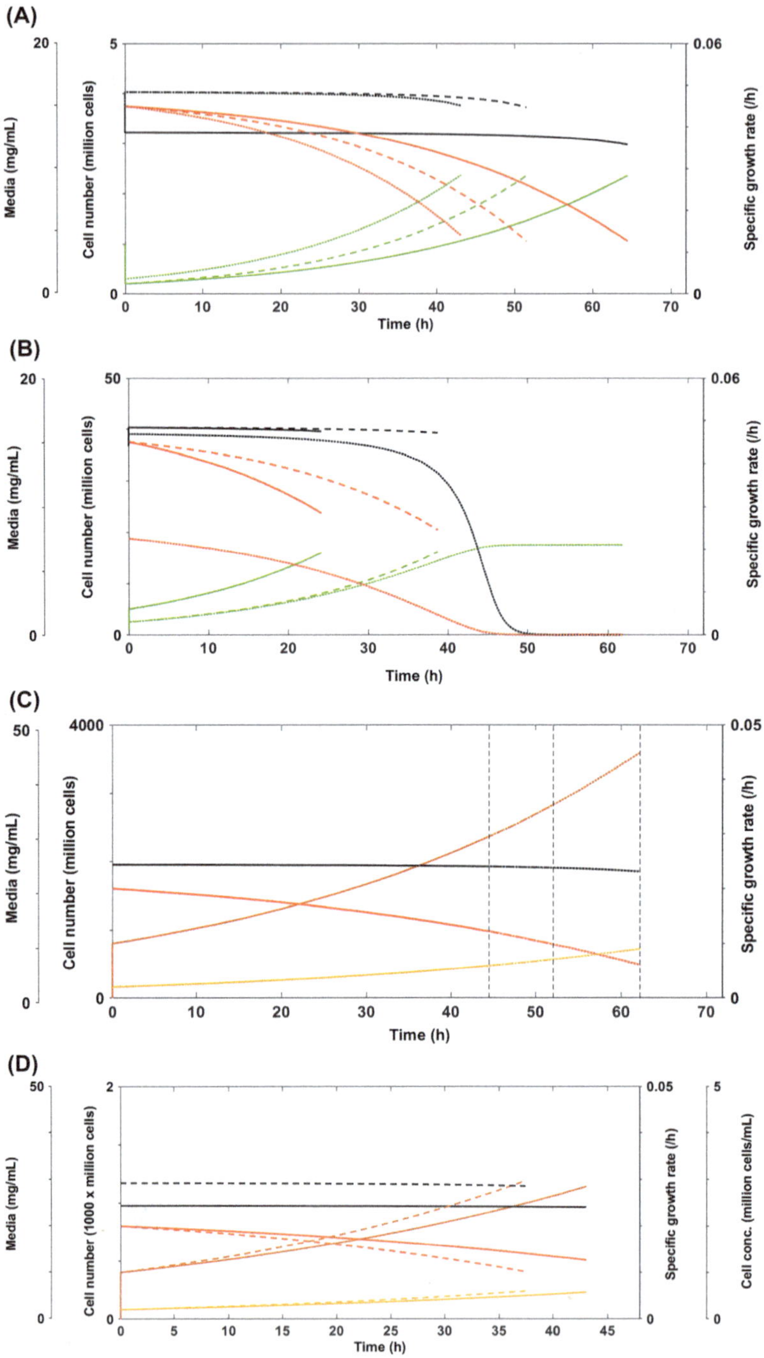

Fig. 10.6 (**a**) Seed vial to T-25 flask. Three conditions are shown: (i) $\mu = 0{,}040\ h^{-1}$; seed 200,000 cells (line plots); (ii) $\mu = 0.050$; seed 20,000 cells (dashed plots); (iii) $\mu = 0.050$; 300,000 cells (dotted plots). (**b**) T-25 flask to T-175 flask. Three conditions are shown: (i) $\mu = 0.040$, seed five million cells, media 15 g/L (line plots); $\mu = 0.040$, seed 2.5 million cells, media 15 g/L (dashed plots); $\mu = 0.040$, seed 2.5 million cells, media 7.5 g/L (dotted plots). (**c**) Spinner flask culture with microcarriers having 0.2, 0.25, and 0.3 mill/cm^2 confluence. (**d**) Single-use bioreactor with microcarriers and PSC with two growth rates and yields

volume is scaled up to 200 L, as in the manual and robotized designs above. At this stage, variation in propagation rate, yields, and potential results from DoE investigations can be tried.

The four diagrams illustrate a few possibilities to use mechanistic models in the assignment. Certainly, equations can be adapted to specific demands and other intended purposes. This could be to reduce the number of stages in the propagation train, shorten the processing time, and show the potential of optimizing the culture media for better propagation and use of the usually quite expensive media components.

10.4 Conclusive Suggestions for *Global Pharma*

Two design alternatives suggested for this assignment are similar in several of the steps from a biological perspective. However, in the *Manual Alternative*, cells are initially grown on culture plates followed by culture flasks, while in the *Robotized Alternative*, robotically handled culture flasks are used. Both alternatives are assumed to have the same production capacity (5–8 billion ventricular progenitors per week), as required in the assignment.

The advantages and disadvantages of the two alternatives can be summarized as:

- The process steps in the cell selection operations are almost the same in both alternatives and scaled up linearly to reach the targeted production capacity.
- For scale-up of the pre-cultivation and differentiation stages, the *Manual Alternative* requires a larger number of pre-cultivation bottles and culture flasks, or larger volumes of each vessel. The *Robotized Alternative* has the advantage of the robotic procedure with higher throughput. This requires additional investment in equipment and installation.
- Economically, the *Manual Alternative* has the advantage of a lower investment cost and consequently requires less risk capital. However, given the prospect of the technology and estimated market, the risk might be worth taking for *Global Pharma*.
- The *Manual Alternative* has a lower operational cost. This may initially allow a competitive sale price.
- The *Robotized Alternative* would benefit from optimization of costs, for example, by reducing labor costs and increasing the throughput of cells.

To the above, it can be added that the highly automated and controlled *Robotized Alternative* reduces the risk of contamination and ensures better quality while requiring more frequent maintenance and repair of systems, which interrupts production. The recommended single-use bioreactor system (e.g., Xcellerex™ X-platform, www.cytivalivescience.com) is not expected to compromise these advantages.

Based on these premises, and its compliance with the assignment objectives and user requirements, *Global Pharma* is recommended to implement the *Robotic Alternative*.

Additional suggestions to *Global Pharma* with potential for enhanced production in the *Robotized Alternative* are:

- To consider redesigning the robotic system further with newer technology such as online sensors and control of the environment.
- To reduce the cultivation time to 2 days per round and batch, which can be seen in simulations (cf. simulation diagrams). The suggestion is valid for both alternatives.
- To optimize MACS cell separation and its use of microbeads, due to its significant effect on capacity and economy. Also, this suggestion is valid for both alternatives.
- To optimize the cell purification to reduce the loss of ventricular cardiac progenitors, by using reprocessing loops in combination with improved process analytics.

10.5 Tutorial Perspectives on the Assignment

The challenge of this assignment is that it concerns a bioproduction that cannot lean much on proven bioprocess design. This results in several questions and hurdles that need attention and are not always easy to provide good answers to:

- In this design training, it is important to pass the conceptual stage relatively shortly and continue to outline the potential solutions using available means for production. The risk is to become too theoretical. Better is to return to the conceptualization structure and reiterate solutions.
- The quantity of cells produced from the starting materials is low (i.e., a straw from a cell bank), sometimes intended just for one personalized treatment. The need for advancing quality control becomes more demanding than in conventional production of biologics.
- A hurdle is to acquire experimental data where only limited access to published data is available. Reasoning on optimization (e.g., DoE) may, in a short perspective, facilitate this, both on a factual and psychological level by structuring biological and process parameters in a DoE plan (cf. Mandenius and Brundin 2008).
- A threshold will be to collect meaningful information on costs and to judge how cost may change under various conditions.
- Another vital issue in the training is to appreciate the potential for improvement in the biological systems for alternative designs. For example, how can novel findings on the efficiency of the cell lines' capacity alter the outcome of the productivity? The access to modelling tools (e.g., kinetic models in MATLAB or

others) could relatively easily outline such impacts, both on productivity and manufacturing costs.

- Another difficulty will be to apprehend the impact of upfront costs, and how to allocate these into the regular production costs. In this assignment, a difficulty is making use of external development assets and how such could alter the outcome of costs. A way to approach this in the training could be to introduce a sub-scenario where external partners could be involved.

The training must adapt to these issues and provide reasonably good background information, preferably from industrial expertise. Consequently, the tutorial actions need to focus on monitoring the progress of the trainees in around directions and appropriately push them into design work leading to seeing these possibilities.

References

Bissoli I, D'Adamo S, Pignatti C et al (2023) Induced pluripotent stem cell-based models: are we ready for that heart in a dish? Front Cell Dev Biol 11:1129263. https://doi.org/10.3389/fcell.2023.1129263

Brereton RG (2003) Chemometrics, data analysis for laboratory and chemical plants. Wiley, Chichester

Cabral J, Da Silva CL, Chase LG et al (eds) (2017) Stem cell manufacturing. Elsevier, Amsterdam

Chien et al (2012) Ventricular induced pluripotent stem (VIPS) cells for generation of autologous ventricular cardiomyocytes and use thereof. (Boston Hospital). US Patent Application 2012/0009158 A1

Conway MK, Gerger MJ, Baley EE et al (2015) Scalable 96-well plate-based iPSC culture and production using a robotic liquid handling system. J Vis Exp 99:e52755. https://doi.org/10.3791/52755

Darkins CL, Mandenius CF (2014) Design of large-scale manufacturing of induced pluripotent stem cell derived cardiomyocytes. Chem Eng Res Design 92:1142–1152. https://doi.org/10.1016/j.cherd.2013.08.021

Eschenhagen T, Weinberger F (2024) Challenges and perspectives of heart repair with pluripotent stem cell-derived cardiomyocytes. Nat Cardiovasc Res 3:515–524. https://doi.org/10.1038/s44161-024-00472-6

Foo KS, Lehtinen ML, Leung CY et al (2018) Human ISL1+ ventricular progenitors self-assemble into an in vivo functional heart patch and preserve cardiac function post infarction. Mol Ther 26: 1644–1959. https://doi.org/10.1016/j.ymthe.2018.02.012

Hammond et al (2019) Compositions and methods for the treatment or prevention of heart failure. (Univ Calif) US Patent Application 2019/0264189 A1

Harrison R, Tood P, Rudge S et al (2003) Bioseparation science and engineering. Oxford University Press, New York

Hashima M, Finklea FB, Hammons H et al (2025) Hydrogel microsphere stem cell encapsulation enhances cardiomyocyte differentiation and functionality in scalable suspension system. Bioact Mater 43:423–440. https://doi.org/10.1016/j.bioactmat.2024.08.043

Heinzle E, Biwer A, Cooney C (2006) Development of sustainable bioprocesses. Modelling and assessment. John Wiley & Sons, Chichester. https://doi.org/10.1002/9780470058916

Hubka V, Eder WE (1988) Theory of technical systems, a total concept theory for engineering design. Springer Verlag, Berlin

Kristiansen B (2006) Process economics. In: Ratledge C, Kristiansen B (eds) Basic biotechnology, 3rd edn. Cambridge University Press, Cambridge, pp 239–252

Lin Z, Pu WT (2014) Strategies for cardiac regeneration and repair. Sci Transl Med 6:239rv1. https://doi.org/10.1126/scitranslmed.3006681

Mandenius CF, Björkman M (2011) Biomechatronic design in biotechnology: a methodology for development of biotechnology products. John Wiley & Sons, New Jersey. https://doi.org/10.1002/9781118067147

Mandenius CF, Brundin A (2008) Bioprocess optimization using design-of-experiments methodology. Biotechnol Prog 24:1191–1203. https://doi.org/10.1002/btpr.67

Manstein F, Ullmann K, Triebert W et al (2021) Process control and *in silico* modeling strategies for enabling high density culture of human pluripotent stem cells in stirred tank bioreactors. STAR Protocols 2:100988. https://doi.org/10.1016/j.xpro.2021.100988

Martins JRRA, Ning A (2021) Engineering design optimization. Cambridge University Press, Cambridge. https://doi.org/10.1017/9781108980647

Mathew R, McGee R, Roche K et al (2022) Introducing mobile collaborative robots into bioprocessing environments: personalized drug manufacturing and environmental monitoring. Appl Sci 12:10895. https://doi.org/10.3390/app122110895

Melocchi A, Schmittlein B, Jones AL et al (2024) Development of a robotic cluster for automated and scalable cell therapy manufacturing. Cytotherapy 26:1095–1104. https://doi.org/10.1016/j.jcyt.2024.03.010

Montgomery DC (2020) Design and analysis of experiments, 9th edn. John Wiley & Sons, New York. ISBN: 978-1-119-63842-1

Nielsen J, Villadsen J, Lidén G (2011) Bioreaction engineering principles, 3rd edn. Springer-Nature, New York

Ochs J, Hanga MP, Shaw G et al (2022) Needle to needle robot-assisted manufacture of cell therapy products. Bioeng Transl Med 7:e10387. https://doi.org/10.1002/btm2.10387

Pahl G, Beitz W, Feldhusen J et al (2007) Engineering design, a systematic approach, 3rd edn. Springer Verlag, Berlin

Park et al (2025) Method for purification and production of ventricular cardiomyocytes (Biofab Co Ltd) Korean Patent Application WO 2025/063371

Peters MS, Timmerhaus KD, West RE (2003) Plant design and economics for chemical engineers, 5th edn. McGraw-Hill, New York

Petrides D (2015) Bioprocess design and economics. In: Harrison RG, Todd P, Rudge SR et al (eds) Bioseparations science and engineering, 2nd edn. Oxford University Press, New York, pp 441–510. https://doi.org/10.1093/oso/9780195391817.001.0001

Ray SC, Chambers RG, Kumbhakar SC (2022) Handbook of production economics. Springer Nature, New York

Saito Y, Nakamura K, Katanosaka Y et al (2025) Specific induction of right ventricular-like cardiomyocytes from human pluripotent stem cells. Stem Cell Res Ther 16:519. https://doi.org/10.1186/s13287-025-04656-0

Sioshansi R, Conejo AJ (2017) Optimization in engineering, models and algorithms. Springer International Publishing, Germany. ISBN 9783319567679

Stacey GN, Cao J, Hu B et al (2022) Manufacturing with pluripotent stem cells: key issues for future research and development. Cell Prolif 55:e13301. https://doi.org/10.1111/cpr.13301

SuperPro Designer (2025) Overview of software. Student version. www.intelligen.com (retrieved Oct 2025)

Ulrich KT, Eppinger SD, Yang MC (2019) Product design and development, 7th edn. McGraw-Hill, New York

Chapter 11
Case 6: Cultured Meat as Novel Food Supply

11.1 Assignment: Background, Description, and Objectives

The aim of this assignment is to develop a new food product that is manufactured in a biotechnical production process, where the main starting material is tissue cells derived from bovine stem cells (Choi et al. 2021). The specific aim of the training is to design a cost-efficient bioprocess for safe large-scale production in commercial quantities as a novel commodity food product (Post 2012).

The aim of this assignment is to develop a new food product that is manufactured in a biotechnical production process where the main starting material is tissue cells derived from bovine stem cells (Choi et al. 2021). The specific aim of the training is to design a cost-efficient and safe large-scale production in commercial quantities as a novel commodity food product (Post 2012).

The assigner is a private startup company, *Food Bioentrepreneurs*, with the ambition to develop and produce alternative food products. Recently, they have specialized in cultured meat because of its ethical and environmental benefits (Nihashi et al. 2019). *Food Bioentrepreneurs* consider starting up production using stem cells from bovine cell sources (myoblasts) (Lindsay et al. 2019). *Food Bioentrepreneurs'* goal is to scale up the production of the product to an economically feasible process using unique 3D bioprinting technology (Boudreault et al. 2001; Bodiou et al. 2020) (Fig. 11.1).

A prerequisite is that the myoblast cells must grow on or inside a matrix that mimics the muscle tissues. If the matrix is edible, the process can be simplified at a lower cost than if the cells must be dissociated from the matrix. Currently, manufacturers of lab-grown meat use microparticles as matrices in standard batch or fed-batch bioreactor systems (Piola et al. 2013). The cells grow on the microparticles, often consisting of collagen, dextran, silicon, or polystyrene. The approach has disadvantages; the cells grow only on the surface of the particles, and the microparticles are not edible (Bodiou et al. 2020).

C.-F. Mandenius, *Bioengineering Design Methodology*,
https://doi.org/10.1007/978-3-032-33940-9_11

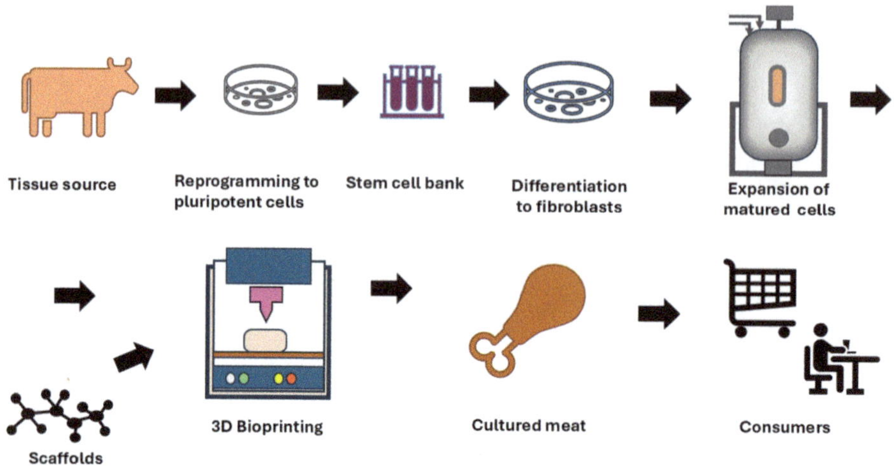

Fig. 11.1 Steps in preparation and manufacture of cultured meat from bovine stem cells. The procedure exploits 3D bioprinted cells in biopolymeric scaffolds

Food Bioentrepreneurs have therefore decided to develop a 3D structure support for the cells that can be manufactured by a bioprinting technique (Guo et al. 2024). Bioprinting exploits 3D printing techniques with biologically derived hydrogels. This so-called bioink is extruded in multilayers with the desired shape and size using special injector devices.

Food Bioentrepreneurs have developed a patent-protected bioink which encapsulates myoblast cells, and two edible hydrogels: hyaluronic acid (HA) and xanthan gum (XG) (Ferreira et al. 2021). Both biopolymers can be produced separately by recombinant bacterial strains. The bioink can be 3D printed into 50–300 μm thin wire-like structures that are perfused by culture media, allowing the myoblasts to grow to a dense meat-like product. The company wishes to optimize the geometry (size and shape) of the printed structures as well as the cultivation conditions in the bioreactor during production.

Food Bioentrepreneurs has the following specified objectives for the assignment:

- Develop a cost-efficient and competitive production process for the cultured bioprinted myoblast product where the patent-protected hydrogel structure is exploited.
- The myoblasts shall be produced from derived bovine stem cells using low-cost culture media.
- To achieve high productivity, the production time must be limited to less than 10 days per batch.
- The design shall ensure Current Good Manufacturing Practice (GMP) for novel food technology.
- The annual production volume of a scaled-up production shall initially reach 5 tons of the cultured meat product. In the second phase, the production volume is expected to increase to 80 tons per year.

- The cost of production, including payback of investments in the manufacturing process, must be less than 50% of the estimated sales price of the cultured meat product.
- *Food Bioentrepreneurs* expects investments to be fully paid back within 5 years.

Food Bioentrepreneurs has the following specific caveats for the assignment:

- The design should included a small-scale test plant aimed at regulatory evaluation of the production. This is motivated by the novelty of cultured meat for which a rigorous regulatory assessment is anticipated.
- Intellectual property rights (IPR) should ensure exclusive access to the production method. The filing and annual costs of the IPR should not exceed 5% of the total investment cost.
- *Food Bioentrepreneurs* accesses user rights to recombinant bacterial strains for production of HA and XG.
- Subcontractors for cell line development, cell line purchase, and procurement of specialized bioprocess equipment could be considered. Costs for such subcontracting should be estimated.

Food Bioentrepreneurs has the following specific caveats for the assignment:

- *Food Bioentrepreneurs* includes design of a small-scale test plant in the assignment, aimed at regulatory evaluation of the production. This is motivated by the novelty of cultured meat, for which a rigorous regulatory assessment is anticipated.
- Intellectual property rights (IPR) must ensure exclusive access to the production method. The filing and annual costs of the IPR are expected to remain under 5% of the total investment cost.
- *Food Bioentrepreneurs* accesses user rights to recombinant bacterial strains for production of hyaluronic acid (HA) and xanthan gum (XG).
- Subcontractors for cell line development, cell line purchase, and procurement of specialized bioprocess equipment could be considered. Costs for such subcontracting must be estimated.

11.2 Training Scenario for the Assignment

The scenario for the trainees is the following:

- The trainees belong to an independent engineering consultancy company that is assigned by *Food Bioentrepreneurs* as described in Chap. 4 (Fig. 4.3). The team of trainees should include 5–6 members preferentially with educational backgrounds in cell biology, bioengineering, food engineering, bioprocess technology, process construction, and materials science. The trainees have access to simulation and modelling tools for bioprocess design and calculations, as well as software for DoE and economic calculations.

- *The Food Bioentrepreneurs* share their know-how about cultured meat technology with the trainees. Internal cost factors for operational costs, including buildings and renting, are provided. Labor costs are based on standard employment agreements and should be added to cost calculations as agreed with *Food Bioentrepreneurs*. *Food Bioentrepreneurs'* insights into IPR questions are shared with the trainees through adjoined industrial experts during the training.
- The R&D unit has previously collaborated with subcontractors for small-scale manufacturing, and experienced expertise is available for the trainees through tutorial experts. The *Food Bioentrepreneurs* accesses internally procured goods such as culture media and growth factors, single-use equipment, and other consumables. The R&D unit has several test benches for investigating prototypes and performing analytical experimentation of plasma samples. The team members are familiar with bioanalytical methods using enzymes and antibodies. If not, experts in training management should support the trainees with advice.
- The trainees' progress report to *Food Bioentrepreneurs* management monthly. The results should be delivered orally and in a written format. The typical time frame for the assignment is in the range of 3–4 months. This can be shortened if lower demand for reporting is expected. Reports should be concise and follow typical company standards (see also Sect. 4.4.7).

11.3 A Recommended Design Approach

11.3.1 Structuring the Assignment and Establishing User Requirements

The assignment from *Food Bioentrepreneurs* covers several novel technologies, including stem cell culturing technology and 3D bioprinting. From the objectives in the assignment, a general structure of *Food Bioentrepreneurs'* meat production can be compiled (Fig. 11.2). A conceptual design approach, as discussed in Chap. 3, must be identified. The following issues are of particular interest to consider in the design work:

- *Supply of stem cell-derived bovine cells:* This must predominantly be myoblasts, which are the main tissue component of meat fibers. Cell lines are available from various sources, whether commercially established or developed in-house.
- *Culture of myoblast cells on microcarrier support:* Several microcarrier types are available on the market. Their functionalities, price, toxicity, and performance in myoblast culture must be understood.
- *Bioprinting technique*: Building 3D structures with a meat-like structure is widely reported as feasible with bioprinting using bioink. The bioink is a polymeric material, compatible with cells such as myoblasts, often suggested to be based on hydrogels and additional supportive structural elements.

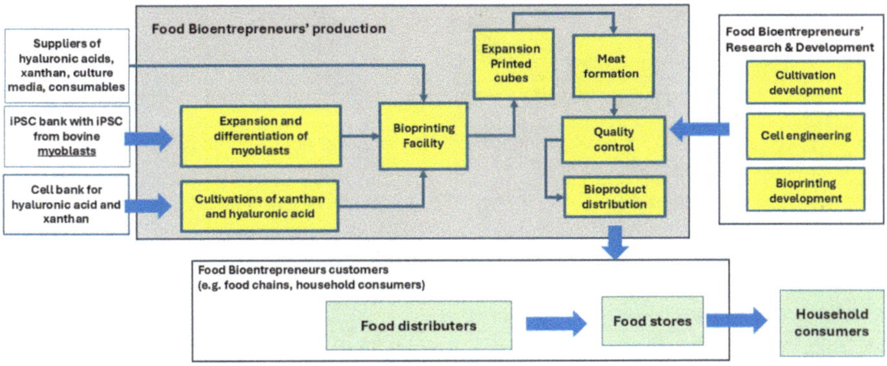

Fig. 11.2 The overall structure for the development and production of cultured meat at Food Bioentrepreneurs. The focus of the design assignment is within the yellow and green boxes

- *Bioink functions*: The bioink is supposed to accommodate a high portion of aqueous media and allow expansion of cells. This should allow a high and controllable content of meat-like cells. Typically, several biocompatible components are blended in the bioink. The blend should facilitate printing in chosen shapes and textures.
- *Recombinant cultures for producing key components in bioink*: Separate bioprocessing of the biopolymeric materials xanthan and hyaluronate carbohydrate polymers is an alternative to purchasing commercial products.
- *Perfusion bioreactors*: The bioprinted structures should be expanded in bioreactors with perfused nutrient media. The bioengineering conditions must be optimal.
- *Formulation of the cultured meat product*: The bioprinted cultured meat has a texture that deviates from the natural product. The alternative to form minced meat seems the easiest alternative. Additives for flavor and texture are components to be added at the late formulation stage.
- Regulatory aspects on good practice must be studied (Coecke et al. 2005).

As for every food product, customer evaluation of the product's texture, flavors, and meat-likeness should influence the production. This could potentially help in reducing production costs.

Several references may provide general facts and state-of-the-art of these technology-related issues (Choi et al. 2021; Nihashi et al. 2019). A thorough analysis of the stakeholders' requirements on the product, its marketing and manufacturing, yielding priorities and target metrics should be carried out (Table 11.1). It is obvious that the assigner, *Food Bioentrepreneurs*, has high expectations of the profitability of the product. It means from a designer perspective that the manufacturing process must be highly streamlined and optimally configured. Reduction of process steps and units will be required, and an efficient scaling up is necessary for attaining a production with acceptable profitability.

Table 11.1 Requirements and target specifications with priorities on Food Bioentrepreneurs production and customers

Requirement	Target specification	Priority
Consumers ofcultured meat		
Market price must be lower than corresponding products (own or competitors)	The reduced price should be in the range 50–90%	Very high
Potential toxic effect must be verified in the formulated cultured meat	No toxic effects acceptable	Very high
Product shelf-life at customers shall be minimized	Shelf-life must be >1 year when refrigerated	Very high
Food Bioentrepreneurs' market requirements		
Scalability of production volume to market demand is required	5000 kg (5 ton/year) to 80,000 kg (80 ton/year) shall be possible	Very high
IPR shall guarantee the product's market position	IPR must cover at least 80% of production process	High
A customer-attractive formulation of the meat product must be accomplished	Meat product formulation alternatives shall be considered	High
The product must be possible to be refrigerated	>1 year	High
Food bioentrepreneurs manufacturing site		
Manufacturing cost of cultured meat product must be considerably lower than market price	<50% at an annual production of 5 tons at market price of 70 EUR/kg	Very high
The manufacturing shall be highly automatized and allow 24-h operation	The plant shall be automized to 70% with ≤3 operators/team	Very high
Plant investments shall be possible to pay back reasonably fast	Payback period <5 year	High
Plant size must be minimized to reduce cost and environmental impact	Process intensification to 50% shall decrease costs by 25%	Medium

11.3.2 Conceptualization of the Assignment

Based on the requirements, priorities, and specifications, a conceptual map can be established, where functional needs for production of cultured meat are conceptually conceived and analyzed according to the principles described in Chap. 3 (Hubka and Eder 1988; Mandenius and Björkman 2011; Pahl et al. 2007; Ulrich et al. 2019) (Fig. 11.3).

The structure of a conceptual map focuses on bioprinting and *Food Bioentrepreneurs'* own intellectual property rights (IPR). The identified biological and technical functions should pave the way for exploiting state-of-the-art bioprocess technology. Thus, biological functions could preferably involve stem cell technology and the use of bioinks and bioprinting techniques. It is obvious that there are many configurative opportunities to manufacture cultured meat with these preconditions while obeying the constraints set by *Food Bioentrepreneurs* and established in the map.

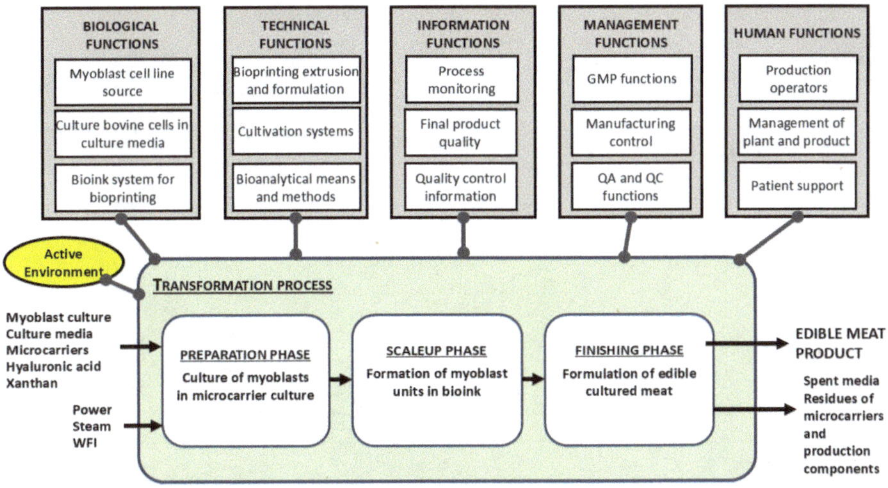

Fig. 11.3 Conceptual functions in the transformation process of the production of bioprinted meat, illustrating the sequence from raw materials to the finished commodity product

The information and managerial functions have key roles in the manufacturing of cultured meat. The final product must undergo extensive quality control and regulatory approval due to novel aspects of the product and the technology used. Thus, the information and management functions must tightly adapt to the new advanced biological and technical functions envisaged to be used.

Furthermore, the human systems, i.e., the operators and process engineers, should be able to handle the advanced and demanding technology in its operation. The customers of the prepared cultured meat must accept and like the quality and form of the product.

The functional map should be used to considerfeasible configurations to produce cultured meat. Six such configurations can be conceived (Fig. 11.4).

A configuration for a small-scale pilot process for testing the manufacturing concepts and to generate basic engineering data for calculation of scale-up opportunities is included in the assignment (Fig. 11.4a). The configuration is characterized by an extensive process, where bioink components are produced in-house, and myoblasts are cultured on microcarriers. The microcarriers must be removed from the myoblasts because they are not edible and are considered safe. Myoblasts are mixed with xanthan and hyaluronic acid into meat units. The units are enlarged on scaffolds placed in a perfusion bioreactor. The enlarged meat units are formulated into a product appealing to the customers.

In a second configuration at pilot scale, the bioink is externally supplied (Fig. 11.4b). The configuration is similar to the previous alternative (A), but the bioink components are procured from external contractors. This means a reduction in the complexity of the manufacturing process but is accompanied by high procurement costs.

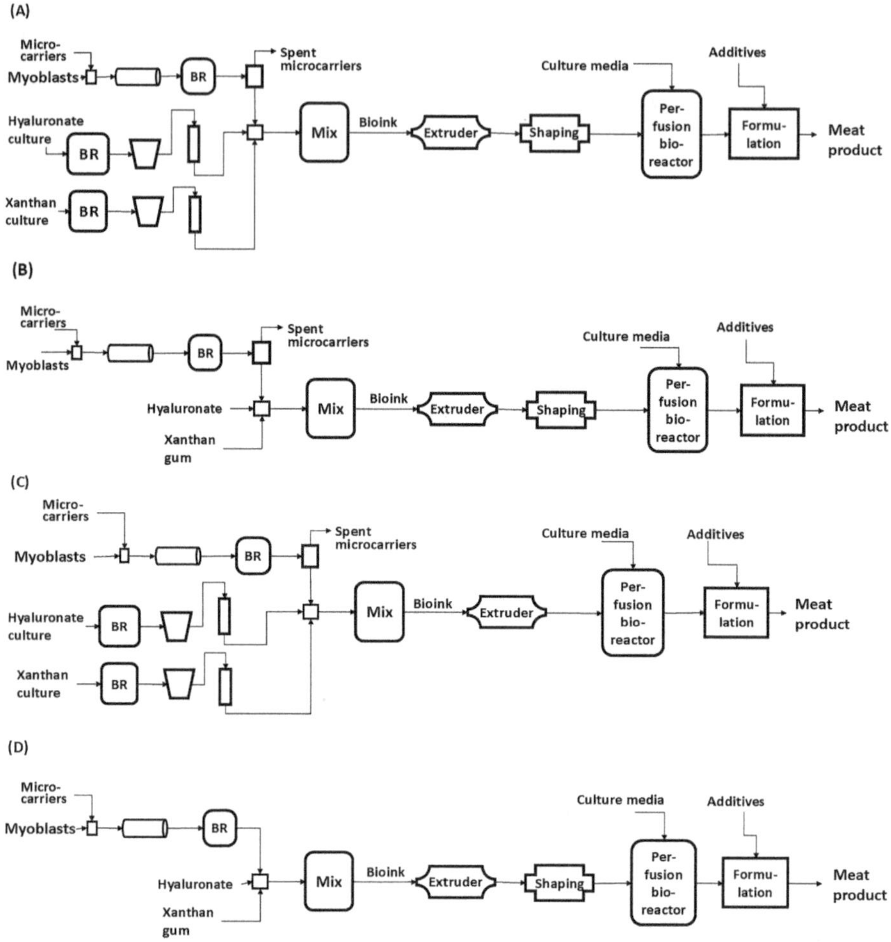

Fig. 11.4 Six process configurations for cultured meat manufacturing. In alternative (**a**), hyaluronate and xanthan are produced in internal bioreactor cultures, and microcarriers are used for myoblast cultivation. In alternative (**b**), hyaluronate and xanthan are acquired from commercial subcontractors, while myoblasts are grown on microcarriers. In alternative (**c**), hyaluronate and xanthan are produced in preceding bioreactor cultures, and myoblasts are grown on microcarriers. In alternative (**d**), the microcarriers are edible and are not separated before mixing with commercially acquired hyaluronate and xanthan to prepare the bioink. In alternative (**e**), the extrudate is formulated directly into a final meat product without post-extrusion shaping or perfusion. In alternative (**f**), commercially acquired hyaluronate and xanthan are combined with edible microcarriers to form the bioink

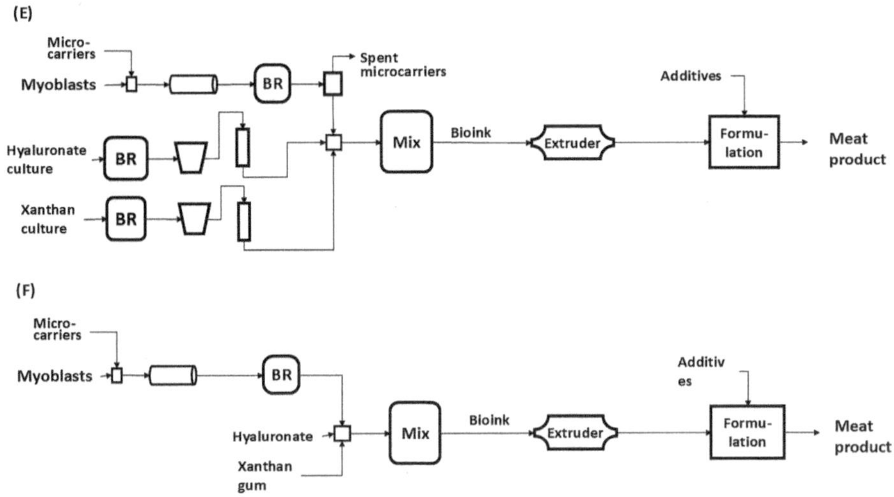

Fig. 11.4 (continued)

In a third configuration, the extruder operation for the bioprinting delivers a composite structure of myoblast bodies that can be expanded in the perfusion bioreactor (Fig. 11.4c). The expanded units are then formulated as above. This is a significant simplification of the production of cultured meat with potential economic benefits.

In a fourth configuration, a degradable, nontoxic microcarrier can safely be used as a part of the bioink (Fig. 11.4d). The microcarriers with myoblasts are mixed with hyaluronate and xanthan components. This simplifies the manufacturing considerably and should be economically more advantageous given that the new microcarrier material fulfills several technical requirements, such as loading capacity, price, and safety. In this configuration, all other steps are unchanged compared to the previous configurations.

In a fifth configuration, the process is scaled up using an internal supply of components (Fig. 11.4e). The configuration is functionally the same as in A, but the extrudate is formulated directly from the effluent. This is a feasible configuration if the first stage can produce larger quantities of cells and bioink and if the extruder step has capacity to process those quantities. The manufacturing benefits are considerable, but technical improvements are necessary. For example, the cell production capacity for the microcarrier culture must be scaled up, and the throughput in the bioprinter step must be increased.

In a sixth configuration, bioink is supplied externally while other conditions are the same as above (Fig. 11.4f). It is assumed that bioink components are delivered by subcontractors and that the bioprinted meat units can be formulated beneficially. If this is possible to accomplish, it seems to be an attractive design solution, due to a smaller manufacturing process, probably easier to manage and control, and to reach regulatory approval.

Three patent applications are potential threats for the configurations (Barzee et al. 2025; Razza et al. 2025; Seok et al. 2025). The IPRs describe cultured meat preparation procedures and the use of 3D bioprinting for cultured meat.

11.3.3 Detailed Design of Selected Conceptual Configurations

Three of the configurations in Fig. 11.4 could be further developed into detailed designs (Fig. 11.5). Attention is given to upcoming techniques, such as new single-use reactors and novel microcarrier materials.

A small-scale pilot process (Fig. 11.5a) is designed according to configuration A in Fig. 11.4. Culturing of myoblasts on microcarriers (e.g., Cytodex™ Microcarriers, www.cytivalifesciences.com) is carried out in single-use spinner flasks of a size of 100–5000 mL. The cells are released from the microcarriers in a mixer to which trypsin is added. The cells and microcarriers are separated by a microfiltration unit with a wide pore size. The separated cells are mixed with hyaluronate and xanthan provided by a subcontractor into a bioink. The bioink is printed and formed in an extruder unit to cubically bodies, which are subsequently expanded in a perfused bioreactor. The high-density cubes constitute the product that will need some further formulation to a final product shape.

For larger-scale manufacturing, a process in a 2000 L bioreactor with disposable culture bags could be designed (Fig. 11.5b). The upscaling is 400-fold from a 5 L bioreactor volume to 2000 L. The preculture is still carried out in a spinner flask of 500 mL. The myoblasts are grown on Cytodex at both stages and are released in a subsequent 2000 L mixing tank and separated by a one-stage microfilter. The process allows a small-scale production for performance testing.

A radical scale-up is carried out where several of the steps in the above alternatives are replaced (Fig. 11.5c). By applying the configuration in Fig. 11.4f a significantly reduced cost is expected. However, two technological improvements are required. First, a microcarrier that is edible (e.g., gelatin-based or alginate-based) must be identified and supplied. Second, the bioprinting capacity must be adapted to a much higher throughput with bigger machines or parallel processing.

11.3.4 Economic Evaluation of the Detailed Designs

The estimated investment costs in the three designs differ considerably, mainly due to the expenditures for microcarrier cultivation and bioprinting equipment (Peters et al. 2003; Kristiansen 2006; Ray et al. 2022). To this, costs for R&D to establish these systems are added. However, a reduction of units in the process will lower costs.

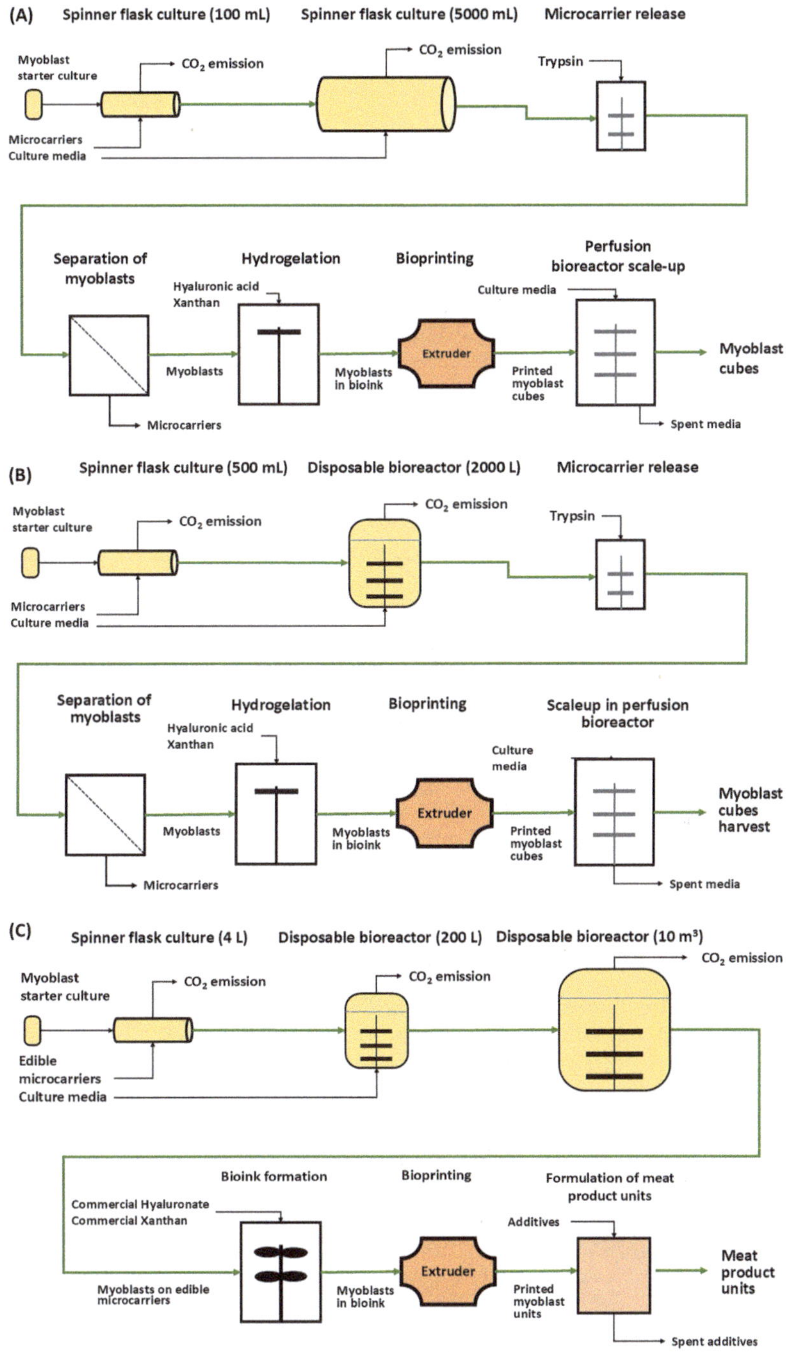

Fig. 11.5 Three detailed designs for cultured meat manufacture. In alternative (**a**), a small-scale process manufactures cultured meat from a myoblast cell line source via cultivation on microcarriers, scaling up, and preparation in a bioink based on hyaluronate and xanthan, followed

The economic evaluation shall answer the following questions:

- Can a realistic market price be reached with the design alternatives, making the myoblast cultured food a sound business project?
- If so, can the optimization options turn the production economy into a net income for *Food Bioentrepreneurs*?
- Can subcontracting lower the costs compared to an in-house production design of myoblast cultured food?

In the design of the small-scale pilot plant for testing (Fig. 11.5a) and the small-scale production plant (Fig. 11.5b) stirred reactor tanks for microcarrier release and microfilters for separation are required. The trypsin cost for release of myoblasts from the microcarriers is considerable. Also, the extruder unit and the perfusion bioreactor are expensive units.

The procurement of dissolvable microcarriers, hyaluronic acid, and xanthan becomes significant. When these components and raw materials are purchased in large quantities, their volumetric prices will be reduced.

The bioprinter equipment is necessary to order from external vendors. The cost will significantly influence the economics for the entire manufacturing process. All costs for unit operation equipment, all auxiliary equipment, such as a pumping system, controller, valve, and piping, should be included in the estimation.

The cost estimation shows that only the large-scale manufacturing process has a good economic prospect to reach *Food Bioentrepreneurs* revenue target at a market price level of 70 EUR/kg cultured meat is set (Table 11.2). A lowering of the market price to 35 EUR/kg would cover the costs at an annual payback time of 5 years. This would be close to a competitive market price.

The economic estimation also shows that investment costs for this advanced processing technology are considerably significantly higher than the operational costs. The exclusive methodology for acquiring cell materials and components as well as the use of production equipment such as bioprinting increases the manufacturing costs. If these costs can be minimized and procurement of raw materials, such as microcarriers and biopolymers, can be minimized, it would be possible to target a production cost level closer to a better competitive bioproduct.

Still, food products for daily consumption have lower market prices than typical biotechnology products, in particular biopharmaceuticals. To reach a revenue on the same level requires a production volume of ton-quantities.

However, a lower cost can be realized by extensive optimization, as further discussed in the next section, based on the following actions:

Fig. 11.5 (continued) by extrusion through bioprinting into meat cubes that are enlarged in a perfusion reactor before formulation into the final product. In alternative (**b**), the process is scaled up to several-fold larger volumes with fewer steps. In alternative (**c**), a further scale-up is implemented where the microcarriers are edible and do not require separation, the bioink is prepared from commercial hyaluronate and xanthan raw materials, and the mixture is bioprinted into meat units that can be formulated directly into an edible product

Table 11.2 Economic evaluation for the three design alternatives for cultured meat production

Type of costs	Small pilot plant (kEUR)	Small production plant (kEUR)	Large-scale production plant (kEUR)
Investment costs			
Upfront production R&D			
Production development	100	200	300
Subcontracted R&D	80	150	200
Total upfront production R&D	*180*	*350*	*500*
Equipment for production			
Cultivation equipment	50	200	2000
Separation units (MC)	20	40	0
Reaction vessels (ink, BR)	40	80	0
Bioprinter unit	100	500	1500
Quality control instruments	80	80	80
Total production equipment costs	*290*	*900*	*3580*
Additional costs for production			
Installation of equipment (×0.5)	370	975	2125
Project planning (×0.3)	222	585	1275
Taxation (×0.1)	174	195	425
Buildings (×0.3)	222	585	1275
Total additional production cost	*348*	*1080*	*4296*
Total investment costs	**818**	**2330**	**8376**
Operational costs (annual)			
Consumables for production			
Consumables (media, raw)	10	30	300
Microcarriers	10	30	200
Bioink components	20	100	400
Consumables quality control	10	10	10
Total consumables for production	*80*	*170*	*910*
Additional operational costs			
Subcontracting of cell line	50	80	100
Labor production (incl QC)	50	200	400
Renting of buildings	10	20	30
Taxation	20	20	20
Management	20	50	50
Additionaloperational costs	*150*	*370*	*600*
Total operational costs	230	635	1510
Annual payback (5 years)	*164*	*466*	*1676*
Total annual production costs	328	1101	3186
Relative production cost per kg meat (EUR)	*500*	*220*	*40*

- Maximizing the cellular growth of myoblasts with an optimized composition of culture media components. This is a feasible design of experiment task, using methods discussed in Chaps. 3 and 4.
- Ensuring that equipment is optimally dimensioned in relation to specific rates in the cultivation stages of the manufacture. Mechanistic modelling could pave the way for this.
- Improvements of the bioprinting equipment based on optimization and better technical design.
- Optimization of printed composite meat units by a better proportion of cells and bioink components.

The distribution of costs shows that a significant part of the expenditure is for the operational costs. This share varies with production volume and affects the share the initial investment costs for the plant (Fig. 11.6). Consequently, the net income is much favored by a larger production for this advanced food product.

11.3.5 Optimization of the Design Alternatives

The three prioritized designs will be optimized by fine-tuning production parameters that directly govern manufacturing costs (Martins and Ning 2021; Sioshansi and Conejo 2017). Table 11.3 identifies high-leverage parameters where minor adjustments offer significant improvements to yields and cycle times. From a technical perspective, applying factorial design and mechanistic modelling allows for a systematic exploration of the design space, ensuring that resource inputs are minimized without compromising output quality. By resolving these technical bottlenecks, the project can maximize productivity and achieve the cost efficiencies essential to the economic objectives of *Food Bioentrepreneurs*. This dual approach ensures that process sensitivities are identified early, preventing costly pilot-scale failures and reducing the time-to-market for new iterations. Ultimately, by establishing a robust, data-driven framework for parameter control, the company can secure a competitive advantage through lower operational costs and more sustainable resource management.

Optimizing the Production Conditions for Myoblast Cultured Meat by Design of Experiments The performances of design alternatives are possible to optimize by design of experiments (DoE) methodology (Brereton 2003; Montgomery 2020; Mandenius and Brundin 2008). Three kinds of optimization objectives should be considered: (1) the medium composition, (2) the conditions during the cultivation, and (3) the growth of myoblast cells. At this stage, it is advantageous to identify factors that seem likely to improve growth rate and yields in cultivations. The application of the DoE methodology should follow its established procedures by studying those factors that are most likely to be associated with improving cellular growth rates and yields (Table 11.4).

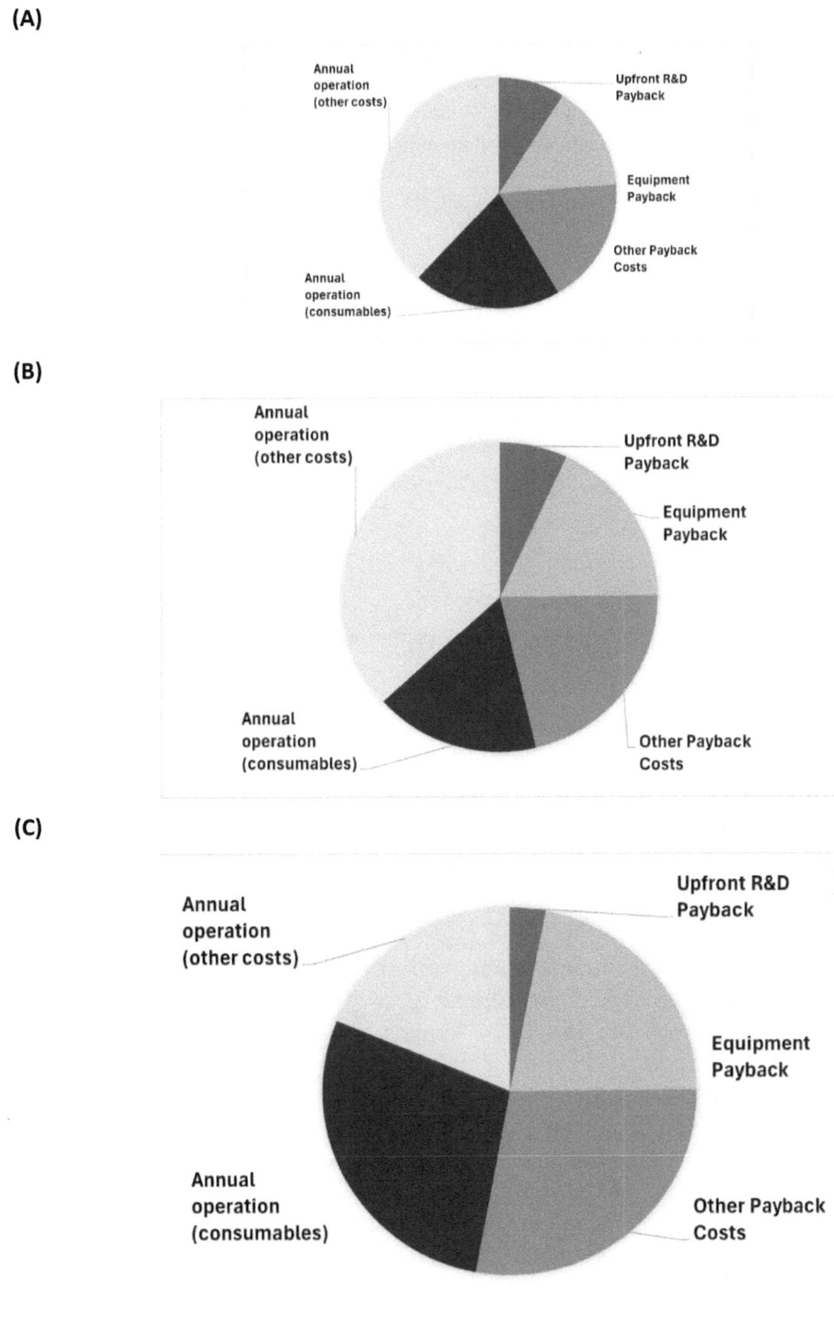

Fig. 11.6 Distribution of costs in the small pilot plant (**a**), small production plant (**b**) and the large plant (**c**). Only annual payback costs are shown

Table 11.3 Parameters of relevance to investigate for optimizing production

Object of optimization	Expected outcome	Applicable optimization technique
Media composition in bioreactors for production of HA and XG	High productivity and shorter production time in the process train of HA and XG	Primarily factorial design of culture media components and levels
Cultivation parameters in HA and XG bioreactors	Increased production rates of HA and XG	Factorial design of controllable parameters such as time, oxygen, and temperature
Myoblast cultivation	Improved productivity	Factorial design of parameters as above
Expansion of myoblasts in bioink by adjusting perfusion culture and rate	Higher density of myoblasts in the composite bioink and faster production rate	Mechanistic modelling
Composite proportion	Quality of product	Factorial design of speed and flow

Factors such as pH, temperature, stirring speed, and inoculation should be investigated for their effect on cellular growth and volumetric productivity. A two-level DoE procedure should be applied with those factors, as described in Chap. 4.

Optimization of the composition of culture media is another opportunity to enhance cell growth. Typically, media factors, such as basic media and additives, are likely to improve growth and yield (Table 11.4).

Another opportunity to optimize the production by DoE is to study the release of myoblasts from the microcarriers. The main factors of interest could be the amount of added trypsin, temperature, stirring of the reactor, and type of microcarriers and their concentration. The obvious responses to measure would be trypsin activity and time, for example, as release rate.

Very challenging would be to optimize the structure of the microcarrier with respect to porosity, size, and surface character. These factors can be systematically investigated in relation to the growth of myoblasts.

Table 11.4 DoE plan for optimization of production of cultured meat

Optimization object	Factors in DoE plan	Responses to measure
Cultivation conditions	pH, temperature, agitation rate, dissolved oxygen Proportion of microcarriers	Growth rate of myoblasts on microcarriers Yield of myoblasts per medium components Release time of myoblasts from microcarriers
Culture media composition	Basal media DMEM Serum FSB and HS	Myoblast density and number in bioink Analytical methods for media components
Release of myoblasts from microcarriers	Trypsin per grafted microcarriers	Myoblast density and number Trypsin activity method
Blending conditions for bioink	Hyaluronic acid, xanthan, crosslinker, myoblasts	Expansion rate of cells in bio-reactors Enzyme-based assays for HA and XG Myoblast density and number
Permeability of bioprinted bodies	Perfusion rate, density of cells in bioink	Myoblast density and number

It would also be of great interest to use DoE to improve the blending of bioink components. The proportion of hyaluronic acid, xanthan, crosslinker, and myoblasts are factors that could be expected to influence the capacity of the bioink. The response parameter would then be to measure the quality properties of the formed bioink, for example, the density of myoblasts.

Finally, the permeability of the bioink bodies would be a parameter strongly related to the productivity of the whole process. Thus, the perfusion rate, culture conditions, and density in the final reactor step and the effect on expansion of myoblasts in the bioink bodies could be studied with DoE.

Optimizing Production of Myoblast Cultured Food by Mechanistic Modelling An alternative approach to optimizing the production of myoblasts and bioprinted meat units is the application of mechanistic modelling (Nielsen et al. 2011; Doran 2013). By utilizing mass balances to map the interrelationships between critical process parameters, this method mathematically defines the mechanisms governing mass conversions and flows across various manufacturing configurations (Fig. 11.5). Implementing a mechanistic framework serves several strategic purposes:

- Scaling Production Intensity: Optimizing throughput by maximizing volumetric productivity and reducing batch cycle times
- Characterizing Myoblast Kinetics: Quantifying the impact of cell growth properties on overall system performance
- Optimizing Microenvironments: Evaluating the influence of cultivation conditions and nutrient distribution within perfused bioprinted units

The mechanistic levels may be the conventional batch bioreactor, where the balances are related to growth kinetics. The models usually assume a Monod-like growth behavior over time, as is illustrated in the diagrams below (Fig. 11.7 and 11.8). These models are useful to dimension the bioreactor size and to predict cell production.

Furthermore, the models can include growth kinetic constraints related to myoblast cells and their characteristic transformations into wrong cell types, as well as their survival in the specific environment of a production process and on the artificial surfaces of microcarriers.

In the subsequent manufacturing step, myoblast cells proliferated within a bioink in the perfused bioreactor. These growth kinetics are influenced and controlled quite differently. The need to understand, model, and predict this cellular growth in the production is as relevant and important as the other production stages.

Several parameters are critical in these stages and influence the mechanisms of conversion and should consequently be included in the models (Table 11.5).

A set of differential equations provides the framework for simulating the mechanisms in simple models (Eqs. 11.1–11.4). Obviously, a few parameters and rates need to be assessed from experiments or literature data to make the modelling trustworthy. A company like *Food Entrepreneurs* usually has laboratory facilities for experimental testing.

Table 11.5 Parameters investigated in mechanistic modelling for optimization

Parameter investigated	Model	Expected outcome
Cell production phase		
Perfusion rate to the continuous perfusion reactor	Kinetic mass balance based on specific growth rate of CHO cells	Productivity timing of operation
Growth rate of myoblasts	Kinetic balance with specific growth and expression parameters	Mab productivity per reactor volume
Volume of culture system	Culture density reached under various volumetric conditions	Optimization of volume of plant in relation to time
Microcarrier loading capacity		
Bioprocessing of bioink scaffolding components		
Rate of component production	Kinetics of component production	Estimation of productivity of dimensioning of process size
Growth of recombinant culture	Kinetics for growth of strains	Total productivity related to downstream steps
Bioprinting phase		
Yield in bioink formation	Mass balance with recycling ratio adjustable	Effect of cell number and MAb conc. In bioreactor effluent
Formulation phase		
Yield of printed approved cultured meat units	Simple factorial effect of centrifuge or filter and columns	Estimation of effect of total yield on productivity of end-to-end system

Mass balance for a batch bioreactor with growing myoblasts on microcarriers could be described according to:

$$\mathrm{d}N_{\mathrm{myoblast}}/\mathrm{d}t = q_{\mathrm{myoblast}} \cdot N_{\mathrm{myoblast}} - k_{\mathrm{binding}} \cdot S_{\mathrm{nutrient}} + k_{\mathrm{binding}} \cdot S_{\mathrm{nutrient}}/V_{\mathrm{bioreactor}} \tag{11.1}$$

Mass balance for release of myoblast cells from microcarriers by trypsin:

$$\mathrm{d}N_{\mathrm{release}}/\mathrm{d}t = N_{\mathrm{myoblast}} \cdot c_{\mathrm{trypsin}} + k_{\mathrm{trypsin}}/V_{\mathrm{bioreactor}} \tag{11.2}$$

Mass balance for bioink production from components:

$$m_{\mathrm{bioink}}/\mathrm{d}t = k_{\mathrm{bioink}} \cdot N_{\mathrm{myoblast}} + k_{\mathrm{mix}} \cdot c_{\mathrm{bioink}}/V_{\mathrm{bioreactor}} \tag{11.3}$$

Mass balance for expansion of myoblasts in bioink units in a perfused system:

$$\mathrm{BI}_{\mathrm{units}}/\mathrm{d}t = k_{\mathrm{myoblast}} \cdot N_{\mathrm{myoblast}} \cdot c_{\mathrm{bioink}} + c_{\mathrm{units}} \cdot F_{\mathrm{nutrient}}/V_{\mathrm{bioreactor}} \tag{11.4}$$

where the key parameters are the myoblast concentration, N_{myoblast}; bioreactor volume, $V_{\mathrm{bioreactor}}$; bioink, BI; number of bioink units, $\mathrm{BI}_{\mathrm{unit}}$; concentration of printed units, c_{units}; perfusion flow rate, F_{nutrient}; kinetic growth rates of the myoblasts (μ); mixing time, t_{mixing}; trypsin rate, k_{trypsin}; bioprinting rate, k_{printing}; and the limiting nutrient media component, S_{nutrient}. Limit constraints for microcarrier numbers in the bioreactor are necessary to include in the model (Fig. 11.7).

With the model equations, critical conditions for the production can be evaluated in the simulations by adjusting kinetic rates and volumes. This could involve the volume of the reactor, specific growth of the cells, and concentrations or amounts of nutrients, microcarriers, and seeding (Fig. 11.8a). The outcome of the evaluation can be used to decide equipment dimensions for assumed specific rates for growing myoblasts on microcarriers, as well as other concentrations and procedures in the reactor operation. The goals of the modelling are to optimize volumes and time in relation to the production target. The model equations could be extended to include myoblast survival on microcarriers, loading capacity of the microcarriers, and the reactor space to accommodate these. The growth is distinguished in three phases: free growth in culture media, growth on a microcarrier surface, and crowding effects on the surface. In the simulation diagram, two specific growth rates of myoblasts and two seeding concentrations are shown for the same reactor volume (Fig. 11.6a) using the equations:

$$k_{\mathrm{growth}} = k_{\mathrm{growthmax}} + S_{\mathrm{nutrient}}/(S_{\mathrm{nutrient}} + K_{\mathrm{S}}) \tag{11.5}$$

$$\mathrm{d}N_{\mathrm{myoblast}}/\mathrm{d}t = k_{\mathrm{growth}} + N_{\mathrm{myoblast}} \tag{11.6}$$

$$\mathrm{d}S_{\mathrm{nutrient}}/\mathrm{d}t = -\left(k_{\mathrm{growth}}/Y_{\mathrm{N/S}}\right) + N_{\mathrm{myoblast}} \tag{11.7}$$

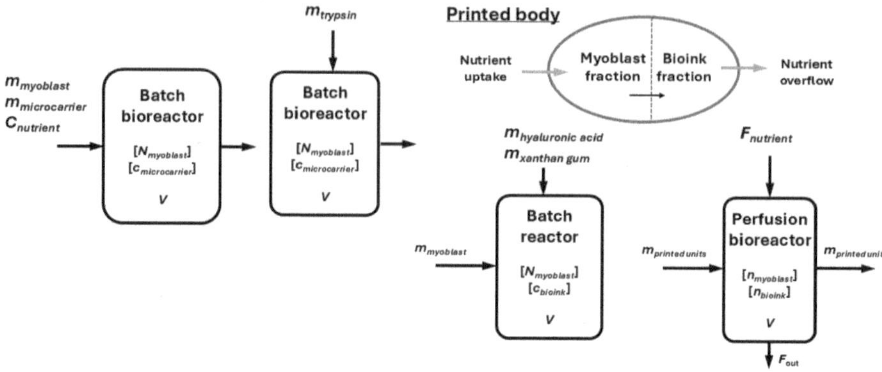

Fig. 11.7 Structure of mechanistic models for the cultured meat manufacturing steps with critical parameters decisive for process performance

$$n_{\text{myoblast}} = V_{\text{bioreactor}} + N_{\text{myoblast}} \tag{11.8}$$

$$n_{\text{conc}} = V_{\text{bioreactor}} + \text{bead} \tag{11.9}$$

$$\text{if } N_{\text{myoblast}} > \text{bead}_{\text{capacity}};\ \text{ then } N_{\text{myoblast}} = \text{bead}_{\text{capacity}} \tag{11.10}$$

where the key parameters are the myoblast concentration, N_{myoblast}; bioreactor volume, $V_{\text{bioreactor}}$; bioink, BI; number of bioink units, BI_{unit}; concentration of printed units, c_{units}; perfusion flow rate, F_{nutrient}; kinetic growth rates of the myoblasts (μ), mixing time, t_{mixing}; trypsin rate, k_{trypsin}; bioprinting rate, k_{printing}; and the limiting nutrient media component, S_{nutrient}. Limit constraints for microcarrier numbers in the bioreactor are necessary to include in the model.

The release of myoblast cells from the microcarriers by trypsin treatment in a batch reactor can also be modelled (Fig. 11.8b). The high cost of the trypsin enzyme motivates optimization of this step. The critical parameters are the amount of trypsin, its enzyme activity (release rate), the mass flow of carrier-bound cells to be processed, and the relation to time and reactor volume. The critical parameters are the trypsin cost, time for processing, and myoblast survival of trypsin treatment, while reactor volume is of less importance due to limited design requirements of agitation and temperature control. In the simulation diagram, the release of myoblasts at two levels of trypsin activity (Fig. 11.6b). The simulations are based on:

$$\mathrm{d}N_{\text{myoblast}}/\mathrm{d}t = k_{\text{trypsin}} + N_{\text{myoblast}} \tag{11.11}$$

$$\mathrm{dCytodex}/\mathrm{d}t = -N_{\text{myoblast}} \tag{11.12}$$

$$\text{if Cytodex} < 0;\ \ \mathrm{d}N_{\text{myoblast}}/\mathrm{d}t = 0 \tag{11.13}$$

where the key parameters are the myoblast concentration, N_{myoblast}; bioreactor volume, $V_{\text{bioreactor}}$; trypsin rate, k_{trypsin}; and the Cytodex microcarrier concentration, *Cytodex*.

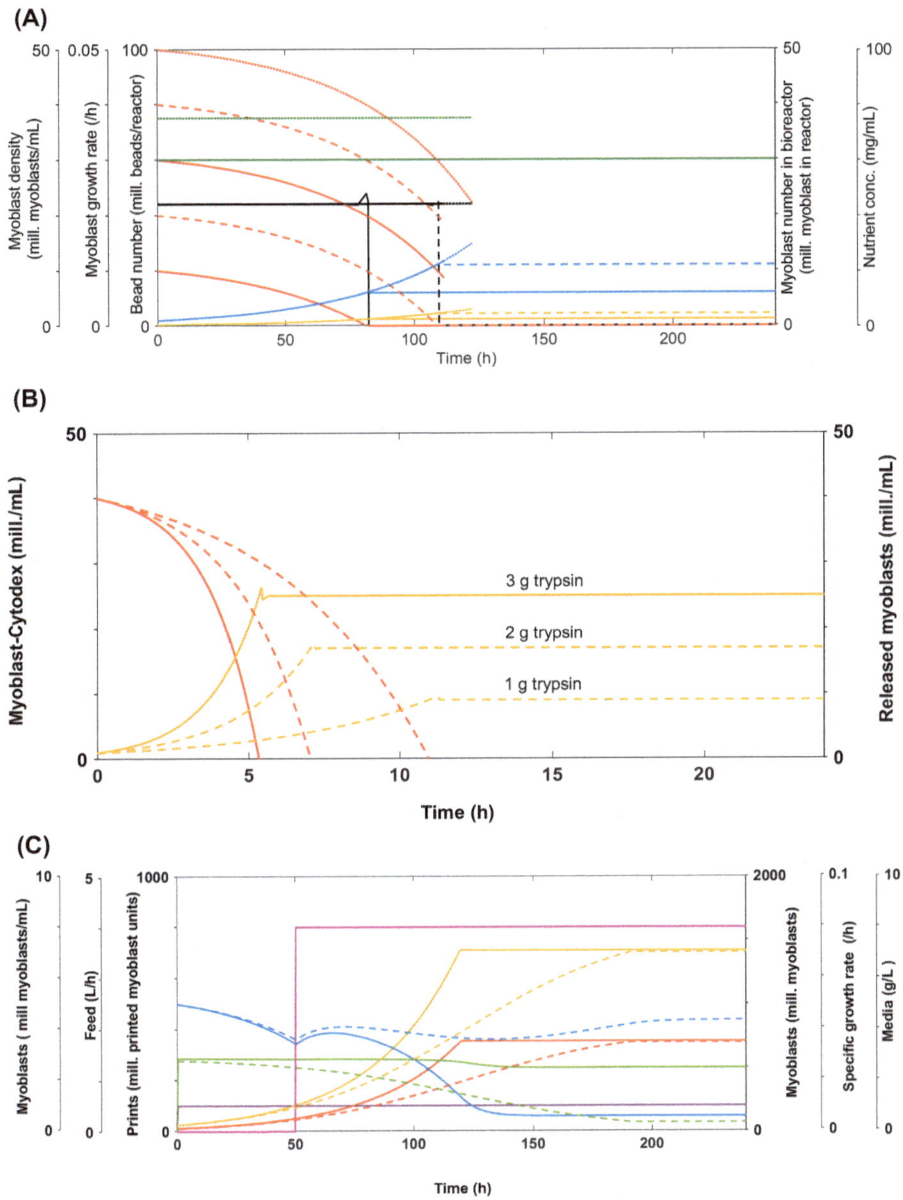

Fig. 11.8 (**a**) Myoblast growth of microcarriers in the first batch reactor stage. The horizontal lines for two loadings of microcarriers (green). The total production of myoblast as microcarrier bound cells (g) are depicted by blue lines at five starting concentrations of nutrient (red). Myoblast growth rates are shown as well (black). (**b**) Release of myoblasts from microcarriers at additions of trypsin (1, 2, and 3 g trypsin). (**c**) Expansion of myoblasts in the bioink bodies in a perfused continuous bioreactor. Density of myoblasts in the bioink print (yellow line), the expansion of myoblast cells in the bioreactor (green line), and perfusion rate at two perfusion rates (L/h or h^{-1})

The expansion of myoblasts in the bioink under perfusion conditions can also be predicted (Fig. 11.8c). Diffusion resistance in the printed myoblast cubes due to the increasing cell density limits the growth and productivity in the final step. The model structure is derived from the mechanistic representation of the cubes (Fig. 11.7). The perfused bioreactor's mass balance equation follows a typical continuous reactor model. The initial number of printed cubes with low myoblast density is continuously flowed with nutrients. The cell growth in the printed cubes will be retarded in the model. When growth is slow in the cubes, they should be harvested. The simulation shows the efficient period in the reactor. The simulation facilitates deciding on the required reactor size and loads in relation to the production target. In the simulation diagram, the time course for growth in the cubes is simulated for set numbers of cubes, nutrient flow rate, and starting conditions (Fig. 11.6c).

The following model equations are useful:

$$\mu_{\text{myoblast}} = \mu_{\text{myoblast}-\text{max}} \cdot S_{\text{media}} \cdot (S_{\text{media}} + K_S) \tag{11.14}$$

$$\mu_{\text{myoblast-effective}} = \mu_{\text{myoblast}} \cdot (N_{\text{myoblast, max}} - N_{\text{myoblast}}) / N_{\text{myoblast- max}} \tag{11.15}$$

$$\mathrm{d}N_{\text{myoblast}} / \mathrm{d}t = \mu_{\text{myoblast-effective}} \cdot N_{\text{myoblast}} \tag{11.16}$$

$$\begin{aligned} \mathrm{d}S_{\text{media}} / \mathrm{d}t = & -(\mathrm{d}N_{\text{myoblast}} / \mathrm{d}t) / Y_{X/C} \\ & + S_{\text{feed}} \cdot F_{\text{perfusion}} / V_{\text{bioreactor}} - S_{\text{media}} \cdot F_{\text{perfusion}} / V_{\text{bioreactor}} \end{aligned} \tag{11.17}$$

$$\text{if } t > 50 \text{ then } F_{\text{perfusion}} = F1 \tag{11.18}$$

$$\text{if } N_{\text{myoblast}} > 7, \text{ then } N_{\text{myoblast}} = 7 \tag{11.19}$$

where the key parameters are the myoblast concentration, N_{myoblast}; bioreactor volume, $V_{\text{bioreactor}}$; bioink, BI; number of bioink units, BI_{unit}; concentration of printed units, c_{units}; perfusion flow rate, $F_{\text{perfusion}}$; kinetic growth rates of the myoblasts (μ); bioprinting rate, k_{printing}; and the limiting nutrient media component, S_{media}. Limit constraints for microcarrier numbers in the bioreactor are necessary to include in the model.

Obviously, the mechanistic modelling allows complementary assessments of the productivity of the production system. This can contribute to reduce costs for equipment investments and make operations more cost-effective in line with the objectives of *Food Bioentrepreneurs*.

11.4 Conclusive Suggestions for *Food Bioentrepreneurs*

For meeting the objectives in the assignment for cultured meat production complex and technically advanced production processes are required. The economic frames are demanding, and it is difficult to accomplish a profitable production.

It is therefore suggested that *Food Bioentrepreneurs* consider the following actions in the design of a manufacturing process:

- Choose a large-scale production design where the production process has as few steps as possible and procure the input raw materials for hyaluronic acid and xanthan from external suppliers and only use their own production process for growing myoblast cells. This has the advantage of reducing the investments in separate lines for hyaluronic acid and xanthan in their own process.
- If successfully applied, the unit production price of cultured meat is considerably reduced. With a scale-up of production, the economic gain is amplified. Going from negative production cost at an assumed market price, the estimated cost of production is reduced, and a net income can be reached at the suggested scale.

This presupposes that the sales during the 5-year period reach at least 20% of the estimated market. If not, three possibilities remain:

- To extend the payback time, e.g., to 10 years, which means that sales volumes or price levels can be lower. If the investors can cope with that, it is a feasible way.
- A lower investment in a new plant may also change the prerequisites. The large-scale production will allow this.
- A further optimization of the biological system's capacity to produce more cells to increase the cell density to enhance the volumetric productivity of the plant.

This would be expected to favor the *Food Bioentrepreneur's* competitive position on the market by being first with the cultured meat product introduction and being able to offer the product at a realistic price to the customers.

11.5 Tutorial Perspectives on the Assignment

Early in the design process, it will become evident that production efficiency is critical to making this biotechnological concept economically viable.

Trainees may require significant tutorial guidance in the following areas:

- Prioritize speed over precision: Avoid getting bogged down in precise rates and prices during early evaluations; use rough estimates to compare alternatives quickly.
- Competitive awareness: Monitor filed patent applications to stay ahead of competitor solutions.

Based on previous experience, trainees require substantial support in the following areas:

- Integration of technical and economic feasibility: A fundamental learning objective is recognizing that technical innovation must be paired with economic feasibility to be commercially viable. Internalizing this early in the process is essential for maintaining the correct strategic direction.
- Conceptual transitions and decision-making: Transitioning beyond the conceptual stage and reaching a consensus on design alternatives represents a significant hurdle. Specifically, students often find it difficult to quantify the economic trade-

offs between procuring commercial-grade xanthan and hyaluronate versus implementing integrated in-process production.
- Data scarcity and iterative methodology: Inadequate experimental data often hinder the decision-making process. For inexperienced team members, the nonlinear, iterative nature of design can lead to confusion during the initial training phases.
- Methodological frameworks*:* The application of structured experimental reasoning, such as factorial design, facilitates collaboration on both a technical and psychological level. Organizing biological and process parameters within a DoE framework (cf. Mandenius and Brundin 2008) provides a robust basis for more streamlined decision-making.

Furthermore, the following strategies are recommended to enhance project momentum:

- Heuristic estimation*:* To maintain progress, trainees should utilize order-of-magnitude estimates for rates and pricing during early-stage evaluations rather than seeking premature precision.
- Expedited conceptualization: Rapid progression through the conceptual phase is necessary to define the scope and technical requirements of a novel continuous process.
- Intellectual property analysis: To ensure competitive differentiation, teams must actively scrutinize the landscape of existing patent applications and prior art.

References

Barzee T et al (2025) Bottom-up approach for sustainable cultivated meat production. US Patent Application US2025/0261665 A1

Bodiou V, Moutsatsou P, Post MJ (2020) Microcarriers for upscaling cultured meat production. Front Nutr 7:10. https://doi.org/10.3389/fnut.2020.00010

Boudreault P, Tremlay JP, Pepin MF et al (2001) Scale-up of a myoblast culture process. J Biotechnol 91:63–74. https://doi.org/10.1016/S0168-1656(01)00291-7

Brereton RG (2003) Chemometrics, data analysis for laboratory and chemical plants. Wiley, Chichester

Choi KH, Yoon JW, Kim M et al (2021) Muscle stem cell isolation and in vitro culture for meat production, a methodological review. Compr Rev Food Sci Food Saf 20:429–457. https://doi.org/10.1111/1541-4337.12661

Coecke S, Balls M, Bowe G et al (2005) Guidance on good cell culture practice: a report of the second ECVAM task force on good cell culture practice. Altern Lab Anim 33:261–287. https://doi.org/10.1177/026119290503300313

Doran PM (2013) Biochemical engineering principles, 2nd edn. Elsevier, Amsterdam. https://doi.org/10.1016/C2009-0-22348-8

Ferreira RG et al (2021) Techno-economic analysis of a hyaluronic acid production process utilizing streptococcal fermentation. Processes 9:241. https://doi.org/10.3390/pr9020241

Guo X, Wang D, He B et al (2024) 3D-bioprinting of cultured meat, a promising avenue of meat production. Food Bioprocess Technol 17:1659–1680. https://doi.org/10.1007/s11947-023-03195-x

Hubka V, Eder WE (1988) Theory of technical systems, a total concept theory for engineering design. Springer Verlag, Berlin

Kristiansen B (2006) Process economics. In: Ratledge C, Kristiansen B (eds) Basic biotechnology, 3rd edn. Cambridge University Press, Cambridge, UK pp 239–252

Lindsay CD et al (2019) Bioprinting of stem cell expansion lattices. Acta Biomater 95:225–235. https://doi.org/10.1016/j.actbio.2019.05.014

Mandenius CF, Björkman M (2011) Biomechatronic design in biotechnology: a methodology for development of biotechnology products. John Wiley & Sons, New Jersey. https://doi.org/10.1002/9781118067147

Mandenius CF, Brundin A (2008) Bioprocess optimization using design-of-experiments methodology. Biotechnol Prog 24:1191–1203. https://doi.org/10.1002/btpr.67

Martins JRRA, Ning A (2021) Engineering design optimization. Cambridge University Press, Cambridge. https://doi.org/10.1017/9781108980647

Montgomery DC (2020) Design and analysis of experiments, 9th edn. John Wiley & Sons, New York. ISBN: 978-1-119-63842-1

Nielsen J, Villadsen J, Lidén G (2011) Bioreaction engineering principles, 3rd edn. Springer-Nature, New York

Nihashi Y, Umezawa K, Shinji S et al (2019) Distinct cell proliferation, myogenic differentiation, and gene expression in skeletal muscle myoblasts of layer and broiler chickens. Sci Rep 9:16527. https://doi.org/10.1038/s41598-019-52946-4

Pahl G, Beitz W, Feldhusen J et al (2007) Engineering design, a systematic approach, 3rd edn. Springer Verlag, Berlin

Peters MS, Timmerhaus KD, West RE (2003) Plant design and economics for chemical engineers, 5th edn. McGraw-Hill, New York

Piola M, Soncini M, Cantini M et al (2013) Design and functional testing of a multi-chamber perfusion platform for three-dimensional scaffolds. Sci World J 2013:123974. https://doi.org/10.1155/2013/123974

Post MJ (2012) Cultured meat from stem cells, challenges and prospects. Meat Sci 92:297–301. https://doi.org/10.1016/j.meatsci.2012.04.008

Ray SC, Chambers RG, Kumbhakar SC (2022) Handbook of production economics. Springer Nature, New York

Razza N et al (2025) Methods and compositions for the preparation of fibrous muscle bundles for cultivated meat production. US Patent Application US2025/0207096 A1

Seok et al (2025) Method for producing cell-based fish containing fish muscle shape-mimicking muscle using 3D bioprinting technology and cell-based fish prepared thereby. US Patent Application US2025234907 A1

Sioshansi R, Conejo AJ (2017) Optimization in engineering, models and algorithms. Springer International Publishing, Germany. ISBN 9783319567679

Ulrich KT, Eppinger SD, Yang MC (2019) Product design and development, 7th edn. McGraw-Hill, New York

Chapter 12
Case 7: Design of a Point-of-Care Diagnostic Device for SARS-CoV-2 Infections

12.1 Assignment: Background, Description, and Objectives

The aim of the training in this assignment is to design a diagnostic device for point-of-care testing of severe acute respiratory syndrome SARS-CoV-2 infection (Krammer 2020; V'kovski et al. 2021). The assignment includes both evaluating different design alternatives for the diagnostic device and an efficient process for its production.

The assigner, *Diagnostic Incorporated*, is a life science company specializing in the development and commercialization of clinical diagnostic instruments and kits. The company operates an R&D facility with 25 employees located within a research park adjacent to a prominent university renowned for its expertise in life sciences, medicine, and bioengineering. Leveraging this proximity, the firm recruits staff directly from the university to ensure a workforce possessing cutting-edge proficiency in life sciences and sensor technologies (Teeparuksapun et al. 2010).

Diagnostic Incorporated has identified the prospect of entering the market with a new point-of-care diagnostic device for rapid testing of SARS-CoV-2 infection. They believe that their know-how in bioanalytical techniques and experiences in marketing diagnostics to the healthcare market favor their premises to launch a competitive product to urgent needs due to the SARS-CoV-2 pandemic. But they also foresee that such a device can easily be converted to other commercial diagnostic targets where point-of-care testing is of great value (Parihar et al. 2025).

The bioanalytical prerequisites for diagnostic covid testing are well-known (Sokolowska et al. 2020). The molecular 3D structure of the virus is characterized, and the potential target structures for biorecognition by immunological or other related methods are known. Performance criteria for assaying are described (Wang et al. 2020; Gluckman et al. 2023). Modern biosensor techniques furnish a variety of measurement approaches, including immunosensors and sensors based on aptameric recognition structures (Gürsan et al. 2023).

C.-F. Mandenius, *Bioengineering Design Methodology*,
https://doi.org/10.1007/978-3-032-33940-9_12

Diagnostic Incorporated has profound technical experiences in diagnostic applications with similar approaches. However, to develop a new product, they need support from external expertise to compare different designs from a quality and production economic perspective. *Diagnostic Incorporated* has therefore decided to assign an external consultancy group to investigate design opportunities and pros and cons for alternative designs. The following objectives of the assignment have been set up:

- Deliver two alternative design solutions for a SARS-CoV-2 diagnostic biosensor based on modern biorecognition principles such as antibodies or aptamers that facilitate large-scale global production and distribution.
- Provide a design that functions as either a platform-based system with exchangeable consumables or a fully disposable unit, ensuring the architecture is easily adaptable to other diagnostic targets.
- Ensure the device is intuitive for home use and self-testing so that operation procedures do not impede marketing or clinical adoption.
- Meet rigorous criteria for sensitivity and selectivity, ensuring that ten repeated tests within 1 h do not deviate by more than 10% in precision using the same batch of consumables.
- Ensure all disposable components maintain a shelf storage life of at least 6 months under standard facility conditions.
- Develop a strategy for an initial volume of 500,000 units per year to capture a 10% market share, with the capacity for a threefold upscaling of production.
- Maintain production costs at less than 50% of revenue, ensuring that any reusable reader device costs less than 50 EUR to manufacture.

The assignment is subject to the following specific caveats:

- The product must be globally protectable through patents, ownership, or formal user agreements.
- The upfront R&D and investment costs must be paid off within 5 years.
- Any requirement for subcontracting separate parts in the design must be clearly justified.
- All solutions must comply with current clinical demands in Europe to allow for CE-certification.

12.2 Training Scenario of the Assignment

For design training of students or other trainees, a scenario should preferably be based on the following prerequisites:

- The trainees are supposed to be a design team belonging to an independent consultancy company (cf. Fig. 4.5). The trainees should form a team composed of 5–6 individuals with backgrounds in biomedical technology, sensor technology, process construction and bioanalytical technology. They have access to digital design tools, simulation and modelling tools for bioprocess design and calculations, as well as software for design of experiments (DoE) and process economic calculations (see also Sect. 3.11). The consultancy company has no own resources for prototyping or testing diagnostic devices, nor does *Diagnostic Incorporated* have access to such but will agree to subcontract such testing and evaluation.

- The trainees should be in close contact with *Diagnostic Incorporated's* own expertise on development and production. In the training scenario, this is realized through external tutorial experts. These experts share their medical and marketing plans with the trainees to the degree necessary for solving the assignment. Internal cost factors for operational costs, including buildings and renting, are provided. Labor costs are based on standard employment agreements and should be added to cost calculations.
- The *Diagnostic Incorporated* has previously collaborated with subcontractors for small-scale manufacturing, and experienced expertise is available for the trainees through tutorial experts.
- The trainees' report to *Diagnostic Incorporated* management on progress and final reports. The results should be delivered orally and in writing. The typical time frame for the assignment is in the range of 3–3 months. This can be shortened if lower demand for reporting is expected. Reports should be concise and succinct and follow typical company standards (see also Sect. 4.4.7).

12.3 A Recommended Design Approach

(i) *Structuring the Assignment and Establishing User Requirements*

From the assignment description and background of *Diagnostic Incorporated*, critical conditions and a general structure of the assignment can be conceived (Fig. 12.1). As evident, development activities and other preconditions are already established at *Diagnostic Incorporated.* Activities in the assignment include the work of identifying potential recognition structures that can mimic the Covid target, how to assemble the device, and how to adapt it to user needs. The sales of the product to the customers are the responsibility of the company's marketing people, and they assess the size of the market and the product price (as given through the assignment). Thus, the focus of the design work should be the following:

- To identify suitable biorecognition structures
- To identify what disposable components of the devices should be accessible and economically possible
- To find realistic continuous production conditions
- To establish process design configurations with these that comply with *Diagnostic Incorporated* production criteria
- To assess and compare the economy of alternatives and compare these with *Diagnostic Incorporated* demands of production volumes and costs.

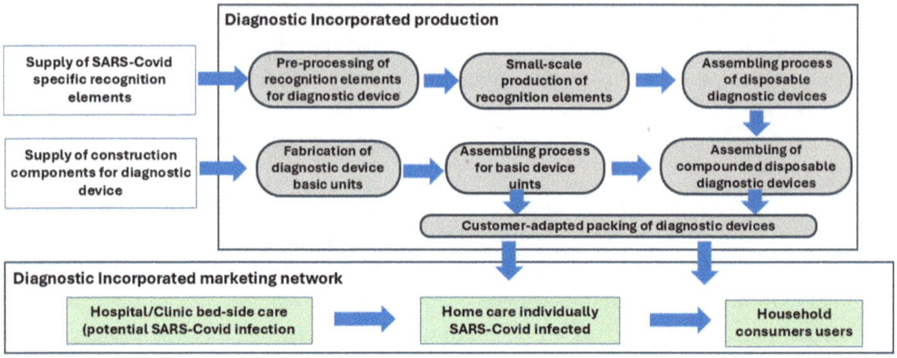

Fig. 12.1 The overall structure of the assignment with important key conditions, factors, and critical issues. Conditions and the general structure for the Covid diagnostic device

- To evaluate the scalability of the alternative designs for a higher production volume.
- To ascertain that prioritized design alternatives comply with regulatory requirements

The design must identify acceptable practice needs for the intended users of Covid testing. This must include the need for healthcare support, specifications, and settings for realistic target values. Moreover, the cost limits for the implementation and production of a device must be assessed in relation to Diagnostic Incorporated's planned market volumes.

To reach the objectives of affordability, optimization should be considered once a feasible detailed design is established. That can preferably be done by statistical experimental methods and mechanistic modelling.

Before conceiving design alternatives, a deeper understanding of user needs is necessary. Product users are considered to include not only those inside the company, such as production personnel, but also those individuals responsible for sales who possess qualified insight into what medical treatment needs. This understanding can be achieved through discussions and interviews with experienced coworkers in the company, with external technical expertise, and, of course, with the clients. This must include representative users, in particular medical doctors responsible for the medical treatment of patients with NHL. From the outcome of the discussions and interviews, each need or requirement is converted into specifications that are either qualitative or quantitative (Table 12.1). These specified needs are ranked based on their criticality, importance, or urgency. These specifications must be agreed upon with Diagnostic Incorporated. It will then be possible to check recurrently during the design work that these needs are met and to the degree expected. Without doubt, these needs and requirements are crucial for the success of the product on the market.

From the framework of the assignment (Fig. 12.1) and the ranked and specified needs and requirements, it is possible to start a conceptualization of the assignment.

Table 12.1 User requirements and specifications with priorities for the Covid diagnostic device

Requirement	Specification	Priority
Patients/healthcare using SARS-CoV-2 testing		
Failure of detection shall be very low	99.9% correct response	Very high
Disposables must be distributed globally and fast	Within 2 days	Very high
Product shelf-life in customer refrigerators shall minimize supply logistics	Storage stability of consumables must exceed 1 year	High
Response time for device should be better than other products	Less than 1 min	Very high
Diagnostic Incorporated's market requirements		
Cost of production versus market price	<50% given at annual production of devices	Very high
IP protection should guarantee no infringement and be easy to protect in court	IPR must cover at least 80% of production	High
Diagnostic Incorporated's production unit		
A tenfold increase in market volume should be possible in the same plant with minor reinvestment	Starting from one million units per year to four million per year. Reinvestment <15% of original investment	Very high
Given 24-h production cost for operation personnel, the cost shall be minimized by a high degree of automation	Operator team shall be less than three operators	High
The environmental impact of waste should not negatively affect the production economy	<2% of production cost must be met (investment and public fees)	High
Production time for one production cycle shall be low	<1 day	High
Campaign production regime should be possible	Start-up and close-down of a campaign shall be <1 week	Medium
Production protocol must be possible to transfer to other plant locations	*Diagnostic incorporated* should be prepared for a transfer	Medium

(ii) *Conceptualization of the Assignment of the Diagnostic Device*

Based on the description of the assignment from *Diagnostics Incorporated*, and the users' specifications and priorities, a conceptual map can be established that shows the functional needs for the design and the fabrication of a SARS-CoV-2-specific diagnostic device (Fig. 12.2). As recommended in Chaps. 3 and 4, the map's functions and systems can be summarized into (Mandenius and Björkman 2011; Hubka and Eder 1988; Pahl et al. 2007; Ulrich et al. 2019):

Biological functions of the diagnostic device for biorecognition elements with a specificity toward SARS-CoV-2 virus biostructures that ensure an accurate response and discriminate the response from other infectious biostructures. The elements must exhibit necessary stability and analytical reproducibility, be easy to fabricate, and have a long product lifetime. The biorecognition element must have a good

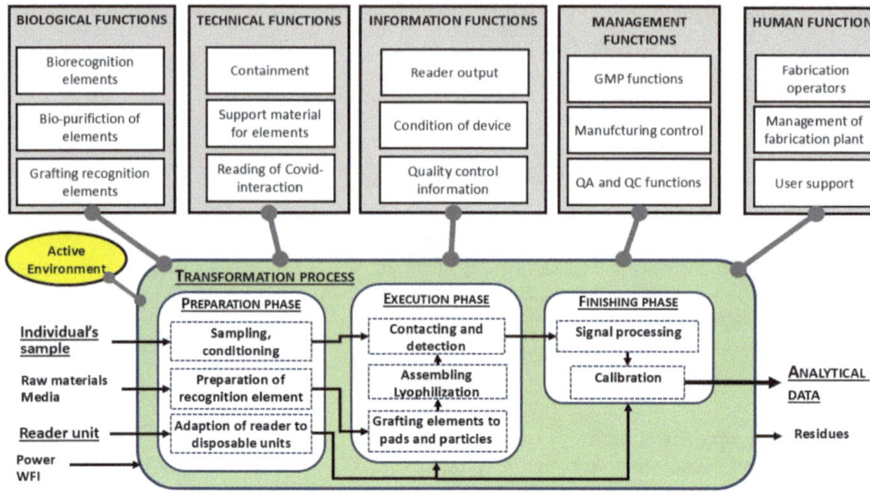

Fig. 12.2 Conceptual functions and transformation process for a diagnostic device for testing SARS-CoV-2 infection

possibility to be attached to disposable units, such as disposable chips or stripes, or in contained disposable units. Those diagnostic elements must be very stable, and pure, to ensure a high degree of reliability when attached to the disposable parts. Thus, the stated objectives of *Diagnostic Incorporated's* assignment define the biological functions of the device.

The technical functions of the device should ensure a functionality that can interact with the attached biorecognition element and deliver an accurate measurement signal. Moreover, the technical functions need to be a confined and encaged detection system for providing a convenient device for the user. The choice of fabrication materials has a key role. It should be durable, allowing conjugation with either a biological recognition element or an element of organic or inorganic origin. The material must be able to cope with the patient sample.

The information functions are influenced by an interaction between the tested material and the sensor device detection unit. This unit should generate a response signal with high reliability. It should be translated to useful numerical values for the users. The device must be possible for its compliance to regulatory or certifying organizations. The reader output must be independent of the device itself so that disturbances or ambient conditions do not bias the reader output. Thus, the information functions are strongly interconnected to the users' needs and requirements as prioritized.

The management functions involve the operation of the device, the control of the production and delivery of the product, and its adaptation to quality criteria in healthcare. These must be investigated and implemented in the design solution. The manufacturing of all parts of the device and its consumables must undergo control and adhere to Total Quality Management. It must reach internal control criteria set by *Diagnostic Incorporated* and its subcontracting companies. International standards for medical devices must be certified.

The human functions involved all people in the production and the use of the device (individuals using the device at home, at bedside, in clinic, by nurses and medical doctors). It includes production personnel (operators, engineers, managers, service personnel), those responsible for convenient and safe operations, in the fabrication plant and in the support chain. The needs of the patient, nurse, medical doctor, or other person using the diagnostic device must be allowed to influence the design to a significant degree. This is part of the assignment objectives and the prioritized user requirements.

The map comprises both the use of the sensor device for testing suspected SARS-CoV-2 infection of individuals and the production of the diagnostic platform, including disposable and reader units (Fig. 12.2). It would be possible to separate the figure into two parts, one for the testing procedure and one for producing the device units. However, given the assignment objectives and the assigner's perspective, it is considered an advantage to put them together in one conceptual map. This simplifies understanding interactions between functions and components for the best design alternatives.

This is true because objectives and user needs appear in all five functional categories. This underscores interactions that appear and contribute to the transformation process.

From studying the functions' adaptability to the specified needs, a variety of biotechnical configurations can be considered to realize the requested functionality. Especially three biorecognition methods can be considered (Fig. 12.3):

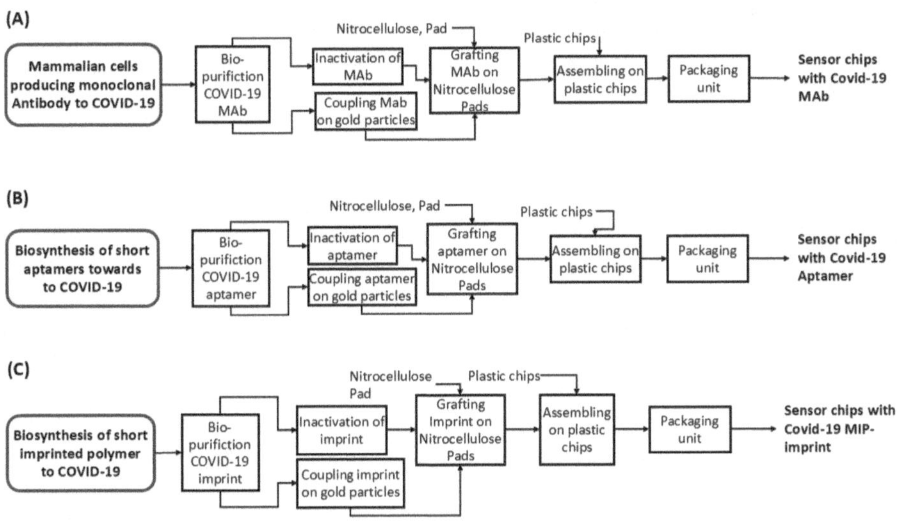

Fig. 12.3 Configurative design alternatives derived from the conceptual map

- Monoclonal antibody for one or more receptor sites with high specificity toward current Covid variants (Rosa et al. 2022; Gürsan et al. 2023)
- Molecular imprinted polymers (MIP) where an engineered recognition site mimics the Covid receptors on the virus capsid (Crapnell et al. 2020; Idila et al. 2017)
- Stable low-molecular aptamers selected by the SELEX technique toward the Covid-target receptors (Zhou et al. 2014; Ning et al. 2020)

These biorecognition possibilities are potential components in the three tentative configurations, showing different combinations with detection methods and other functions from the conceptual map (Fig. 12.2). Importantly, the configurations allow mass production, in their own facilities or by subcontractors, where recognition elements should comply with *Diagnostic Incorporated*'s objectives.

From these configurations, based on reasoning from known prerequisites, two alternatives can be selected for a more detailed design.

The configurations should be judged from their ability for:

- Compliance with the objectives of *Diagnostic Incorporated* and identified user needs
- Preserving stability of recognition elements in the device
- Assumptions of fabrication cost and cost-effective scale-up and mass production of the parts of the diagnostic device

(iii) *Detailed Design of the Conceptual Alternatives of the Diagnostic Device*

Two configurations are particularly relevant for comparison regarding their technical equipment and material flows (Fig. 12.3). This evaluation should be guided by the functional frames and objectives of the assignments (O'Brian 2019). Furthermore, these configurations should be discussed with experts at *Diagnostic Incorporated* to weigh their pros and cons. This will facilitate establishing design priorities and specifically determining whether to utilize antibody or aptameric recognition elements for the SARS-CoV-2 target.

The priorities should concern the following considerations:

- Aptamers are attractive due to their stability as organic molecules.
- Aptamers may be produced cost-effectively due to fewer reaction steps, modest cost of raw materials, and a small-scale facility for production.
- Monoclonal antibodies are attractive due to their established derivation methods and production methods.
- Monoclonal antibodies are believed to have the best credibility on the market due to their widespread use in diagnostic applications.
- Aptamers require, however, more quality testing due to being unproven for the application.
- Aptamers may have long-term potential and durability for forthcoming products on the same platform.
- Both alternatives are feasible in miniature device formats, which is an advantage for the intended application.

A design based on a SARS-CoV-2-specific antibody expressed in a cell culture, purified and attached to a nitrocellulose pad results in a production process with 15 units (Fig. 12.4a). A part of the antibody is inactivated and is used as an internal reference. The active and reference antibodies are assembled on a plastic strip which forms the user chip. Gold particles are used to amplify the detection of target binding. The chips are to be used with a detector unit delivered by a subcontractor.

In the other detailed design, the antibody ligand is replaced by a SARS-CoV-2-specific aptamer and a non-specific aptamer (Fig. 12.4b). The procedure to attach the aptamers is comparable with the antibody attachment procedure. The subsequent fabrication of the plastic chips remains unchanged. The detection is also based on a detector amplified by gold particles.

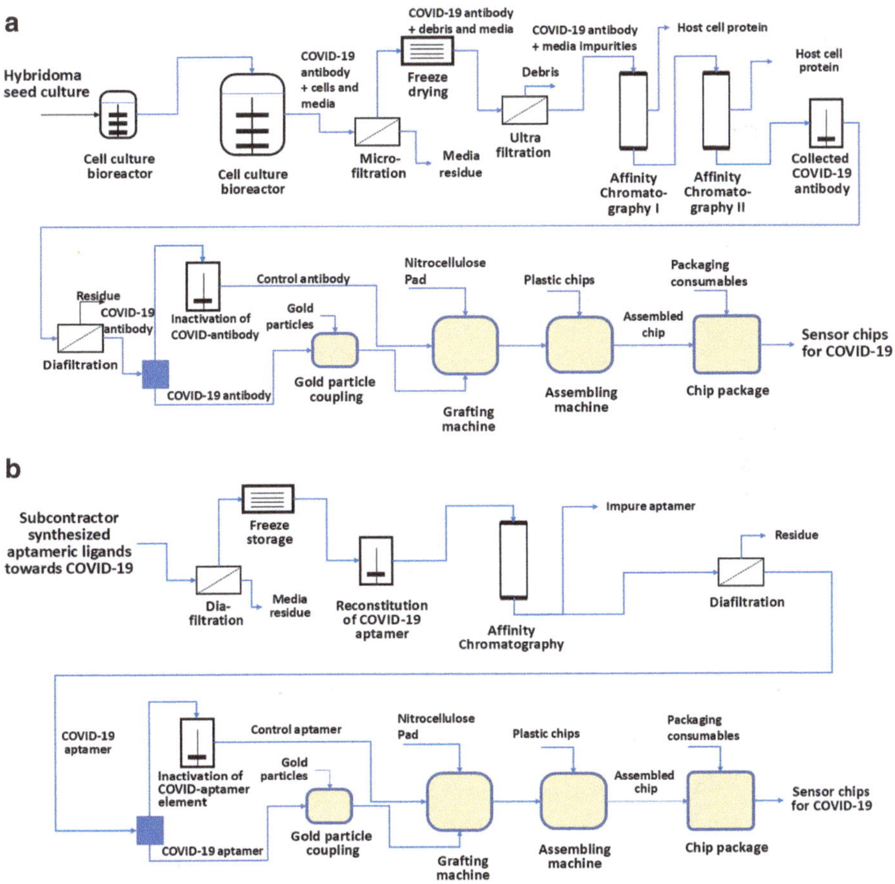

Fig. 12.4 (**a**) Detailed design for a process for fabrication of chips based on using a monoclonal antibody specific to SARS-CoV-2. (**b**) Detailed design for a process for fabrication of chips based on using a synthesized aptamer specific for SARS-CoV-2

The main difference between the two designs is that the specific aptamer components are developed, screened, and delivered by a subcontractor while the specific antibody is produced at small scale by *Diagnostic Incorporated*. This is motivated by the size of production, small enough to be performed in 10–50 L bioreactors with conventional culture techniques. However, the development of a specific antibody-expressing cell line is commissioned to a subcontractor. These differences will influence the economy of production. It is obvious from the design that this requires resources in the form of competence, small-scale processing equipment, and technical skills. The advantage is that it is under *Diagnostic Incorporated's* full control; the disadvantage is that it is a vulnerability for the company, which may be a too large risk-taking.

For both designs, a reusable handheld detector device is employed. The provision of the detector is subcontracted based on proven techniques.

(iv) *Production Economic Evaluation of the Detailed Designs*

The evaluation of production economics should reveal where critical costs are generated in the designs and if *Diagnostic Incorporated's* assignment objectives are covered and compatible with these costs (Peters et al. 2003; Ray et al. 2022).

The development, implementation, and production costs for the two prioritized alternatives are usually assessed at a precision level of 15–25%. It should be emphasized that the evaluation does not aim to show the precise costs per se but to provide a cost structure that shows where the economic risks are found. This will in this case especially concern:

- The balance between costs for subcontracting and in-house production
- The cost for reaching the required quality
- The mass production implications on costs

The costs for production between the alternatives differ to some extent (Table 12.2).

The expenditure that deviates substantially between the alternatives is the *upfront R&D and subcontracting costs*. For the antibody in-house production alternative, the cell line for the specific SARS-CoV-2 antibody must be established and banked (Master Cell Bank), and a method for antibody production must be developed. For the aptamer production, the SARS-CoV-2-specific aptamer must be established and produced. This work can be subcontracted by external research and development services and/or developed in the company. Here, it is chosen to use subcontracting external services for establishing the cell line and the aptamer structures.

Also, the mass fabrication of chips by assembling the antibodies or aptamers with chips must be developed by a combination of external and internal upfront R&D.

Finally, the reader device needs to be developed.

All upfront R&D costs are here estimated to be 800 kEUR for the antibody alternative and 900 kEUR for the aptamer alternative. It should be added that the uncertainty of these assessed costs is relatively high.

The *chip fabrication plant* requires substantial investment in both alternatives. This includes fabrication equipment (assembly machines with strip cutter, cassette

Table 12.2 Summary of the cost evaluation for the two recommended design alternatives

Type of costs	Diagnostic device with antibody (kEUR)	Diagnostic device with aptamer (kEUR)
Investment costs		
Upfront production R&D		
Upfront internal R&D	500	500
Upfront external R&D (reader device)	200	200
Upfront external R&D (aptamer)	–	200
Upfront external R&D (antibody)	100	–
Total upfront production R&D	*800*	*900*
Equipment and instruments		
Bioreactor units	150	–
Separation units, freezer unit	100	–
Auxiliary units Equipment for chip fabrication	50 200	– 200
Packaging machine	100	100
QC lab instrumentation	50	50
Total equipment and instrumentation costs	*650*	*350*
Other production expenditures		
Validation of plant	100	100
Installation of equipment (× 0.5)	325	450
Project planning of plant (× 0.3)	195	270
Taxation (× 0.1)	65	90
Buildings (× 0.3)	195	270
Total additional production expenditures	*880*	*1180*
Total investment costs	**2330**	**2430**
Operational costs (annual per targeted production volume)		
Consumables for production		
Consumables for chip fabrication	20	20
Consumables for antibody production	60	–
Consumables for quality control	20	20
Total production consumable	*100*	*40*
Additional operation expenditures		
Labor in production (incl. QC)	100	50
Renting of buildings	100	100
Taxation	25	25
Subcontracting of cell line/aptamers	75	75
Maintenance of plant	150	50
Management	50	50

(continued)

Table 12.2 (continued)

Type of costs	Diagnostic device with antibody (kEUR)	Diagnostic device with aptamer (kEUR)
Total additional operation expenditures	*500*	*350*
Total operational cost	*600*	*390*
Annual payback of investments (5 years)	*466*	*486*
Total annual production cost	**1066**	**876**

presser, sample pad strip cutter and conjugate pad strip cutter) assessed to 1000 kEUR.

The in-*house antibody production* requires additional equipment investment (for cultivation, recovery, purification and process analysis) assessed to amount to 300 kEUR.

With the installation and validation, the total investment costs for production, including the upfront R&D costs, amount to 2330 kEUR for the antibody alternative and 2430 kEUR for the aptamer alternative.

The *operational costs* include culture media, other consumables for production, salaries for production personnel, QC costs, and other indirect costs that are proportional to the annual production volume. It is likely that some of these costs can be squeezed down due to the size of the procured quantities of consumables and subcontracted materials. The annual cost for operation amounts to 600 kEUR for the antibody alternative and 380 kEUR for the aptamer alternative.

The *total annual production cost* with the same payback period for both alternatives (5 years) is estimated to 3430 kEUR for the antibody alternative and 2830 kEUR for the aptamer alternative.

Decisive criteria for the overall economy are the number of chips consumed annually per patient user and the potential net income per chip. It is assumed that one customer uses one reader device. The strategy is to generate income from the sale of disposable chips while supplying the users with the reader device for free. The economic risk of this marketing strategy is further evaluated in the modelling part below.

A strategical expenditure is the reader unit for the chips. In the economic evaluation, the same type of chip reader is assumed for both alternatives, thereby causing no difference in the cost analysis. A chip reader cost through subcontracting of 50 EUR per reader unit, user, and year is assumed.

Sales volume will influence the net income. Net income at the same price favors the antibody device and allows a more competitive price setting. Here, a yearly sale of 500,000 chips is assumed, which will result in a favorable overall economy.

The circle charts show the distribution of costs for the antibody and aptamer alternatives (Fig. 12.5). As seen, the proportion of investments favors the antibody device. As this leads to faster payback to investors, it is likely that this option is also preferable for that reason.

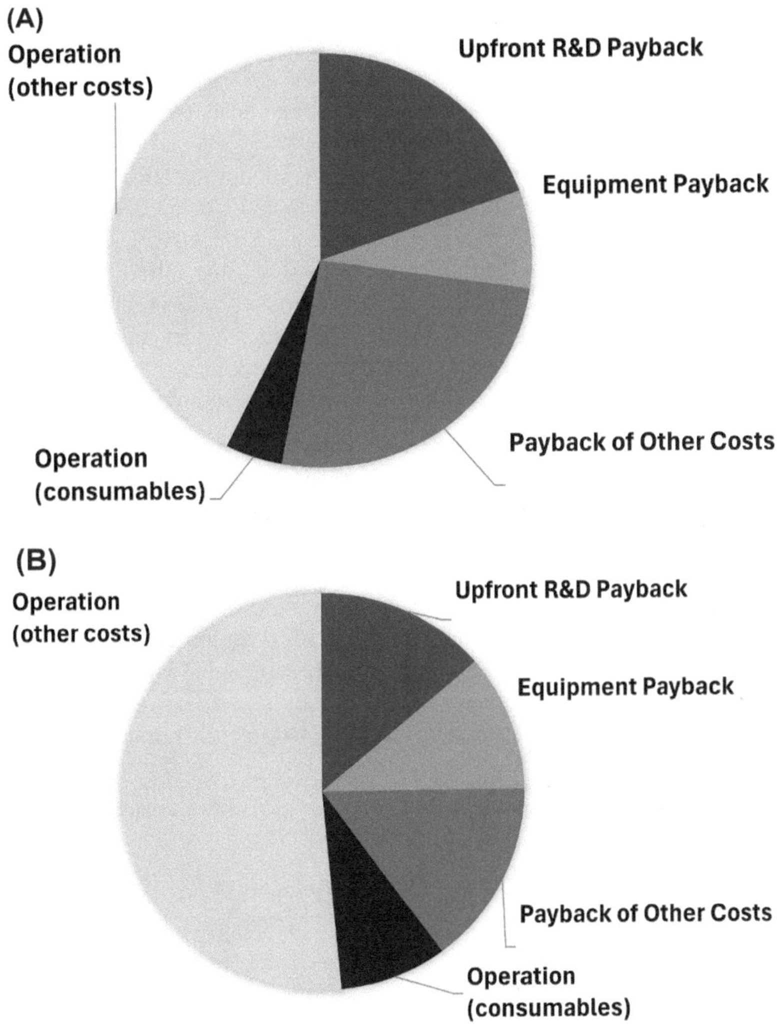

Fig. 12.5 Comparison of distribution of cost for production of the antibody (**a**) and aptamer (**b**) alternatives

It is assumed that a company like *Diagnostic Incorporated* will negotiate purchases in the procurement process to improve the economy. The assignment about that, but to grasp the interconnectivity of costs and design options, and to integrate quality into the design at an affordable cost.

(xxii) *Optimization of the Design*

Once it is decided which design alternatives are to be prioritized, their performance and production economy can be optimized using established optimization methods (Martins and Ning 2021; Sioshansi and Conejo 2017). The design alternatives discussed under section (iv) present distinct opportunities for improving both operational performance and cost-efficiency. Consequently, specific optimization targets must be prioritized and selected based on their likelihood of yielding successful results, weighed against the resources and costs required to perform the optimization.

Table 12.3 summarizes several viable options for optimization, alongside their applicable optimization techniques and potential benefits or outcomes. The overall goals of these optimization actions are to maximize productivity and yields while reducing resource utilization and overall processing time, all of which directly contribute to a positive impact on the long-term production economy.

The optimization work must preferably be executed at a later stage of product and production development. It is crucial that these activities are strategically prioritized so as not to delay or retard the eventual marketing and commercial launch of the product.

Optimizing the production of SARS-CoV-2 chips by design of experiments technique: *Diagnostic Incorporated* should use the design of experiments (DoE) technique to optimize primarily to improve the analytical performance of the chip as advised (Table 12.3).

Several parametrical factors are potential candidates for DoE investigation (Mandenius and Brundin 2008; Montgomery 2020; Brereton 2003). The procedure described in Chap. 3 should be used, based on screening and two-level experiments. Commercially available programs are recommended for such investigations. It is up to *Diagnostic Incorporated* to decide how far it is worthwhile pursuing these efforts.

Table 12.3 Objects that can enhance production by using optimization techniques

Object of optimization	Intended outcome	Applicable optimization technique
The design of the chip in terms of biorecognition elements and size	A more geometrically compact chip with better performance	Factorial design of experimentally available parameters
The performance of the aptamer element in terms of specificity, stability, and yield of attachment	Minimizing the number of aptamer elements without compromising diagnostic performance	Factorial design of selected parameters
The time for diagnosis at the user end	Shortening the delay of diagnostic response rendering a more competitive product	Factorial design and structured modelling
Production time for the chip and device	A lower production cost per chip unit	Structured modelling
Prolonging the storage time	Extended storage time with unchanged performance will make the product more competitive	Factorial design of stabilizers and storage conditions
Assembling times and lags in production	Shorter total production time and higher throughput and productivity	Mechanistic modelling and factorial design

Table 12.4 Objects for design of experiments to optimize in the SARS-CoV-2 chips

Objects for optimization	Factors in DoE plan	Responses to measure
Choice of chip fabrication materials	Chip materials Chip surface treatment methods	Attached aptamers Attached antibodies
Choice of chemical linkage structure of ligand (aptamer or antibody)	Chip ligand structure	Attached aptamers Attached antibodies
Choice of ligand immobilization method on chip	Attachment methods	Attached aptamers Attached antibodies
Packaging of ligands on each chip	Number of recognition elements per chip	Attached aptamers Attached antibodies
Influence of media in the fabrication methods	Testing different media	Binding of target
Occupation of fabrication machine in plant	Time for attachment in production	Number of attached aptamers Attached antibodies
Necessary number of aptamers to attach per chip	Attachment number of aptamer	Number of attached aptamers per chip Analytical response of each chip

The factors suggested in Table 12.4 are examples, and other factors can be considered for DoE optimization. At the prototype stage of the design, it is advisable to vary the factors experimentally and to measure responses and effects on a test bench that realistically mirrors the usage of the device.

Some of the factors are qualitative measures. This could aim to compare differences between chip surfaces that the investigator chooses. For example, three to four surface materials considered economically feasible can be selected for comparison. The same can be done with respect to chemically different ligand structures and attachment methods. The DoE responses should then be: (i) the number of attached aptamers, which will require some type of marker, and (ii) the activity or availability of the aptamer of the fabricated chip, which will require a marked test virus that represents the SARS-CoV-2 virus.

Quantitative DoE factors should be studied at two or three levels of concentrations or numbers. Here, the same response measurement methods can be used.

Other DoE options of interest could be:

- The geometric dimensions of the chip and equipment can lead to improved performance of reaction efficiency, reaction time, and use of construction material and consumables. All of them have a potential impact on unit production costs.
- The sensitivity of the assay may also be optimized by dimensional aspects of the sensor device. As specified, the sensitivity must reach a set value and be validated. A sensitivity margin for the assay should be ascertained, which ultimately is a design matter.

Performing these experiments will require considerable time, effort, and cost, so prioritizing the DoE work is very recommendable. Long-term and short-term impacts of the design due to the optimization should guide the DoE plan. Most likely, factors that are easy to control are feasible to include. Reaction components at high and low concentrations, amounts of reagents and samples, when a device, antibody in or added per unit, and size of unit are such parameters that are wise to select. Responses such as stability or variability, assay response time, costs of goods and services, number of assays per time, are examples of parameters of interest to assess.

For performing the experimental work of the DoE, first-version prototype devices should be constructed with the main purpose of performing the experiments. A dedicated lab allowing parallel experiments would make it possible to carry out DoE within a relatively short period at a reasonable cost. The foreseeable impact of the sensor device's performance could potentially be in the order of 100–200%. The win would primarily be the cost of goods and the competitive edge over alternative devices on the market.

The focus of the DoE plans should be on:

- Sample volume and sensitivity
- Device size and response time
- Cost per test and production cost of antibody

Here, parameters for an aptamer-based device are discussed, including such costs as provision and production of aptamers, which is highly decisive for the economy. If this is replaced by another recognition system, the outcome will certainly be affected, for the better or worse. This emphasizes the importance of performing these calculations as an early step of the development process to exclude uneconomical alternatives. However, in the early stage, this is not easy due to the prediction of cost for newly invented reagents and their procurement.

Optimization by SARS-CoV-2 chip production by mechanistic modelling: Preferences should be given to parameters that can be related to the performance of the sensor device and the production economics (Table 12.3). The response time of the diagnostic sensor is possible to model by differential equations from critical cost-related variables (Doran 2013; O'Brian 2019; Nielsen et al. 2011). Certain redundancy with results from DoE may be expected. However, mechanistic modelling results will be more accurate and can facilitate maximization of analytical performance and dimensioning of the chips.

Sensitivity of detection, volume of sample per test, assay response time, and total assay time are good candidates for structured and mechanistic modelling, especially if these can be associated with construction and operation. The time variable in the differential equations (dX/dt) can be replaced with, for example, the sample volume (dX/dV) or assay cost ($dX/d€$), and their relation to critical parameters in the model equations. Considering the form and structure of such relationships will actively support the detailed design. Several parameters related to the sensor device are of interest and possible to use in the models (Table 12.5).

Table 12.5 Variables for mechanistic modelling in the aptamer and antibody alternatives

Parameter investigated	Model variables	Expected outcome/ information value
Production time	Number of chips produced production cost (total) production cost (per unit)	Ligands immobilized per chip Aptamer immobilized chip MAb immobilized per chip
Surface area of chip	Detection reading	Reader performance data
Production time per chip	Assembling steps	Defined downstream machines
Cost of production	Assembling steps Type of assembling machines	Best economy
Production time in upstream stage (cultivation)	Upstream production of MAb Upstream production cost	Best design alternative due to cost of upstream choice

Three main modelling approaches can be considered: (i) to address the design of the chip itself, (ii) to maximize the production capacity of the chip fabrication plant, and (iii) to minimize the cost for production of chips. The three simulations below exemplify how the models can be structured and used, and what outcome that can be anticipated.

In the *first example*, the total annual production volume of chips in relation to the design of the chip fabrication plant is modelled. The simulation shows how the production throughput is maximized by reducing the number of antibody molecules or aptamer molecules on each chip (Fig. 12.6a).

The simulation is based on the following equations:

$$\mathrm{Prod}_{\mathrm{chip}} = N_{\mathrm{lines}} t_{\mathrm{chip}} \tag{12.1}$$

$$\mathrm{Lig}_{\mathrm{annual}} = \mathrm{Prod}_{\mathrm{chip}}\ C\ \mathrm{Lig}_{\mathrm{chip}} \tag{12.2}$$

$$r_{\mathrm{ligand}} = k_{\mathrm{ligand}}\ A_{\mathrm{chip}} \tag{12.3}$$

where $\mathrm{Prod}_{\mathrm{chip}}$ is the annual production of chips (chips/year), N_{lines} is the number of production parallel fabrication machines in the plant (number of lines), t_{chip} is the time for fabricating each chip (h), $\mathrm{Lig}_{\mathrm{annual}}$ is the annual consumption of ligand (mg antibody or aptamer), and $\mathrm{Lig}_{\mathrm{chip}}$ is the number of ligands on each chip (mg/chip).

In the simulation, a limiting attachment rate of ligands, r_{ligand} (ligands/s), to the chip surface, A_{chip}, is assumed (Eq. 12.3). The rate is characterized by a rate constant k_{ligand} (ligands/cm^2 h).

Obviously, a too low fabrication rate can be compensated for by a parallel number of machine lines. The graphs show how the annual production capacity of chips depends on processing time for each chip and the number or size of machines of the fabrication plant. Moreover, the graphs relate this to the consumption of ligands.

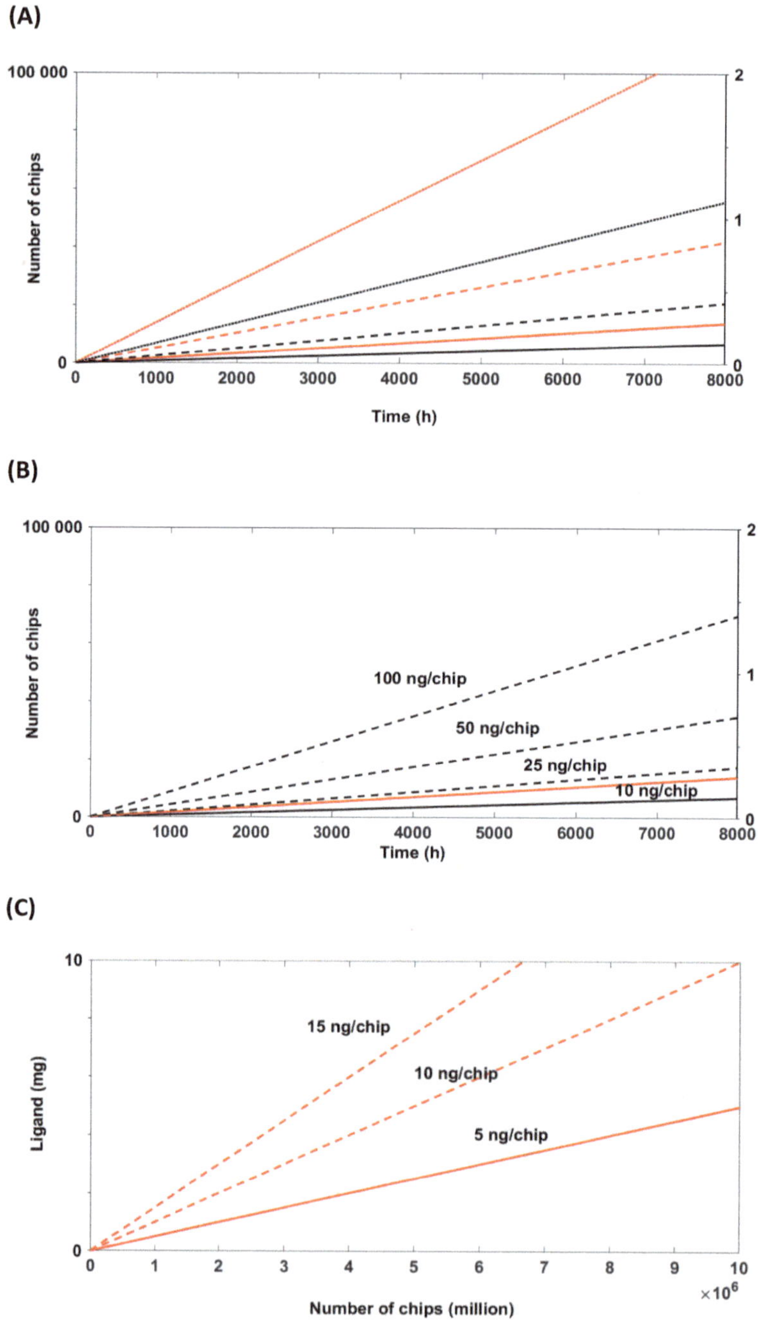

Fig. 12.6 (**a**) Annual chip production with time at defined processing conditions per chip (red, number of chips; black, number of ligands consumed). (**b**) Production performance at varying ligand loading per chip related to ligand consumption (black) and number of chips (red). (**c**) Ligand consumption at increasing production of chips at three ligand loadings per chip (red)

The simulation helps to predict the necessary size of the plant to reach the production goals set in the assignment and the impact of shortening the attachment procedure of ligands and the preparation of chips.

If motivated, a parallel graph to estimate the economic consequence on production by these modifications of the production method can be set up.

In the *second example*, the design of each SARS-CoV-2-specific chip is modelled. The purpose is to study how to maximize the assay sensitivity in relation to the number of ligand molecules per chip. The simulation shows how the assay response increases with assay time in the direction of the detection limit, which must be reached (Fig. 12.6b). These levels are indicated in the simulation diagram. The model equations include the rate of affinity binding of the ligand (antibody or aptamer) and the number of ligands and surface area of each chip.

The simulation uses the following model equations:

$$\mathrm{Prod}_{\mathrm{chip}}/dt = S_{\mathrm{covid}} \times k_{\mathrm{ligand}} \tag{12.4}$$

$$k_{\mathrm{ligand}} = A_{\mathrm{chip}} \times \mathrm{Lig}_{\mathrm{chip}} \tag{12.5}$$

$$\mathrm{Resp}_{\mathrm{chip}}$$

where $\mathrm{Resp}_{\mathrm{chip}}$ is the response of the assay related to the binding of the SARS-CoV-2 target (mg target); S_{covid}, the number of target molecular structures in the assayed sample (target/sample); k_{ligand}, the association rate of SARS-CoV-2 targets to the ligand on the chip (mg target/s/ligand); A_{chip}, the area of the chip (cm^2); and $\mathrm{Lig}_{\mathrm{chip}}$, the amounts of ligands on each chip (mg/chip).

The simulation graphs show how the assay time depends on the size of the chip (in terms of its area and number of ligands), and the association rate of the chosen ligand (antibody or aptamer).

The simulation helps to predict the necessary size of the chip used in the assay to reach the set detection limit and its margin. Furthermore, it indicates the potential to select and develop ligands to maximize response and detection time. By that, cues for further development of the assay components are designated.

In the *third example*, the production cost of SARS-CoV-2-specific chips is modelled, whether the ligand is an antibody or aptamer. The simulation shows how the production throughput of chips influences the total annual cost (Fig. 12.6c). The ligand cost (antibody or aptamer) depends on expenditure for procurement from subcontractors. In the simulations threshold price levels subcontracting-based procured volume of ligands. This is compared with in-house production of the ligands. Of course, in-house provision of these also equipment costs influence this.

The simulations in this example use the following model equations:

$$\mathrm{Prod}_{\mathrm{annual}}/\mathrm{dLig}_{\mathrm{covid}} = \left(\mathrm{Lig}_{\mathrm{covid}} \times \mathrm{Cost}_{\mathrm{ligand}} \times \mathrm{Lig}_{\mathrm{chip}}\right) + \mathrm{Cost}_{\mathrm{operations}} \tag{12.6}$$

$$\text{Tot-Cost}_{\text{ligand}} = \text{Cost}_{\text{ligand}} \times \text{Lig}_{\text{covid}} \tag{12.7}$$

where $\text{Prod}_{\text{annual}}$ is the total annual production cost (k€/year), $\text{Lig}_{\text{covid}}$ is the consumed amount of ligands per year (mg/year), $\text{Cost}_{\text{ligand}}$ is the procurement cost (or internal production cost) of ligands (€/mg ligand), Lig_{chip} the number of ligands on each chip (mg/chip), and $\text{Cost}_{\text{operation}}$ is the annual costs for other operations in the production (k€/year).

The ligand procurement cost is constrained to a quantity where the unit cost is lowered by 20% when exceeding a one-million-unit quantity. By this, the gain or advantage of producing larger quantities of the product is seen and facilitates to foresee the potential of increasing the market share of the product. It shows the leverage of investing time in refining the design of the assay product toward a lower price setting.

Thus, the mechanistic model provides complementary information to the statistical optimization. In particular, the mechanistic model can address *how many ligands need to be produced* for a certain number of chips. Therefore, it is appropriate to use the mechanistic model once the number of ligands per chip is established in the DoE optimization study.

12.4 Conclusive Suggestions for *Diagnostic Incorporated*

Two design solutions have been identified that align with the project objectives and prioritized user requirements. The design process focused on delivering superior diagnostic performance and robustness while maintaining low total production costs. Success depends on addressing several critical factors:

- Securing competent subcontractors at competitive rates for both design alternatives
- Ensuring all stages of the production chain are scalable to high volumes
- Efficiently coordinating the manufacturing and integration of sensor chips and reader devices

If these factors are effectively managed, the aptamer-based design is recommended for the following reasons:

- Aptamers offer superior stability, which is essential for a product distributed globally across diverse environmental conditions.
- The platform is easily adaptable to other diagnostic targets with minimal development costs, provided molecular screening of aptamer structures is successful.
- The aptamer production line is less sensitive than antibody-based alternatives, particularly during the assembly and ligand-attachment phases.
- Scaling production through parallel lines or relocating to alternative manufacturing sites is economically feasible.

- The design meets all internal objectives for sensitivity, reproducibility, response time, and shelf-life.
- Launching the device for benchtop use initially is recommended, with home care and bedside applications serving as secondary markets.
- The annual production target of 500,000 chips is realistic for this design. However, reliance on subcontractors for key components will significantly impact profit margins, and future scaling will require substantial investment in machinery.

One identified risk is that aptamer sensitivity may be insufficient for certain viral stages; however, this can be mitigated by increasing the density of aptamer ligands on each chip.

The primary external threat is the likelihood of competitors developing similar devices at lower price points with enhanced performance. Economic analysis further indicates that labor costs—both internally and at the subcontractor level—will exert significant influence on the final production costs.

Ultimately, the aptamer-based platform is the superior strategic choice for Diagnostic Incorporated due to its environmental resilience, manufacturing scalability, and long-term versatility across diverse diagnostic targets. By prioritizing this design, the company can meet its rigorous performance and shelf-life requirements while establishing a robust foundation for global distribution. To ensure a successful launch, the company must focus on securing high-value subcontracts and optimizing the unit-cost-to-revenue ratio, thereby mitigating competitive pricing threats and ensuring the investment is fully amortized within the targeted 5-year window.

12.5 Tutorial Perspectives on the Assignment

The primary challenge of this assignment lies in balancing biological complexities with the engineering requirements necessary to create a viable, economically realistic medical device. A significant hurdle is the strategic trade-off between the recurring income from consumables and the cost coverage of non-disposable hardware. While this is a business-driven decision, it is essential for bioengineering designers to understand how this dynamic influences the integration of hardware and sensor chips.

It is critical that trainees recognize that the biological aspects of this project operate across five distinct levels:

- The biomolecular nature of the viral disease
- The biological specificity of recognition required for clinical sensitivity and precision
- The comparative advantage of biological recognition over alternative methods
- The optimization of these elements from an engineering perspective
- The determination of what is economically feasible

A common pitfall for trainees is becoming preoccupied with biological uniqueness at the expense of production economy and actual user needs. Regarding the engineering perspective, trainees often require guidance to deepen their understanding of fabricating and assembling non-biological components. As this typically falls outside their prior experience, insightful mentorship is necessary to help them integrate these components into the final device design.

Tutorial actions should emphasize the following:

- Maintain a constant focus on the end-user's specific needs and requests.
- Reinforce the value of SWOT analysis. While trainees are often familiar with the concept, they rarely apply it effectively to fine-tune a design.
- Address the natural preference for biological solutions by consistently referring back to the original functional requirements, which are often neglected during the later stages of development.
- Lower the threshold for considering subcontracting. Trainees often assume that production must remain entirely in-house for exclusivity; however, they should be encouraged to view subcontracting as a strategic tool, supported by thorough cost calculations and a clear description of subcontracting premises.

The potential biological elements available are diverse, yet experimental data remains sparse. Consequently, early experimental verification is required to select or exclude alternatives with certainty. Since standard design tools offer only a rough evaluation of these possibilities, the project benefits significantly from rigorous conceptual structuring.

In the final stages of training, tutors should suggest the use of DoE. Developing a preliminary experimental plan through DoE promotes higher-quality work and allows trainees to judge which design alternatives hold the greatest potential, significantly increasing the overall learning outcome.

References

Brereton RG (2003) Chemometrics, data analysis for laboratory and chemical plants. Wiley, Chichester

Crapnell RD, Dempsey-Hibbert NC, Peeters M (2020) Molecularly imprinted polymer based electrochemical biosensors: overcoming the challenges of detecting vital biomarkers and speeding up diagnosis. Talanta Open 2:100018. https://doi.org/10.1016/j.talo.2020.100018

Doran PM (2013) Biochemical engineering principles, 2nd edn. Elsevier, Amsterdam. https://doi.org/10.1016/C2009-0-22348-8

Gluckman JP, McGill SG, Kalivretenos AG et al (2023) The use of molecularly imprinted polymers for the rapid detection of emerging viral outbreaks. *US Patent Application* US2023/0103369

Gürsan E, Sentürk MH, Yildiz E et al. (2023) Impediometric immunosensor for the diagnosis of Covid-19. Patent application WO 2023/091119 A1

Hubka V, Eder WE (1988) Theory of technical systems, a total concept theory for engineering design. Springer Verlag, Berlin

Idila N, Hedström M, Denizlid A et al (2017) Whole cell based microcontact imprinted capacitive biosensor for the detection of *Escherichia coli*. Biosens Bioelectron 87:807–815. https://doi.org/10.1016/j.bios.2016.08.096

Krammer F (2020) SARS-CoV-2 vaccines in development. Nature 586:516–527. https://doi.org/10.1038/s41586-020-2798-3

Mandenius CF, Björkman M (2011) Biomechatronic design in biotechnology: a methodology for development of biotechnology products. John Wiley & Sons, New Jersey. https://doi.org/10.1002/9781118067147

Mandenius CF, Brundin A (2008) Bioprocess optimization using design-of-experiments methodology. Biotechnol Prog 24:1191–1203. https://doi.org/10.1002/btpr.67

Martins JRRA, Ning A (2021) Engineering design optimization. Cambridge University Press, Cambridge. https://doi.org/10.1017/9781108980647

Montgomery DC (2020) Design and analysis of experiments, 9th edn. John Wiley & Sons, New York. ISBN: 978-1-119-63842-1

Nielsen J, Villadsen J, Lidén G (2011) Bioreaction engineering principles, 3rd edn. Springer-Nature, New York

Ning Y, Hu J, Lu F (2020) Aptamers used for biosensors and targeted therapy. Biomed Pharmacother 132:110902. https://doi.org/10.1016/j.biopha.2020.110902

O'Brian D (2019) Engineer 4.0: life science handbook for medical devices and biopharmaceuticals. Kindle ISBN-13: 978-1795753340

Pahl G, Beitz W, Feldhusen J et al (2007) Engineering design, a systematic approach, 3rd edn. Springer Verlag, Berlin

Parihar M, Sahana NWN, Biswas R et al (2025) Point-of-care biosensors for infectious disease diagnosis: recent updates and prospects. RSC Adv 15:29267. https://doi.org/10.1039/d5ra03897a

Peters MS, Timmerhaus KD, West RE (2003) Plant design and economics for chemical engineers, 5th edn. McGraw-Hill, New York

Ray SC, Chambers RG, Kumbhakar SC (2022) Handbook of production economics. Springer Nature, New York

Rosa BG, Oluwatomi EA, Guo X et al (2022) Multiplexed immunosensors for point-of-care diagnostic applications. Biosens Bioelectron 203:114050. https://doi.org/10.1016/j.bios.2022.114050

Sioshansi R, Conejo AJ (2017) Optimization in engineering, models and algorithms. Springer International Publishing. ISBN 9783319567679

Sokolowska M, Lukasik ZM, Agache I et al (2020) Immunology of COVID-19, mechanisms, clinical outcome, diagnostics, and perspectives. A report of the European Academy of Allergy and Clinical Immunology (EAACI). Allergy 75:2445–2476. https://doi.org/10.1111/all.14462

Teeparuksapun K, Hedström M, Mattiasson B (2010) Immunochemical binding assays for detection and quantification of trace impurities in biotechnological production. Trends Biotechnol 28:20–27. https://doi.org/10.1016/j.tibtech.2009.10.002

Ulrich KT, Eppinger SD, Yang MC (2019) Product design and development, 7th edn. McGraw-Hill, New York

V'kovski P, Kratzel A, Steiner S et al (2021) Coronavirus biology and replication: implications for SARS- CoV-2. Nat Rev Microbiol 19:155–170. https://doi.org/10.1038/s41579-020-00468-6

Wang MY, Zhao R, Gao LJ et al (2020) SARS-CoV-2: structure, biology, and structure-based therapeutics development. Front Cell Infect Microbiol 10:87269. https://doi.org/10.3389/fcimb.2020.587269

Zhou W, Huang PJJ, Ding J et al (2014) Aptamer-based biosensors for biomedical diagnostics. Analyst 139:2627–2640. https://doi.org/10.1039/c4an00132j

Chapter 13
Case 8: A Bedside Sensor for Blood Glucose Testing of Diabetic Patients

13.1 Assignment: Background, Description, and Objectives

The aim of this training is to develop a convenient diagnostic sensor device, based on proprietary technology, for use in diabetic care in the clinic and in home care (Willis et al. 2025). The sensor device has a multimillion-dollar global market, and several competitors are marketing functionally comparable devices (Bode et al. 2021; Saha et al. 2023). The goal is to design an updated model that outperforms the competitors' devices in convenience and cost-effectiveness while maintaining rigorous standards of precision and reliability (Freckmann et al. 2019; Weinstock et al. 2020; Khanwalker et al. 2022).

The assigning company, *Medtech Sensorics*, has for more than 10 years successfully developed a series of small homecare instruments for blood testing.

The sensor devices utilize a three-enzyme process to process blood cells and convert plasma glucose into a colored by-product (Sanchis-Gomar et al. 2012). A photometric detector then measures this by-product within a disposable cuvette, translating the light absorption into a digital glucose reading via a calibration equation. The enzymes are provided by a larger enzyme manufacturer, and the disposable cuvettes and the reader device are manufactured by subcontractor firms.

The competitors to *Medtech Sensorics* have increased their share of the diabetic care market with inexpensive glucose sensor devices (Jonsson et al. 2015; Drucker et al. 2010; Vreeke et al. 2002; Klintmose 2001; Skyggebjerg and Hillerod 2008; Sabu et al. 2019). It is necessary for *Medtech Sensorics* to strengthen its competitive edge toward these other products by offering a new sensor product at a lower price and with better performance.

Medtech Sensorics has therefore commissioned its development department to reengineer its present sensor device according to the following objectives:

- The basic bioanalytical principle of measurement should be unchanged to rely on existing Intellectual Property Rights (IPR), manufacturing experience, and production logistics.

C.-F. Mandenius, *Bioengineering Design Methodology*,
https://doi.org/10.1007/978-3-032-33940-9_13

- A new detection principle for the device should be considered to reach the above criteria, or the existing enzyme method with photometric absorption measurement should be redesigned.
- The new design must reduce manufacturing costs by 50%, excluding R&D costs and necessary IPR actions.
- The new design must ensure at least comparable precision when measuring blood glucose, according to what is already clinically acceptable, or possibly increase the precision.
- The new device shall allow use under varying conditions, such as varying ambient temperatures and higher storage temperatures. It should also eliminate the need for refrigerated storage of disposable cuvettes.
- The consumables (e.g., flow cells, cuvettes, or chips) of the device must have an increased shelf life.
- The new device should be smaller in size and utilize fewer consumables.
- The device should be easier to operate and handle for both patients at home and nurses in clinics.

The following caveats have been added to constrain the design possibilities:

- *Medtech Sensorics* maintains the right to utilize all current subcontractor products.
- Existing IPRs remain valid for another 10 years. If a new detection principle is adopted, new IPR must be secured; *Medtech Sensorics* is prepared to cover these costs up to 200 kEUR.
- Regulatory filings and annual IPR fees for the new device must not exceed 150 kEUR.
- *Medtech Sensorics* requires a detailed risk analysis alongside a credible mitigation plan.
- The new device is not expected to generate net income during the first 5 years of production.
- The production of consumables must be transferable to other countries while remaining compliant with local regulatory and validation requirements.

13.2 Training Scenario of the Assignment

For design training of students or other trainees, a scenario should preferably be based on the following prerequisites:

- The trainees are allocated to the R&D unit of *Medtech Sensorics*. The R&D unit has dealt with sensor device engineering for more than 10 years.
- The assigned design team has five members with backgrounds in mechanical engineering, measurement technology, biochemical engineering, electrical engineering, and computer programming.

- The R&D unit has several test benches for investigating prototypes and performing analytical experimentation of plasma samples. The team members are familiar with bioanalytical methods using enzymes and antibodies. If not, experts in training management should support the trainees with advice.
- The R&D unit has previously collaborated with subcontractors for sensor device fabrication and small-scale manufacturing, and experienced expertise is available for the trainees through tutorial experts.
- The trainees have access to computer-aided design (CAD) tools, simulation, and modelling tools for bioprocess design and calculations, as well as software for design of experiments (DoE) and process economic calculations (see also Sect. 3.11). They also have access to in-house information about purchase and procurement agreements for the existing glucose sensor product.
- *Medtech Sensorics* accesses internally procured goods such as culture media and growth factors, single-use equipment, and other consumables.
- Internal cost factors for operational costs, including buildings and renting, are provided by *Medtech Sensorics*.
- Labor costs are based on standard employment agreements and should be added to cost calculations as agreed with *Medtech Sensorics*.
- The trainees' progress report to *Medtech Sensorics* management monthly. The results should be delivered orally and in writing. The typical time frame for the assignment is in the range of 3–4 months. This can be shortened if lower demand for reporting is expected. Reports should be concise and succinct and follow typical company standards (see also Sect. 4.4.7).

13.3 A Recommended Design Approach

(i) *Structuring the Assignment and Establishing User Requirements*

From the description of the assignment and background of *Medtech Sensorics*, the general conditions of the assignment can be structured (Fig. 13.1). Several upfront activities have taken place, and other preconditions are settled. This includes the work with establishing methods for acquiring the analytical biosystem and how to assemble the bioproduct components at the scale required for global distribution. Thus, the design tasks for the trainees are the following:

- To secure a low-cost production of a bioanalytical recognition element based on antibodies or enzymes
- To identify design options for the parts of this multicomponent product
- To assemble these optional parts favorably
- To consider how the dimensions of the device components can be minimized
- To assess and compare the economic outcomes of configurations and compare these with *Medtech Sensorics* demands for production volumes and costs.
- To evaluate the scalability of the alternative designs at a higher production
- To ascertain that prioritized designs comply with regulatory requirements

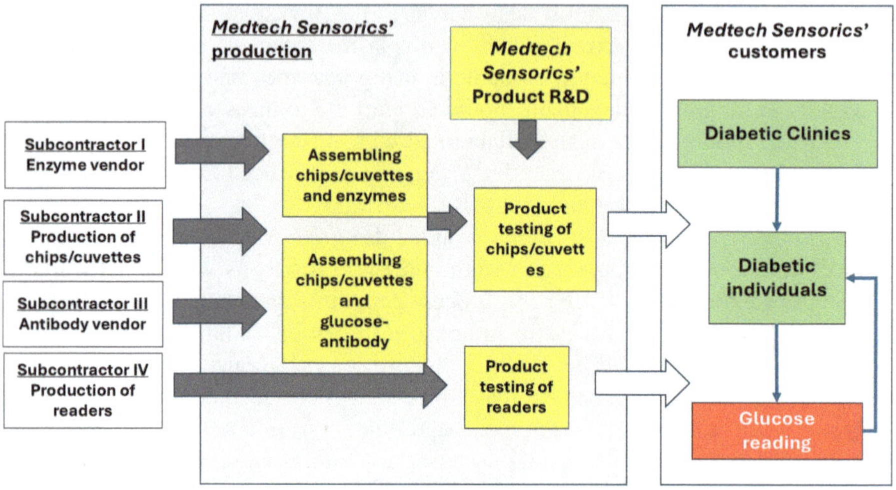

Fig. 13.1 Activities at Medtech Sensorics and subcontractors to the company for development and production of blood glucose devices to clinics and customers

- To carry out a risk analysis for the product and competition strength from a longer perspective

Medtech Sensorics has already provided cost frames for IPR costs and subcontracting to the economic evaluation, while other preliminary cost figures need to be assessed from information obtained from in-house or public sources. The cost estimates are at this stage important at relative levels. It may also be assumed that for a development unit within the company, specific costs are mostly known.

(ii) *Conceptualization of the Assignment*

Based on the assignment, its objectives, and user requirements, a conceptual map can be drawn (Fig. 13.2). The map depicts the functions necessary for performing the transformation process in the sensor device to be designed (Mandenius and Björkman 2011; Hubka and Eder 1988; Pahl et al. 2007; Ulrich et al. 2019). The functionalities of the systems can be summarized into:

- Biological functions for disrupting the blood cells in the patient sample, mixing assay reactants and reactive biomolecules (enzymes or antibodies), and enough conversion activity (catalytical or immunological reactivity) to transform blood glucose into a detectable marker
- Technical functions to contain or delimit the blood sample, a system for detecting the marker, a system for converting the detector signal for transformation into a reading, and a digital system for computing signals and displaying computed values

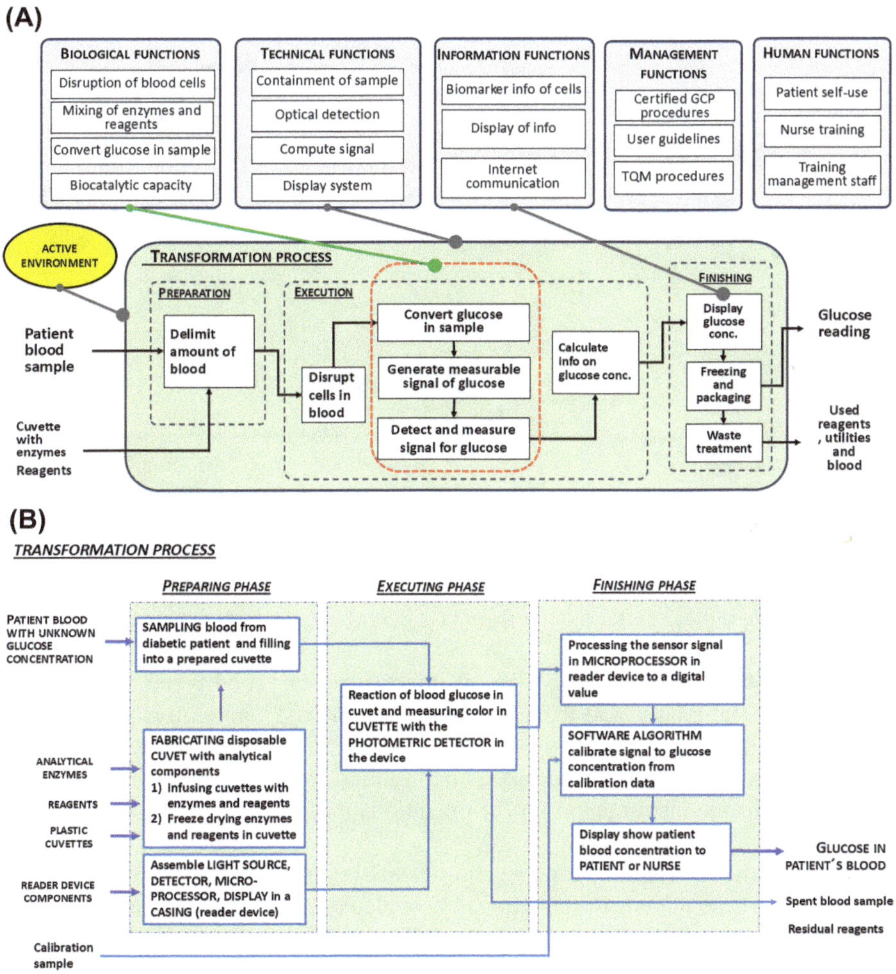

Fig. 13.2 (**a**) The overall conceptual map for the glucose sensor device, and (**b**) detailed for the transformation process

- Systems for transforming signals to clinically useful information, inputs to the device and display for the user to communicate with the device, and a system for exchange of information on digital communication systems
- Management of the device for applying Good Clinical Practice, quality management of the production and distribution of the device to users, and management of certification of the sensor device by external organizations.
- Functions for providing humans involved (patients, doctors, nurses, marketing, and service personnel) with guide instructions, training, and support.

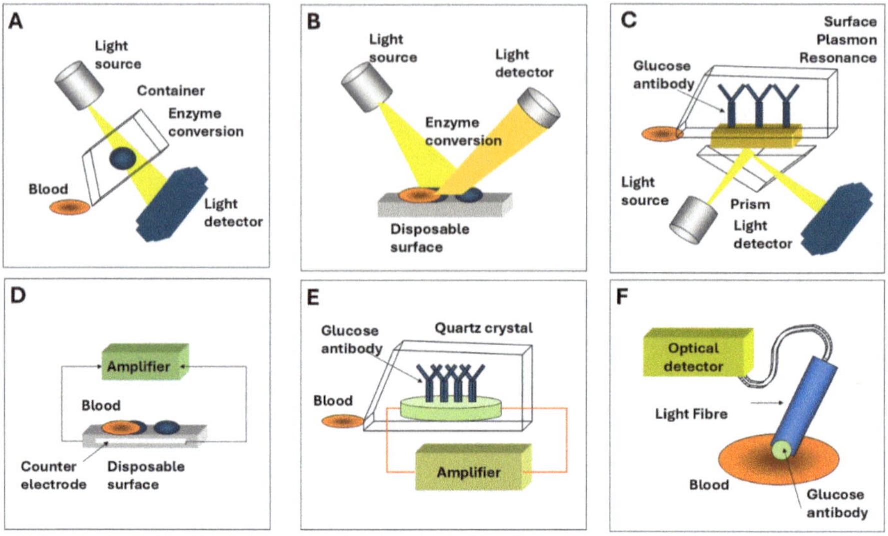

Fig. 13.3 Six configurations for blood glucose sensor devices with potential for further development and design

The transformation process can at this stage be subdivided into phases (Fig. 13.2b). The phases and their operations are ordered consecutively in the map and connected to the functional systems involved in these phases. As is obvious, the biological functions are key for conversion in the transformation process, while the other functions are instrumental for the operation and controlling the transformation in the device.

Based on the conceptual map, several potential configurations can be conceived (Fig. 13.3). These adhere to the expressed objectives, requirements, and priorities stated above. Basically, these involve the following aspects:

- The blood sample from tested individuals shall be volumetrically contained or in other ways delimited for the analytical conversion (A–F).
- The interaction shall take place in a small volume, a cuvette (A, C, E) or a droplet (B, D, F), where glucose is transformed into a detectable marker.
- The marker shall be detected by interaction either with light, in the visible range (A, B, E, F), gravity oscillations of surface electromagnetic waves (C, D), or electrochemical shifts (D).
- The source of signals and its detector unit are interfaced with the volumetrically contained or limited blood sample but are non-disposable, reusable parts of the sensor device (A–F).
- Disposable low-cost units such as cuvettes with disposable and optically active surfaces are key components of the sensor (A–F).

These configurations are likely to realize the targeted priorities by applying state-of-the-art biological and sensor technologies (Table 13.1).

Table 13.1 The users' requirements, the requirements' target specifications and their priority in the design

User requirements	Target specification	Priority
Fast response after injection to inform patients directly	45 s	Very high
Sensor should be of pocket size with low weight allowing patients to be able to handle sensor units at home	<15 × 5 cm and 300 grams	Very high
Convenient for diabetes patients to take samples	Easy-to-read display, <two push-buttons	Very high
Possible to preserve sensor cuvettes in fridge for facilitating their distribution	6 months at +8 °C	High
Longevity of consumables to the sensor device	6 months at +8 °C	High
Profit only on disposable cuvettes to ensure a low price per sensor unit	Fabrication price <30% of sale price	Medium
Sensor devices should have a high longevity to reduce logistics distribution	More than 2 years	High

The alternatives must be constrained within the abovementioned assignment objectives and expressed user needs and adapted to the diversity of techniques shown. In two of the optional alternatives, the enzymatic analytical techniques are again exploited, while in the other four, antibodies toward glucose are used. Different measurement principles are employed using photometry, electricity, gravimetry, fiber optics, and plasmonic spectroscopy. Solid-phase and liquid-phase analyte conversion and detection are applied. Contained and non-contained designs of sample handling are considered in the alternatives.

(iii) *Detailed Design of the Selected Conceptual Configurations*

Based on the priorities in Table 13.1, configurations A and F (Fig. 13.3) are the most feasible for detailed design. These setups allow for both enzymatic and glucose-specific antibody recognition. The flow schemes in Fig. 13.4 outline the full process, from the fabrication of disposable units to the testing of sampled blood.

One feasible design approach is to source the biological components (glucose oxidase, peroxidase, mutarotase, and reagents) from external suppliers and outsource the cuvette fabrication. Following the process in Fig. 13.4a, these components are mixed, filled into cuvettes, and lyophilized before packaging. Patients then use these disposable units to collect blood samples, which react to form a colored marker measured by a handheld reading device. The reading device's microprocessor converts the reading to a glucose concentration, which is displayed on the device. The device is regularly calibrated with standard cuvettes provided to the user. The design alternative requires a limited number of fabrication units and could be scaled up with parallel production lines. Suppliers and subcontractors for biological and plastic components are relatively uncomplicated. It is easy to find alternative suppliers, and the subcontracted fabrication of plastic cuvettes can be carried out by many. However, quality control is a necessity that should not be underestimated.

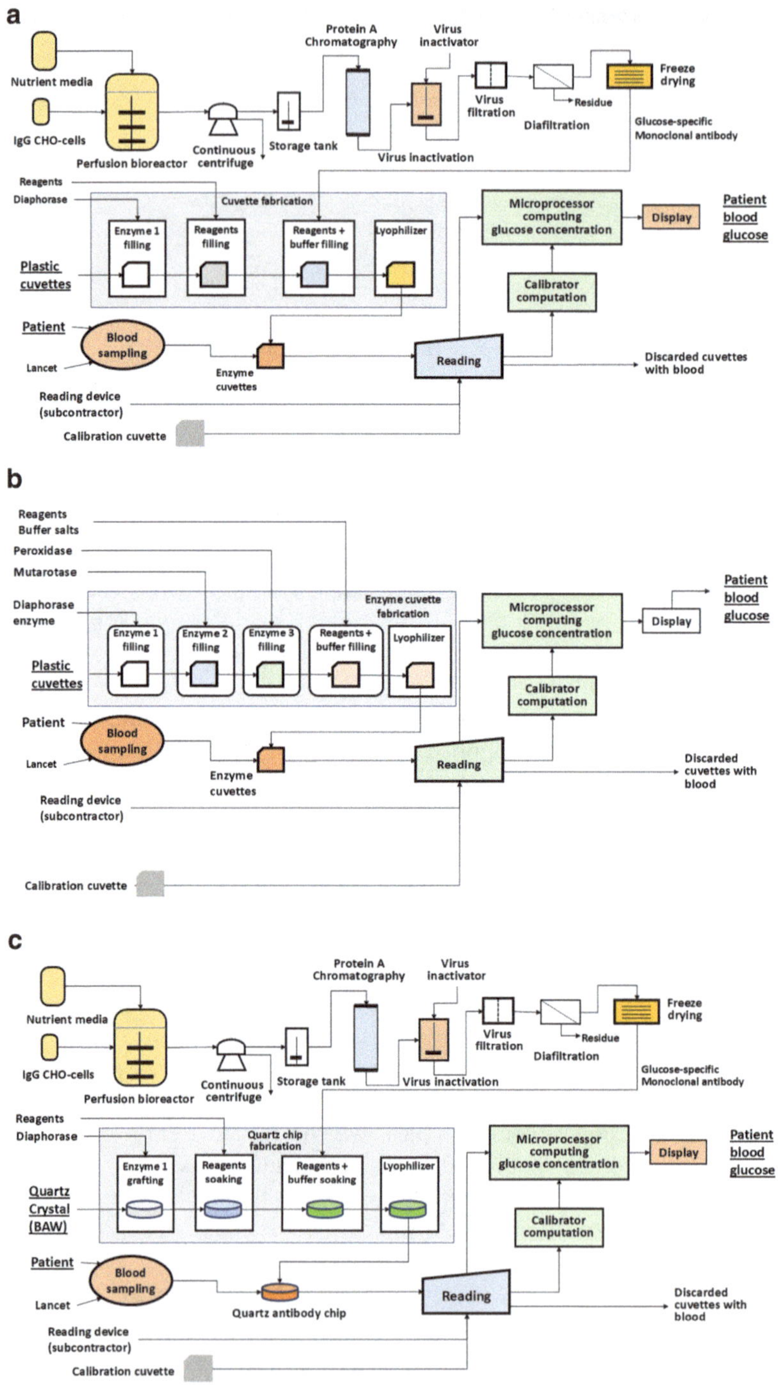

Fig. 13.4 Detailed designs of selected configurations in the conceptual analysis. (**a**) Alternative with enzyme cuvette and photometric detection. (**b**) Alternative with antibody cuvette and photometric detection. (**c**). Alternative antibody and mass balance detection

An alternative is to fill the disposable cuvettes with a glucose-specific antibody (Fig. 13.4b). This can be done with the same or a similar filling equipment. The other steps remain unchanged. The reader device must be adapted to detect the cuvette with other calibrations. This will be an upfront R&D effect, but, in the end, a similar reader device will be delivered to the users. It is an option here to produce the antibody in-house in a small-scale cultivation facility. This has the advantage of better control of antibody supply and scaling up of the production of disposable units.

A different design is required for a sensor device, where the antibody is attached to a gravimetric sensor (Fig. 13.4c). Also here, the remaining scheme can be the same as previously. The gravimetric unit with bound antibodies will be a disposable unit. This design alternative seems technically possible but will require additional R&D work, other components, and a different reader unit and verification of the sensitivity and reliability of the sensor principle.

Especially three patents may infringe on the design or risk infringing on these. Those are a patent on a blood glucose tracking apparatus (Drucker et al. 2010), another method for analyte determination in blood (Jonsson et al. 2015), a lancet-based strip for blood analysis (Klintmose 2001; Vreeke et al. 2002), and a method for glucose in blood (Skyggebjerg and Hillerod 2008). The IPR applications are some of them close to expiring, while some require attention.

(iv) *Production Economic Evaluation for the Detailed Designs*

The evaluation of production economics should focus on three aspects:

- Effect on the total costs by subcontracting of disposable units and reader device
- Effect on the total costs due to development and investments in production equipment
- Estimation of the difference in production costs between the two biological systems used for the detection of glucose

The development and production costs for the design alternatives differ. Costs for subcontracting and for subcontracted supply of components and raw materials have a decisive effect on the total costs and consequently on the market price (Peters et al. 2003; Kristiansen 2007; Ray et al. 2022). The choice of suppliers and subcontractors, in-house production alternatives, and number of fabricated units have a profound effect on the costs (Table 13.2). An important difference between subcontracting and purchase cost is that the subcontracted parts or units could be contracted exclusively to *Medtech Sensorics* and not sold to any others, such as competitors. Common enzymes and media (as used in the enzyme design alternative) can be provided to other customers, while glucose-specific antibodies could be exclusive products but with higher prices. This must be considered in the economic evaluation of the alternatives.

The investment and operational costs are assessed under the assumption that all or a selection of subcontracted components are acquired as suggested in the alternatives (Table 13.3).

Table 13.2 Comparison of estimated subcontracting costs for the design options and in-house production of recognition elements

Subcontractor or vendor procurement	Enzyme device (kEUR)	Antibody device (kEUR)	In-house enzyme production (kEUR)
Enzymes for 5,000,000 disposable units	500	–	–
Glucose-specific antibody for 5,000,000 disposable units	–	200	–
Plastic cuvettes (empty) (5,000,000 units)	50	50	50
Hardware reader device (5000 units = 40 EUR/reader unit)	20	20	20
Software in reader device (5000 units)	10	10	10
Fiberoptic reader probe (5000 units)	10	10	10
Total	**590**	**280**	**80**

Table 13.3 Economic evaluation for enzyme and antibody devices at two market sizes

Total costs	Enzyme device (kEUR)		Antibody device (kEUR)	
Market size	5 mn chips	10 mn chips	5 mn chips	10 mn chips
	3700	*7400*	*4880*	*9760*
Investment cost	2200	1800	2200	1800
Payback (5 years)	440	440	360	360
Total operational cost	860	1720	560	1020
Annual production (incl. payback)	1300	2160	920	1380
Thereof subcontracting	*700*	*2100*	*000*	*000*
Cost of sales/support/admin (10%)	130	216	92	138
Total cost	1400	2366	1012	1418
Annual per customer (5000 or 10,000 customers)	280 EUR	240 EUR	200 EUR	142 EUR

Since *Medtech Sensorics* has no facilities for production of biologics, such as bioreactors and downstream processing equipment, these must be purchased and installed. The impact of this cost is favored by increasing production volume. The initial commercial production volume has been limited to 5000 reader devices per year (i.e., 5000 diabetic users) with an average consumption of 1000 disposable tests per year. Thus, the initial investment is dimensioned for that volume.

The two biological alternatives, glucose detection based on enzymes or antibodies, have a relatively modest effect on the total production cost (Table 13.3). These costs are, as described above, intertwined with how these detection systems are acquired. Instead, the decisive effect is caused by product development, fabrication systems, and strategy.

The total production costs differ therefore between the alternatives. As a result, the potential net income will be higher for the antibody alternative (~11%) at the targeted production volume (5000 users). As this is a low number, the impact of scaling up production is of great interest to look at. The numbers in the table are estimates and depend on volumes and other conditions. Of interest at this stage is the distribution of costs, which indicates where further design efforts could influence the total costs (Fig. 13.5). For example, operational costs seem to dominate and would be worth optimizing further.

The impact of sales volume on the alternatives is a factor of interest to estimate (Table 13.4). It seems that the antibody alternative has also at a larger production an advantage.

(xxii) *Optimization of the Design Alternatives*

Optimization of design parameters offers many opportunities for maximizing the analytical performance and scalable production capacity of sensor devices (Martins and Ning 2021). When successfully applied, this systematic approach yields refinements across the entire developmental spectrum. These improvements range from the microscale characteristics of disposable components, including the optimization of cuvette fluidic geometries, the enhancement of sensor chip surface morphology, and the fine-tuning of biorecognition element binding kinetics, to the macro-scale integration of optoelectronic reader units and the streamlining of underlying fabrication workflows (Table 13.5).

However, because comprehensive optimization demands exhaustive empirical studies and significant resource allocation, a targeted prioritization strategy is essential to manage developmental costs. By identifying and focusing on parameters "critical to quality"—specifically those with the most profound influence on signal-to-noise ratios and manufacturing reproducibility—developers can strategically minimize the use of experimental resources. This focused methodology ensures that the final device meets stringent technical specifications while remaining viable for high-volume commercial production.

Optimization of the glucose sensor design by design of experiments (DoE) technique: Factorial design with DoE can be applied with several parameters in the design alternatives (Brereton 2003; Mandenius and Brundin 2008; Montgomery 2020) (Table 13.6). A set of design factors can be associated with the production of ligands in the cuvettes. If the ligands are supplied by subcontractors, it is not an issue for *Medtech Sensorics*, but it is still justified when considering costs between alternatives for a future in-house production. It may indicate that one of the alternatives has a pronounced advantage. The kind of factors to be included would not differ much from those discussed in previous application cases (Case 1–7). What may require special attention is the need for purification of ligands to reach analytical grade.

Reagents are another set of factors of high relevance. The choice of reagents with costs might be critical for glucose test performance. Here, a combination of discrete choices is to be combined with the levels of reagents added per cuvette.

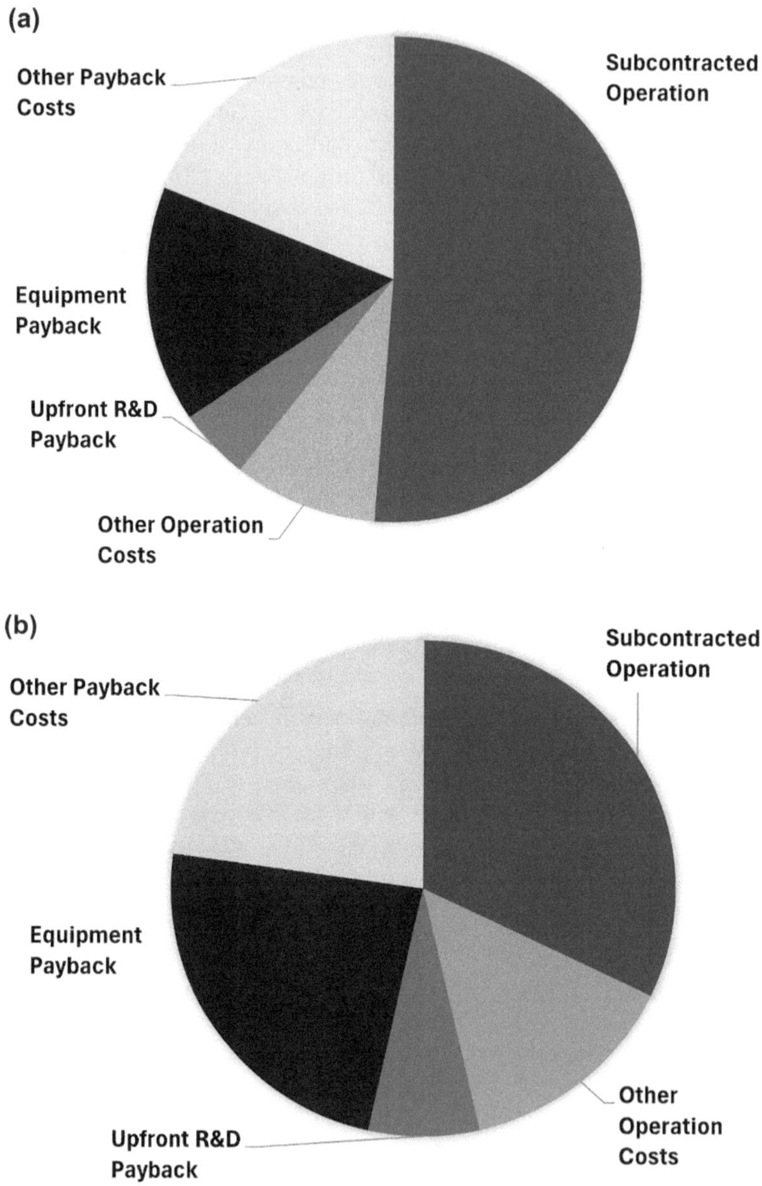

Fig. 13.5 Distribution of costs with the two design alternatives for production of five million disposable units

The choice of plastic materials in the cuvette can be assumed to influence stability and performance of testing. Again, it is discrete factors to be investigated versus responses that are quantitative.

Table 13.4 Investment and operational costs for the enzyme and antibody device options with subcontracting

Cost item	Enzyme sensor (kEUR)	Antibody sensor (kEUR)
Investment costs		
Upfront R&D		
External subcontracted R&D (reader device) Internal development of cuvette	150 100	150 100
IPR development and filing	50	50
Total upfront R&D cost	*300*	*300*
Equipment and instruments		
Assembling machines	400	400
Basic production units (tanks, lyophilizer)	300	300
Reader device prototyping (subcontracted)	200	200
Microprocessor prototyping (subcontracted)	100	100
Total equipment and instrumentation costs	*1000*	*1000*
Additional production costs		
Installation of equipment (× 0.5)	500	400
Buildings (× 0.30)	300	240
Taxation (× 0.1)	100	80
Project planning (× 0.3)	300	240
Total additional expenditures	*1200*	*960*
Total investment costs	2500	2060
Operational costs (annual for 5 mill disposable units)		
Consumable costs		
Enzymes (subcontracted)	590	50
Antibody (subcontracted)	–	160
Consumables fabrication (analytic reagents)	10	10
Designed cuvettes/chips (subcontracted)	50	50
Total consumables for production	*650*	*270*
Additional annual operational costs		
Labor costs (incl. QC)	50	50
External maintenance	10	10
Renting of buildings	10	10
Taxation	20	20
Management	20	30
Annual IPR expenditure and licenses	10	10
Additional costs for operation	*120*	*120*
Total operational costs	**860**	**560**
Annual payback of investment (5 years)	500	420
Total annual production cost	1360	980
Production cost per chip (EUR)	*0,27*	*0,20*

Table 13.5 Parameters considered for optimization of the glucose sensor device

Object for optimization	Expected outcome	Applicable optimization techniques
Geometry of flow cell/chip	The dimensions (aspect ratio) may influence analytical performance	Factorial design
Size of assembling machine	The machine productivity can be optimized	Mechanistic modelfactorial design
Immobilization method	The composition of reagents will influence the yield of binding	Factorial design
Proportion of enzymes	The proportion of sequential enzymes can be optimized	Kinetic model
Volume or area flow cell/chip	The volume or area determines the time of analysis	Mechanistic model
Activation time of coupling	Yield of binding depends on activation time	Factorial design

Table 13.6 A suggested plan for performing optimization using factorial design according to DoE methodology for the glucose sensor

Object of optimization	Factors in DoE plan	Response to measure
Production of enzymes	Culture media, pH, temperature, purification	Enzyme activity
Production of antibody	Culture media, pH, temperature, purification	Antibody activity
Reagents	*Sensitivity, amounts, alternatives*	Sensitivity, stability
Cuvette materials	Plastic materials	Stability, activity
Preservation	Amount of freezing medium, temperature	Expiry, activity

Finally, conditions for preservation of cuvette consumables are important for distribution of products. This will mostly concern temperature span but also involve packaging materials and conditions. Probably it is of high priority in DoE planning.

Most of the responses are measured by activity assays. This is the key parameter for assessing the product's analytical capacity. The activity assays should therefore be very reliable and properly validated. It is recommended to have more than one single assay to rely on.

There are other potential applications of DoE that could improve the performance of the testing. For example, the geometry of the cuvette can be optimized for improving the path length of the absorbance measurement, the surface area available for grafting of enzymes or antibodies, or the measurement volume.

Moreover, the same assays for response measurement can be useful in the mechanistic modelling for generation of data.

Optimization of the design of the glucose sensor by mechanistic modelling: Mechanistic modelling (Nielsen et al. 2011; Doran 2013; O'Brian 2019) allows for the optimization of glucose sensor design by simulating device performance and production requirements (Table 13.6). For instance, these models can determine how enzyme proportions within the cuvette influence glucose conversion in blood samples. They are also instrumental in analyzing how cuvette volume and loading affect analytical response, ultimately linking physical design parameters to economic outcomes.

The reaction dynamics taking place in a cuvette when converting glucose enzymatically can easily be visualized by a set of time-dependent (Eqs. 13.1, 13.2, 13.3, 13.4, 13.5, and 13.6) when consecutively converting glucose:

$$dG_{\text{cuvette}}/dt = -k_{\text{enzyme1}} \times G_{\text{patient}} \tag{13.1}$$

$$k_{\text{enzyme1}} = k_{\text{enzyme}-\max 1} \times G_{\text{patient}}/(K_{\text{MM1}} + G) \tag{13.2}$$

$$k_{\text{enzyme2}} = k_{\text{enzyme}-\max 2} \times G_{\text{patient}}/(K_{\text{MM2}} + G) \tag{13.3}$$

$$dI/dt = k_{\text{enzyme1}} \times G_{\text{patient}} - k_{\text{enzyme2}} \times I \tag{13.4}$$

$$dP_{\text{col}}/dt = k_{\text{enzyme2}} \times I \tag{13.5}$$

$$\text{ABS} = e \times P_{\text{col}} \tag{13.6}$$

where G_{patient} is the patient's concentration of glucose in the sampled blood; G_{cuvette} is the concentration of released glucose in the cuvette after action of the diaphorase enzyme; I is the concentration of the intermediate reaction product after conversion of the released glucose; P_{col}, the concentration of the colored reaction product after enzymatic conversion of the intermediate; ABS, the photometric absorption measured by the sensor detector; and e, the extinction coefficient in the cuvette. Rate constants in the model can be adjusted when applying the model ($_{\text{kenzyme-n}}$, specific enzyme reaction rates; K_{MMn}, Michaelis-Menten saturation constants).

The model can be used to investigate the effect of enzyme loading and enzyme activity in the cuvette (Fig. 13.6a). This may indicate the amounts of enzymes to be used in each cuvette to ensure proper response. In the simulation diagram, ranges for detection limits can be introduced (upper as well as lower limits). In the model, the enzymatic conversion of the glucose sample (e.g., by diasporas) can be adapted as desired:

$$dG_{\text{cuvette}}/dt = k_{\text{enzyme}} \times G_{\text{patient}} \tag{13.7}$$

It is of interest to compare the dynamics in the cuvette with a single-step antibody reaction for glucose detection after the conversion to glucose in the cuvette (Eqs. 13.7, 13.8, 13.9, and 13.10).

$$k_{\text{A}} = k_{\text{Amax}} \times G_{\text{patient}}/(K_{\text{A}} + G_{\text{cuvette}}) \tag{13.8}$$

$$dG_{\text{cuvette}}/dt = -k_{\text{A}} \times G_{\text{cuvette}} \tag{13.9}$$

$$dP_{\text{A}}/dt = k_{\text{A}} \times G_{\text{cuvette}} \tag{13.10}$$

where k_{A1} and k_{A1} are the specific association and dissociation rates for the glucose-specific antibody and P_{A}, the concentration of the antibody-glucose complex.

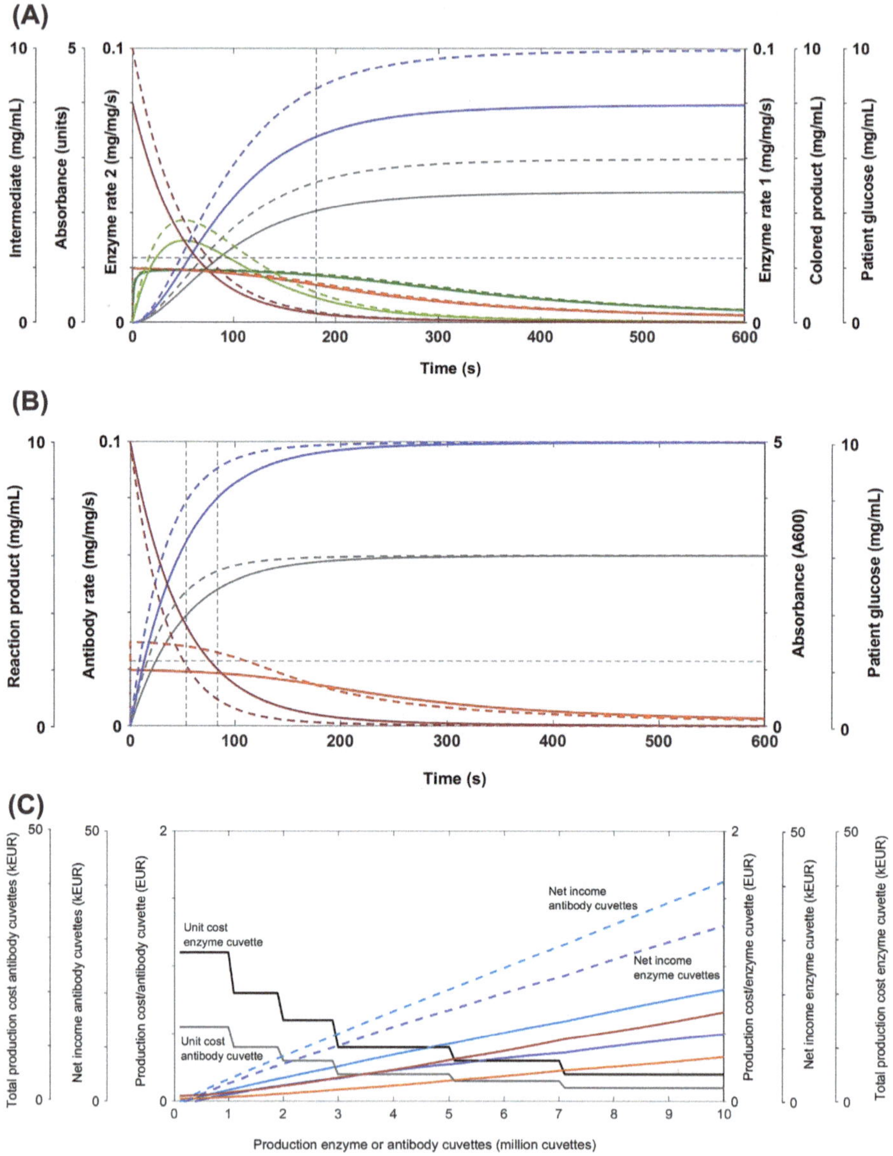

Fig. 13.6 (**a**) Response in a three-enzyme cuvette. Detection limits for glucose in blood (horizontal dashed lines). Two activities compared (line/dashed). (**b**) Comparison with antibody cuvette. (**c**) Net income for the antibody (light blue) versus enzyme cuvette (dark blue) at varying total (dark and light brown) and unit production (black, gray) costs. Dashed lines show net income at an increased sales price from 4 to 6 EUR/unit

Simulations of the model equations allow comparison of critical design parameters between the enzyme and antibody alternatives (Fig. 13.6b). Of special interest are the amounts of enzyme or antibody in the cuvette, the blood sample volume collected in each assay, and the enzyme or antibody rates to react with or associate with glucose and intermediates.

The most critical parameters to determine are those related to detection, i.e., the lowest concentration of the reaction product that is possible to detect. Of importance is also to determine the highest blood glucose concentration that can be detected. The cuvette volume and amounts of acting enzymes or antibodies can be dimensioned from the simulations.

If the sensitivity is not high enough for the photometric sensing, a trade-off between sensitivity and response time can be investigated. There are possibilities to compensate for this by increasing the volume of the cuvette or the amount of enzyme or finding an antibody with a high on-rate. This can be shown in the model by additional simulations with higher constant values in the model equations. Thus, the mechanistic modelling helps in dimensioning the setting of the parameters and then assessing the pros and cons of this.

A larger cuvette volume allows more enzyme/antibody molecules to be contained in the cuvette. This either speeds up the reaction or extends the measurement range.

These values provide the basis for detailed economic investigations into cuvette fabrication, specifically regarding raw material consumption, production time, and manufacturing costs. Comparing the economic impact of various design alternatives is paramount (Fig. 13.6c). A critical factor is determining the production scale, specifically the annual volume of cuvettes manufactured and sold. The simulations enable an analysis of the relationships between production capacity, equipment costs, material consumption, and negotiated purchase prices, utilizing Eqs. 13.11, 13.12, 13.13, 13.14, and 13.15.

$$\text{Cost}_{\text{prod}} = \text{Cost}_{\text{cuvette}} \times n_{\text{cuvette}} \tag{13.11}$$

$$d\text{Cost}_{\text{cuvette}}/dn_{\text{cuvette}} = \text{Cost}_{\text{equip}}/n_{\text{cuvette}} + \left(\text{Cost}_{\text{consum}} + \text{Cost}_{\text{ligand}}\right) \times n_{\text{cuvette}} \tag{13.12}$$

$$dP_{\text{income}}/dn_{\text{cuvette}} = P_{\text{cuvette}} \times n_{\text{cuvette}} \tag{13.13}$$

$$P_{\text{antibody}-\text{cuvette}} = P_{\text{cuvette}} \times \text{Ab} \tag{13.14}$$

$$\text{Profit}_{\text{tot}} = (n_{\text{cuvette}} \times P_{\text{cuvette}}) - \text{Cost}_{\text{prod}} \tag{13.15}$$

where $\text{Cost}_{\text{prod}}$ is total production cost for cuvettes; $\text{Cost}_{\text{cuvette}}$, cost per cuvette; n_{cuvette}, the number of cuvettes produced during a period; $\text{Cost}_{\text{eqip}}$, the total investment cost in equipment; $\text{Cost}_{\text{consum}}$, the cost for consumables per cuvette except the ligand costs; $\text{Cost}_{\text{ligand}}$, the cost for ligands (enzymes or antibodies) per cuvette; P_{income}, the total sales income at the given market price P_{cuvette}; Ab, the percentage of lower production cost of antibody*;* $\text{Profit}_{\text{tot}}$, total net income of cuvette sales*; and* $P_{\text{antiboby-cuvette}}$, the total income of sales of antibody cuvettes.

Equations 13.12, 13.13, 13.14, and 13.15 compute the total cost with increasing production number of cuvettes. New investments in machines are added in the simulation when production volume exceeds 500,000 cuvettes per year. n subcontractors.

The simulation model estimates that the cost for enzyme cuvettes (P_{cuvette}), or antibody cuvettes ($P_{\text{antibody-cuvette}}$), does not differ much in production costs (Fig. 13.6c). However, changes in procurement costs and machine capacity may change these relationships considerably, as simulations predict. It tells when or how *Medtech Sensorics* ought to devote efforts to try to lower the purchase of cuvettes in relation to sales volume.

In the economic estimations, it is of special interest if there are jumps in the purchase costs. The model can easily take this into account by adding new investment costs, i.e., additional machines, when production volume exceeds certain numbers.

These conditions are included in the recommendations given to *Medtech Sensorics*.

13.4 Conclusive Suggestions for *Medtech Sensorics*

The two evaluated alternatives, one utilizing a glucose-specific antibody and the other a three-enzyme sequence, are both viable and capable of resulting in a successful product.

Several rationales and specific suggestions support this:

- Producing analytical proteins internally at Med*tech Sensorics'* facilities is advantageous to ensure deliverability and facilitate in-house scaling. Both options allow for scaling with a sub-linear increase in production costs. The relatively low volume of protein production is logistically feasible and presents no significant regulatory or IPR complications.
- Production costs for both alternatives are comparable. By reducing these costs, the company can offer a lower unit price to customers.
- Protecting the technology through exclusive technical design is crucial. The chip construction represents the most easily defensible component for both designs.
- Financial evaluations support these findings, with net income projected to increase substantially after 4–5 years based on anticipated market demand.
- Scaling production volumes will likely allow for the negotiation of lower subcontractor rates, further improving production economics.
- There is significant potential to optimize the analytical performance of both systems.

The following risks should also be considered:

- Subcontractors should be utilized sparingly and only when necessary. While initial start-up volumes might favor subcontracting, anticipated long-term sales volumes make in-house production more attractive.

- The diabetes sensor market is highly competitive; notably, some pharmaceutical companies may subsidize testing devices for their customers.
- While design standards for certification are manageable, they must be strictly maintained throughout the sensor's development.

Although the alternatives are similar, the antibody-based approach is prioritized for the following reasons:

- The antibody device is easier to produce as it requires only a single biological component.
- With fewer processing steps, the risk of production interruptions is reduced. Additionally, the market is well-acquainted with immunoassay concepts, though the performance of antibody-based glucose assays must be rigorously verified.
- Replacing an antibody for the same or different assay targets is more straightforward than modifying multi-enzyme systems.

13.5 Tutorial Perspectives on the Assignment

The suggested approach accomplishes this by using day-and-night end-to-end continuous manufacturing processing at a relatively modest scale and using single-use equipment in about half of the units. This strategy facilitates reaching global production targets while reducing costs through smaller equipment footprints and lower personnel and maintenance requirements.

The primary challenges for the trainees in this assignment are:

- To identify and apply state-of-the-art sensor technology and bioanalytical techniques to create an economically feasible product without compromising diagnostic quality.
- To recognize the potential for improving biological systems by leveraging active molecules, such as enzymes and antibodies, in alternative designs. For instance, exploring how novel enzymological findings can alter productivity. Utilizing modelling tools (e.g., kinetic models in MATLAB) can help visualize these impacts on analytical performance and manufacturing costs.
- To master the identification and acquisition of these emerging techniques. This requires trainees to understand how to scout for and secure new technologies, a critical phase where conceptualization is particularly beneficial.

The assignment involves certain risks that trainees must gradually identify and manage, primarily related to:

- Developing a broad perspective early in the process to understand how various constraints influence design alternatives. Trainees must maintain an open mind toward alternative solutions and analyze how specific requirements—such as a minor technical adjustment to improve precision—translate into manufacturing changes.

- Understanding the impact of subcontracting costs and how to allocate them within standard production expenses. Trainees often struggle to utilize external development assets and assess how they affect project outcomes and costs. Introducing sub-scenarios with a variety of external partner options can help address this.
- Navigating the lack of initial experimental data, which can significantly hamper decision-making. For inexperienced trainees, iterative design can be confusing; however, introducing experimental reasoning (e.g., factorial design) can provide both factual and psychological support. Structuring biological and process parameters within a DoE plan (cf. Mandenius and Brundin 2008) will lead to more straightforward decision-making.

A few additional pitfalls that are likely to appear:

- The training can benefit considerably if the trainees are not trapped in finding precise rates and prices and instead run the evaluation of the alternatives conceived with rough estimates. This will accelerate the speed of work and save time.
- It is important to be able to pass the conceptual stage relatively shortly and continue to outline the potential possibilities using the available means for continuous processing. The risk is to become too theoretical. Better is to return and reiterate the conceptualization structure based on reality.
- Neglecting existing designs already known. This means to actively scrutinize that state of filed patent applications and technical and scientific publications and whether these are in the process of IPR processing.

The tutors' essential actions should be to monitor the progress of the trainees in these directions and appropriately push them into design work by disclosing these possibilities.

- Tutors should frequently monitor the direction in the trainees' design work by asking questions about alternatives and risks.
- A SWOT-related perspective can preferably be used in the tutors' guiding actions.
- Tutors should attentively ensure that trainees are not trapped in searching for minor issues and "a needle in a haystack"; instead, focus on critical questions.

References

Bode B, King A, Russell-Jones D et al (2021) Leveraging advances in diabetes technologies in primary care: a narrative review. Ann Med 53(1):805–816. https://doi.org/10.1080/07853890.2021.1931427

Brereton RG (2003) Chemometrics, data analysis for laboratory and chemical plants. Wiley, Chichester

Doran PM (2013) Biochemical engineering principles, 2nd edn. Elsevier, Amsterdam. https://doi.org/10.1016/C2009-0-22348-8

Drucker S, Liamos CT, Colman FC et al (2010) Blood glucose tracking apparatus and methods. Patent application US 2010/0068796

Freckmann G, Pleus S, Grady M et al (2019) Measures of accuracy for continuous glucose monitoring and blood glucose monitoring devices. J Diabetes Sci Technol 13(3):575–583. https://doi.org/10.1177/1932296818812062

Hubka V, Eder WE (1988) Theory of technical systems, a total concept theory for engineering design. Springer Verlag, Berlin

Jonsson M, Riabova E, Eriksson H et al (2015) Device and method for determination of an analyte in blood. Patent application US 2015/03779913

Khanwalker M, Fujita R, Lee J et al (2022) Development of a POCT type insulin sensor employing anti-insulin single chain variable fragment based on faradaic electrochemical impedance spectroscopy under single frequency measurement. Biosens Bioelectron 200:113901. https://doi.org/10.1016/j.bios.2021.113901

Klintmose LP (2001) Disposable lancet combined with a reagent carrying strip and a system for extracting and analyzing blood in the body utilizing such a disposable lancet. Patent application US 2001/0027277 A1

Kristiansen B (2007) Process economics. In: Ratledge C, Kristiansen B (eds) Basic biotechnology, 2nd edn. Cambridge University Press, Cambridge, pp 239–252

Mandenius CF, Björkman M (2011) Biomechatronic design in biotechnology: a methodology for development of biotechnology products. John Wiley & Sons, New Jersey. https://doi.org/10.1002/9781118067147

Mandenius CF, Brundin A (2008) Bioprocess optimization using design-of-experiments methodology. Biotechnol Prog 24:1191–1203. https://doi.org/10.1002/btpr.67

Martins JRRA, Ning A (2021) Engineering design optimization. Cambridge University Press, Cambridge. https://doi.org/10.1017/9781108980647

Montgomery DC (2020) Design and analysis of experiments, 9th edn. John Wiley & Sons, New York. ISBN: 978-1-119-63842-1

Nielsen J, Villadsen J, Lidén G (2011) Bioreaction engineering principles, 3rd edn. Springer-Nature, New York

O'Brian D (2019) Engineer 4.0: life science handbook for medical devices and biopharmaceuticals. Kindle ISBN-13: 978-1795753340

Pahl G, Beitz W, Feldhusen J et al (2007) Engineering design, a systematic approach, 3rd edn. Springer Verlag, Berlin

Peters MS, Timmerhaus KD, West RE (2003) Plant design and economics for chemical engineers, 5th edn. McGraw-Hill, New York

Ray SC, Chambers RG, Kumbhakar SC (2022) Handbook of production economics. Springer Nature, New York

Sabu C, Henna TK, Raphey VR et al (2019) Advanced biosensors for glucose and insulin. Biosens Bioelectron 141:111201. https://doi.org/10.1016/j.bios.2019.03.034

Saha T, Del Caño R, Kuldeep M et al (2023) Wearable electrochemical glucose sensors in diabetes management: a comprehensive review. Chem Rev 123:7854–7889. https://doi.org/10.1021/acs.chemrev.3c00078

Sanchis-Gomar F, Cortell-Ballester J, Pareja-Galeano H et al (2012) Hemoglobin point-of-care testing: the Hemocue system. J Lab Autom 18(3):198–205. https://doi.org/10.1177/2211068212457560

Skyggebjerg O, Hillerod K (2008) System and method for estimating the glucose concentration in blood. Patent application US 2008/0249384 A1

Ulrich KT, Eppinger SD, Yang MC (2019) Product design and development, 7th edn. McGraw-Hill, New York

Vreeke MS, Charlton SC, McCleary AR et al (2002) Sensor with integrated lancet for monitoring blood by colorimetric or electrochemical test method. Patent application NZ 20030526334

Weinstock RS, Aleppo G, Bailey TS et al (2020) The role of blood glucose monitoring in diabetes management. American Diabetes Association. https://doi.org/10.2337/db2020-03

Willis HJ, Asche SE, McKenzie AL et al (2025) Impact of continuous glucose monitoring versus blood glucose monitoring to support a carbohydrate-restricted nutrition intervention in people with type 2 diabetes. Diabetes Technol Ther 27(5):341–353. https://doi.org/10.1089/dia.2024.0406

Chapter 14
Case 9: Design of a Novel Hemodialysis System

14.1 Assignment: Background, Description, and Objectives

The aim of this assignment is to develop the next generation of commercial hemodialysis systems. Extracorporeal artificial kidneys for removing uremic toxic components from the blood have been used for several decades, helping millions of people living with impaired kidney function (Daugirdas et al. 2007). These systems have exploited capillary hollow-fiber dialysis membranes in a circulating flow from and to the patient (Fig. 14.1).

The assigning company, *Dialytica*, is a global leader in medical technology. Dialytica has a market share of 30% and €4.5 billion annual revenue within the kidney care segment. They focused on hemodialysis systems using machines for continuous renal replacement therapy (CRRT) in intensive care settings and advanced hemodialysis systems for chronic clinical care. Building upon more than a decade of expertise in small-scale homecare diagnostics and glucose monitoring, the company is now pivoting toward the next generation of extracorporeal blood purification technology (Gura et al. 2016; Ashby et al. 2019).

Despite the maturity of current systems, significant challenges remain regarding accessibility, patient autonomy, implantability, and personalized treatment (Penny et al. 2021; Kim et al. 2023; Gauly et al. 2022; Meidert and Saugel 2018). There is a critical need for systems that can meet the demands of public healthcare markets over the next 15 years while reducing the burden on clinical infrastructure. These systems can advance hemodialysis systems with respect to autonomy, home care, capacity, and performance to a varying degree. Therefore, *Dialytica* devotes considerable efforts to developing new dialysis products and has assigned its R&D department to develop a new system based on novel technology that can meet new market challenges in the forthcoming years. (Tsuge et al. 2019; Vega-Vega et al. 2023; Mirakhorli et al. 2026). The objectives of the assignment are the following:

- Present new designs for a new low-budget dialysis system for the public healthcare market. The designs should strengthen the competitive edge over

C.-F. Mandenius, *Bioengineering Design Methodology*,
https://doi.org/10.1007/978-3-032-33940-9_14

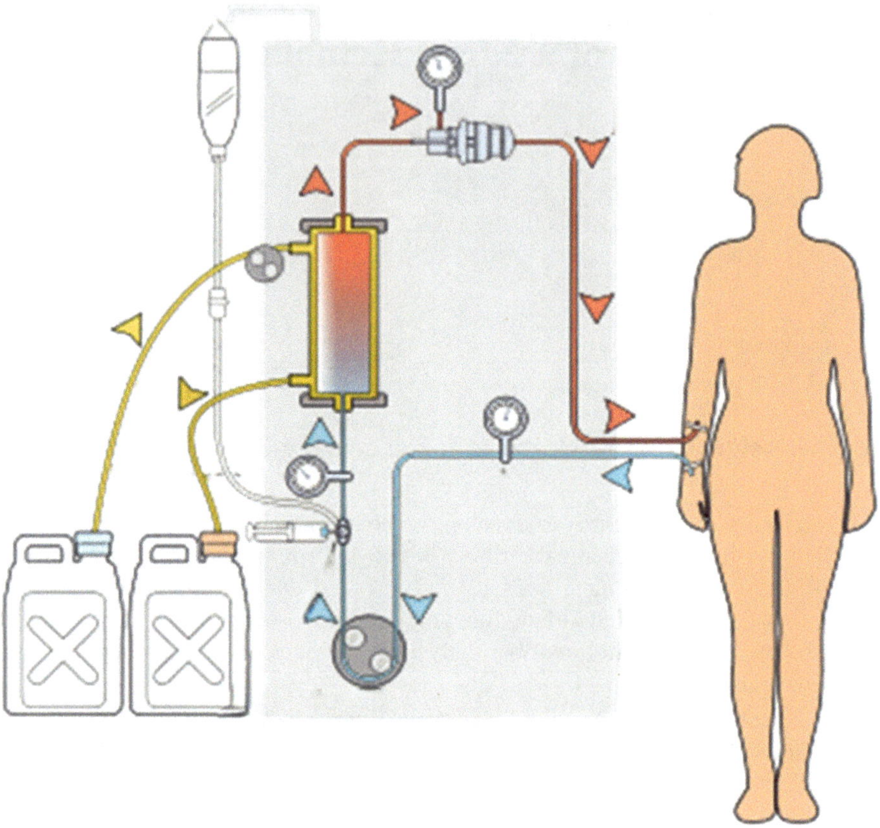

Fig. 14.1 A common extracorporeal dialytic system from major commercial providers. The external dialyzer unit with more than 1000 hollow-fiber capillaries removes the toxicants in the patient's blood. Heparin is infused into the circulation to avoid blood clotting. Flow meters and pressure gauges control the operation of the system. (Permission to reproduce the graphic from NephCure)

other similar products by offering the customers a product at a lower price and with better performance.

- Provide capacity of the extracorporeal systems to efficiently remove middle and low molecular weight components below 45 kilodaltons.
- Ensure that these designs can be managed by the patients themselves without daily support from medical healthcare personnel.
- Provide design solutions resulting in a product that is wearable.
- Ensure that the product is adapted to the patients' individual conditions using advanced artificial intelligence and real-time sensor technology.
- The design solutions must be possible to protect by strong Intellectual Property Rights (IPR).

- The manufacturing costs of the new designs should aim to be reduced by 30%. This should not include additional upcoming R&D costs for the development and necessary IPR actions.

The following caveats have been added that constrain the design possibilities:

- Presently, *Dialytica* controls the IPRs for exclusive parts of their hemodialysis products that are manufactured and provided by their subcontractors. This condition should also prevail for new products.
- *Dialytica* is prepared to cover that cost for new IPRs up to a total cost of 200 kEUR.
- *Dialytica* also wishes to see an elaborate risk analysis with a credible mitigation plan.
- The production of consumables for the device must be possible to move to other countries and cope with regulatory demands and validation requirements at that place.

14.2 Training Scenario of the Assignment

For design training of students or other trainees, a scenario should preferably be based on the following prerequisites:

- The trainees are allocated to the R&D unit of *Dialytica*. The R&D unit has dealt with sensor device engineering for more than 10 years.
- The assigned design team has five members with backgrounds in mechanical engineering, measurement technology, biochemical engineering, electrical engineering, and computer programming.
- The R&D unit has several test benches for investigating prototypes and performing analytical experimentation of plasma samples. The team members are familiar with bioanalytical methods using enzymes and antibodies. If not, experts in training management should support the trainees with advice.
- The R&D unit has previously collaborated with subcontractors for sensor device fabrication and small-scale manufacturing, and experienced expertise is available for the trainees through tutorial experts.
- The trainees have access to computer-aided design (CAD) tools, simulation and modelling tools for bioprocess design and calculations, as well as software for design of experiments (DoE) and process economic calculations (see also Sect. 3.11). They also have access to in-house information about purchase and procurement agreements for the existing sensor product.
- *Dialytica* procures culture media and growth factors, single-use equipment, and other consumables at prices provided to the trainees.
- Internal cost factors for operational costs, including buildings and renting, are provided by the tutors.

- The trainees' progress report to *Dialytica* management monthly. The results should be delivered orally and in writing. The typical time frame for the assignment is in the range of 3–4 months. This can be shortened if lower demand for reporting is expected. Reports should be concise and succinct and follow typical company standards (see also Sect. 4.4.7).

14.3 A Recommended Design Approach

(i) *Structuring the Assignment and Establishing User Requirements*

From the description of the assignment and background, the general conditions of the assignment can be structured (Fig. 14.2). Because of *Dialytica's* position as a globally established provider of dialysis equipment and devices, their technological and medical know-how makes it possible to outline a structure for the development work with new designs.

Given the objectives given to the development department, a collection of decisive design issues that need to be solved can be conceived:

- To secure a low-cost production of an extracorporeal device based on the separation capacity of toxic or otherwise harmful blood components
- To take *Dialytica's* current product concept further to a personalized product that adapts to the patient's actual conditions

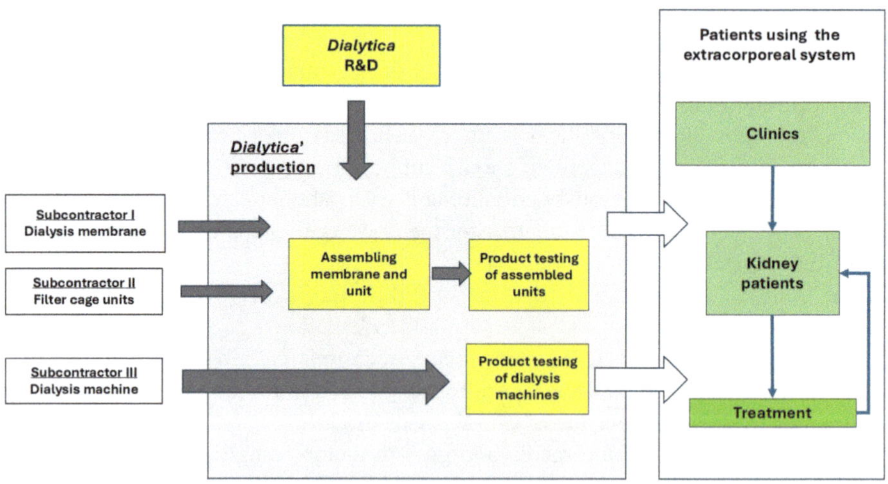

Fig. 14.2 Flowchart shows the activities at Dialytica for the development and production of a new extracorporeal hemodialysis purification system as assigned in the design case. The structure allows flexibility in the choice of internal versus subcontracting product development as well as of procurement of parts of the hemodialysis system

- To develop a device that is directly integrated with the patient, preferably portable or wearable, and possible to operate by the patient himself
- To identify design options for the various parts of this multicomponent product and to assemble these parts favorably
- To consider how the dimensions of the product's components can be minimized
- To assess and compare the economic outcomes of various design configurations and compare these with the intended production volumes and costs
- To evaluate the scalability of the alternative designs at a higher production level
- To ascertain that prioritized designs comply with regulatory requirements
- To carry out a risk analysis of the product and the competitive strength of the designs from a longer perspective

Dialytica has already provided cost frames for potential subcontracting and IPR. The accurate cost estimates are at this stage important at relative levels. It may also be assumed that for a development unit within the company, the costs for most of the components in a hemodialysis system are known.

(ii) *Conceptualization of the Assignment*

Based on the assignment, its objectives and user requirements, a conceptual map can be drawn (Fig. 14.3). The map depicts the functions necessary for performing the extracorporeal dialytic transformation of the patient's blood under controlled conditions (Hubka and Eder 1988; Pahl et al 2007; Mandenius and Björkman 2011; Ulrich et al. 2019). The functionalities of the systems can be summarized into:

- A separation of blood components, mainly small molecules, from blood plasma without negatively affecting the purity of the patient's blood, meaning that the blood may interact with a separation medium, such as a dialysis membrane or ultrafilter, or other physical separative force.
- Extend the dialytic separation to diversified biological components by allotting the device a size- or charge-dependent discrimination functionality.
- Technical functions to contain or delimit the flowing blood, through the separating medium or device, without endangering the blood's biological constituency.
- Technical functions to transport the blood from the body blood circulation and back without damaging the biological function of the blood.
- Technical and informative functions of the extracorporeal circuit with the purpose of ensuring stability and consistency of the dialytic function of the extracorporeal device or system.
- Technical functions that permit the patient to wear the extracorporeal system close to the patient daily in a way that is convenient to the patient's life conditions.
- Management of the device according to Good Clinical Practice, quality management of the production and distribution of the device to users, and allowing certification of the device by external organizations.
- Functions for providing humans involved (patients, doctors, nurses, marketing, and service personnel) with guide instructions, training, and support.

The transformation process can be shown in a conceptual diagram either for the process of the hemodialysis system during operation or the transformation process

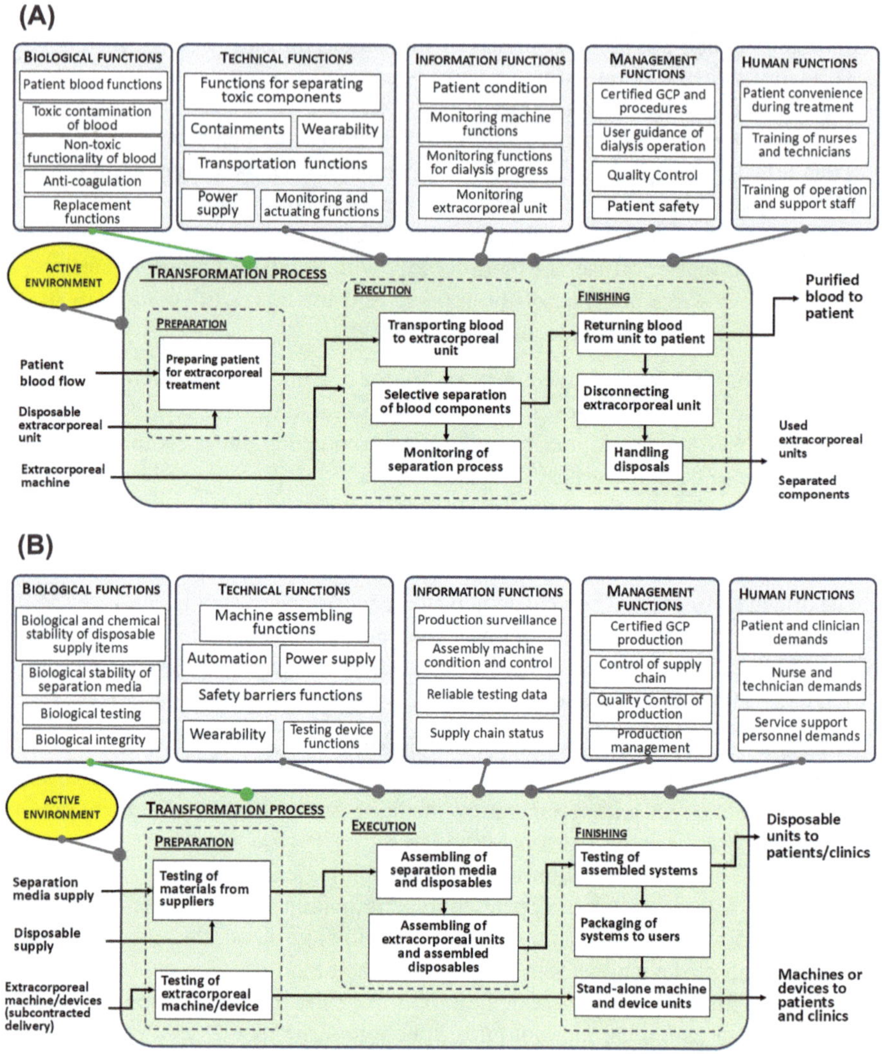

Fig. 14.3 Overall conceptual depiction of hemodialysis systems. (**a**) Depiction showing the operation of the hemodialysis system. (**b**) Depiction showing the manufacture of the hemodialysis system. Several of the functions coincide in the two depictions

for the manufacture of a hemodialysis system at the company (Fig. 14.3). These transformations can be staged into subphases as shown.

For the case of operation of the hemodialysis system, the primary inputs are the patient's blood flow, single-use dialysis separators, anti-blood clotting reagents, other liquids, and the dialysis machine. The primary output is purified blood to the patient, spent liquids, and used separator units. The phases of the treatment are the configuration of the system to the patient, the separation and the return of the purified blood to the patient, and finally, the de-connection of the patient from the system (Fig. 14.3a).

For the case of the manufacture of the hemodialysis system, the inputs of components, their assembly into a system product, the quality testing of the parts of the system, and finally the delivery of the system, either to a clinic or directly to a patient (Fig. 14.3b).

For effectuating the transformation processes, functional systems are required: biologically active functions for separation of toxic blood components, media for negating clotting of blood; technical functions for transportation of blood, dialysate and other liquids, containment cages, and sensors and actuators for controlling the system; information functions for monitoring of conditions of the system and alerts; management functions for system control and operations; human functions related to patients, nurses, doctors, and service personnel.

For the manufacturing case, there must be a production system for assembling the hemodialysis system, quality testing and control functions, packaging, delivery, and customer support functions.

The phases and their operations are ordered consecutively in the map and connected to the functional systems involved in these phases. As is obvious, the biological technical functions are key for the conversion in the transformation process, while the other functions are instrumental for operating and controlling the transformation in the extracorporeal unit and for the convenience of the patient.

The active environment refers to the conditions prevailing during the treatment or manufacture. For example, the ambient temperature will influence the transfer in the dialysis unit and the stability of the dialysis membranes during storage.

Based on the functions of the conceptual map, several potential configurations can be conceived. The scope for new designs or redesigning of existing products as expressed in the objectives of *Dialytica* indicates that a multitude of possibilities are conceivable (Fig. 14.4 showing the main directions of potential configurations). Most of these adhere to the expressed objectives, requirements, and priorities stated above. Basically, these involve the following aspects:

- The patient's blood flow is purified in an extracorporeal unit where the porosity of hollow-fiber dialysis membrane(s) allows smaller toxic molecules (<40 kilodaltons) to be ultrafiltered, while larger blood components are returned to the patient under controlled conditions. The membrane is structured so that its area is large and distributed in a compact caged enclosure.
- The patient's blood flow is purified in an extracorporeal unit where forces other than molecular size separate toxicants, plasma, and blood cells under controlled conditions. The unit is structured so that it can be caged in a disposable unit.
- The separating membrane or other separating device is structured so that its area is large and distributed in a compact caged enclosure.
- The patient's blood flow is purified in an extracorporeal unit where sequential dialysis membranes of varying porosity allow molecules of a span of selected molecular sizes to be filtered and where the blood returned to the patient at

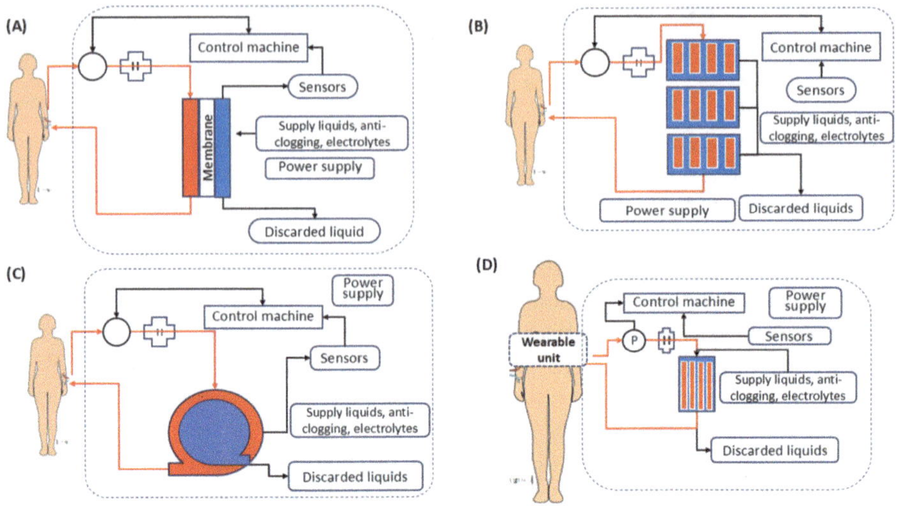

Fig. 14.4 Four configurations for extracorporeal systems with potential for further development and design. (**a**) An optimized conventional dialysis using capillary fibers for separation of toxic molecular components. (**b**) Sequential separation with a filter of different properties. (**c**) Separation of molecular components from the blood is achieved by other molecular forces. (**d**) Hemodialysis system where the previous systems are wearable and miniaturized, making them convenient for the patient to carry and handle

controlled conditions. The ultrafiltration sequence is structured so that its area is large and distributed in a compact caged enclosure.

- The configurations must be realistic to economically manufacture at varying scales.
- If the convenience of the patient substantially benefits from a wearable hemodialysis system and this can be economized, it should be given high priority.
- The necessary development efforts required for a product safe for the patients and regulatory acceptability must be possible to frame in this, whether it is based on external or internal procedures.
- The final product design must be possible to protect legally by new or acquired IPRs.

These frames require a trade-off between further product development, a product adapted to high customer convenience, product performance, and quality. Furthermore, the design space must reconcile cost-efficient manufacturing with the optimized allocation of internal and external resources, as well as securing robust intellectual property protection in parallel with realistic market strategies.

All this should comply with the targeted priorities (Table 14.1) and exploit and apply state-of-the-art technologies. It is inevitably a fact that more profound new designs are required for development efforts, for the product performance itself, and for the manufacturing and supply of safe and approved construction components. However, at this stage it is difficult to rank the strengths of potential design

Table 14.1 Priorities of users and values of specifications

Requirements	Target specification	Priority
Clinicians at hospitals		
Regulatory approval of the dialysis system	Approval	Very high
Repeatable performance of processing	<5% deviation	High
Low unit cost	Disposal extracorporeal unit <100 USD for healthcare provider	High
Patients		
Safety and no side effects	Approval and certification	Very high
High accessibility to treatment	Treatment center reachable within 1 h	High
Short processing time	<20 min	High
Hemodialysis system that is portable	Safety and no side effects are not accepted.	Medium
Hemodialysis system that is wearable	Safety and no side effects are not accepted. Substantially more convenient to use	Medium
Production at dialytica		
Automation in manufacturing	Covers 2/3 of operations	High
Stability of operational steps	Deviation from QC limits 1/1000	High
High delivery by subcontractors	2 weeks hold time	High
Subcontractors		
Subcontracting should be a long-term commitment	At least for 3 years	Very high
Products should have long storage time to facilitate logistics at the subcontractor	>4 months	High
Significant volumes for delivery	>500 extracorporeal units	Medium
Low stock volume	500–1000 units	Medium

alternatives. The economic impact, upfront costs, and long-term effects of production costs are difficult to assess.

The alternatives must be constrained within the abovementioned assignment objectives and expressed user needs and adapted to the diversity of techniques shown. In two of the optional alternatives, the enzymatic analytical techniques are again exploited, while in the other four, antibodies toward glucose are used. Different measurement principles are employed using photometry, electricity, gravimetry, fiber optics, and plasmonic spectroscopy. Solid-phase and liquid-phase analyte conversion and detection are applied. Contained and non-contained designs of sample handling are considered alternatives.

The configurations based on wearable systems will require (i) substantial development, (ii) testing, (iii) regulatory verification, (iv) new supply chains and customer support, and (v) securing intellectual property rights, either by filing new patent application(s) or acquiring user rights to existing IPRs. The manufacturing must either rely on in-house production, or subcontracted fabrication of parts of systems,

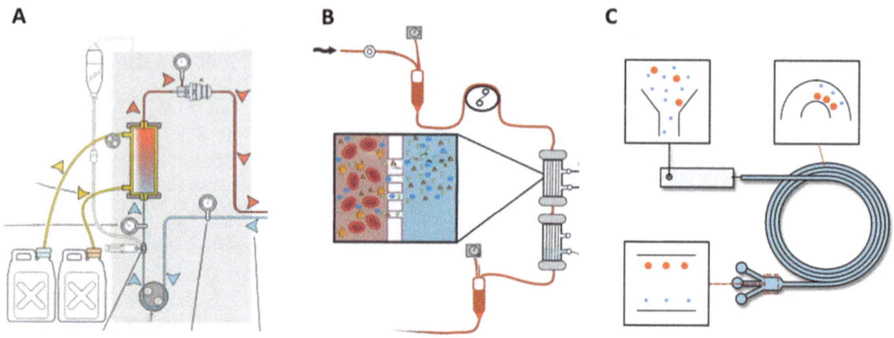

Fig. 14.5 Separation principles used in the designs. (**a**) Hollow-fiber dialyzer unit with auxiliary equipment for extracorporeal treatment at a clinic. (**b**) A sequential separation with ultrafiltration treatment. (Adapted from Bieber et al. 2013). (**c**) Separation of toxicants by other forces, e.g., centrifugal or absorptive treatments. (From Pasitka et al. 2018)

or a combination of these. These premises indicate a costly route for presenting a next-generation of hemodialysis systems. However, existing hemodialysis systems or moderately updated systems also have these requirements.

(iii) *Detailed Design of the Selected Conceptual Configurations*

Based on *Dialytica's* objectives and the priorities outlined in Table 14.1, the four configurations in Fig. 14.4 represent feasible candidates for novel product designs. However, the R&D efforts required for these configurations vary significantly.

Configuration A (Fig. 14.4a) closely resembles current hollow-fiber dialysis systems. Performance gains could be achieved through new membrane materials and optimization (Lee and Hong 2022; Vega-Vega et al. 2023), as illustrated in Fig. 14.5a. While this path requires navigating regulatory requirements and updating supply lines and production facilities, it demands relatively low additional R&D investment.

Configuration B (Fig. 14.4b) introduces more complex and diversified separation sequencing. This approach utilizes alternative diafiltration arrangements and new, optimized separation materials (King et al. 2019). Consequently, this configuration would necessitate greater R&D efforts and the development of new logistical solutions (cf. Fig. 14.5b).

Configuration C (Fig. 14.4c) explores novel separation methods aimed at faster, more efficient removal of toxic components. Proposed techniques include absorptive sieving (Fissell et al. 2009; Tsuge et al. 2019; Nareboina et al. 2025), microfluidic separation (Pasitka et al. 2018), or other nanomolecular solutions (cf. Fig. 14.5c). While promising, this path involves substantial R&D risks. It requires extensive verification, the adaptation of novel production methods, and the challenge of establishing market feasibility. Furthermore, the incremental value for the end customer remains uncertain.

Configuration D (Fig. 14.4d) anticipates the demand for wearable dialysis systems to improve patient convenience. While any of the previous configurations could

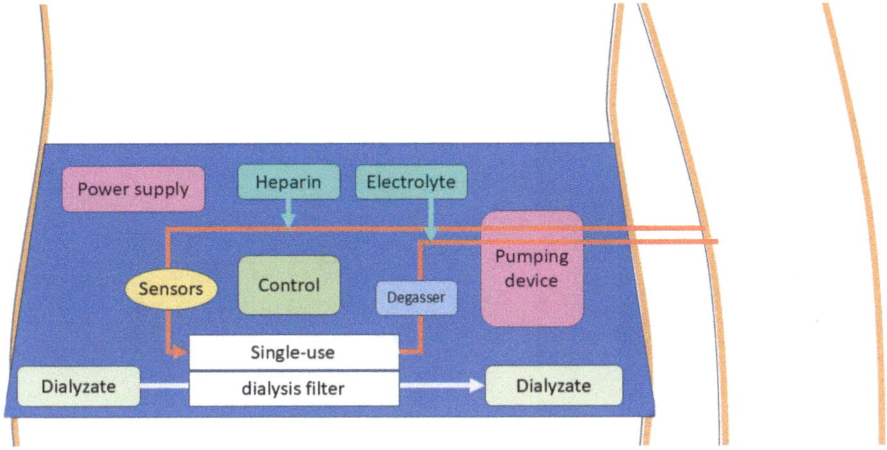

Fig. 14.6 Overall design of a wearable dialysis system basically as previously suggested or protected designs (Fulkerson and Joseph 2009; Gura et al. 2016)

potentially be integrated into a wearable format, designing a compact system that maintains functionality, reliability, and cost-effectiveness is highly challenging (cf. Fig. 14.6). Emerging technologies, such as miniaturization, 3D printing, and integrated control functions, may simplify fabrication and improve reliability, yet this path still requires a profound redesign and a complete overhaul of current manufacturing methods.

Beyond design feasibility, the project must navigate a complex intellectual property landscape. Five existing patent applications from established companies present potential infringement risks or legal challenges for the proposed configurations. These include a foundational patent on general kidney dialysis methods and apparatus (Hogard et al. 2001), as well as specific frameworks for extracorporeal blood treatment devices and procedures (Pouchoulin and Chevallet 2011). Furthermore, the transition toward portability is complicated by established patents on wearable dialysis methods and devices (Fulkerson and Joseph 2009). Finally, more recent intellectual property, covering novel hemodialysis systems and methods (Ebara et al. 2016; Wilt et al. 2019), further constrains the development of next-generation solutions.

The three flowcharts in Fig. 14.7 delineate the fabrication routes for disposable dialysis units and dialysis machines. The dialysis hardware equipment, either machines for use in the clinic or as wearable devices, is fabricated separately by subcontractors.

The first flowchart (Fig. 14.7a) shows fabrication of the established hollow-fiber unit device with minor modification and improvement. It comprises a dialysis fiber product with a better dialysis membrane (e.g., new materials to Cuprophan©; cutoff in the 20 kD range opens for renewed selectivity of dialysis separation of small molecules from the extracorporeally shunted blood stream. The cutoff of the dialysis filter is chosen for removal of low-molecular components in the blood and is

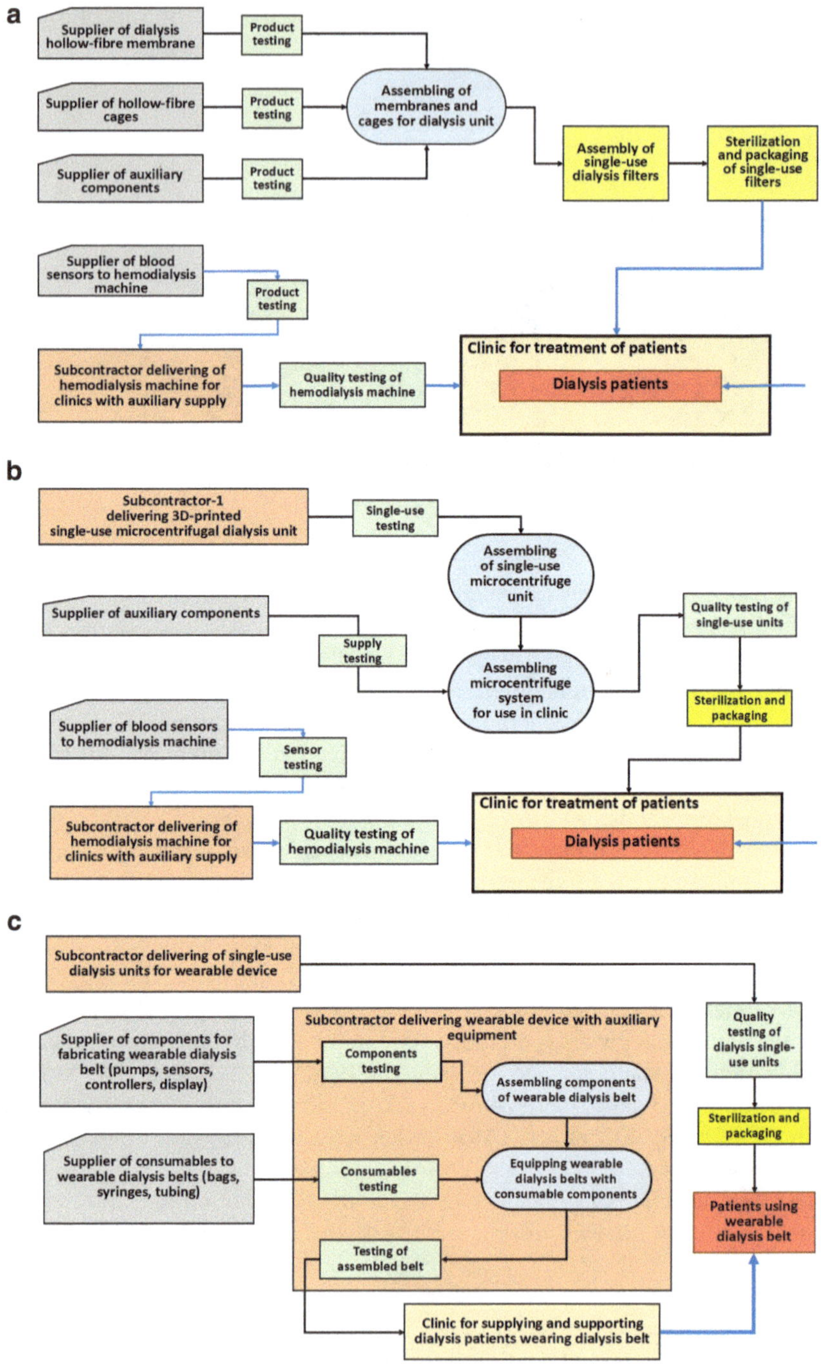

Fig. 14.7 Detailed design of production lines of an extracorporeal hemodialysis system comprising both single-use units and auxiliary dialysis machines or wearable equipment. (**a**) Production of an extracorporeal system with optimized hollow-fiber units for clinical use. (**b**) Production of a novel extracorporeal hemodialysis system intended for treatment in a clinic. (**c**). Production of an extracorporeal wearable hemodialysis unit, based on dialysis technology as suggested in Fig. 14.6, for home care treatment

subsequently followed by a second dialysis filter with a higher cutoff range for filtering medium-sized biopolymeric molecules. Fabrication of hollow fibers into bundles placed in the plastic flow-through cage can be further adapted to mass production. Additional auxiliary components of the dialysis system of improved quality could be procured from a variety of novel external suppliers.

The second flowchart (Fig. 14.7b) shows the fabrication of a more advanced solution based on recent progress with absorptive nanofiber materials (Tsuge et al. 2019) filling the single-use units.

The third flowchart (Fig. 14.7c) shows the fabrication of a wearable hemodialysis device (Fulkerson and Joseph 2009). In this, any of the abovementioned systems can be considered. The assembling of the filters into cassettes is caged into the wearable system, which is also provided with sensor technology for controlled operation. As shown, a dialysis clinic is involved in supporting the patient and providing the dialysis equipment. As in the previous design, the production line includes extensive testing and quality control of the dialysis units and systems.

An additional design possibility involves micro-centrifugation utilizing spiral-shaped microfluidic channels (Park et al. 2024; Pasitka et al. 2018). Originally developed for cell-size separation, such as isolating tumor cells, these miniaturized components are well-suited for high-volume fabrication by specialized subcontractors. When combined with 3D printing and sensor-controlled systems, the development and production costs are projected to be moderate. However, rigorous quality control remains a prerequisite for regulatory acceptance and successful healthcare integration.

Each configuration relies on a robust supply of specialized components, including plastic disposable filters, connectors, tubing, and anticoagulants. To optimize production, *Dialytica* should leverage subcontracting, particularly for electrical hardware, pumps, and pressurized flow circuitry. While subcontracting unburdens internal design efforts, it necessitates stringent quality assurance protocols. Conversely, core separation units may require joint R&D and specialized fabrication facilities.

As apparent in Fig. 14.7, drawings assembling machines and quality testing equipment are required, and probably specially designed equipment is needed.

Substantial parts of these items require acquisition or filing of intellectual property rights (IPR) or, alternatively, securing exclusivity.

(iv) *Production Economic Evaluation for the Detailed Designs*

The evaluation of production economics should focus on comparing the following four aspects for the designs investigated:

- How will *new design alternatives* influence the development and verification costs of dialysis systems?
- How will *additional development* costs for new designs, either by in-house development of new products and production lines, influence the cost structure?
- How will extensive *subcontracting* of dialysis filter units and control devices affect the potential income?

- Provide realistic estimations of the *differences in operative production* costs between the envisaged dialysis systems.

Decisive criteria in evaluation are as follows: (i) the degree of advancement of the design, either previous design solutions or going for radically new designs; (ii) if new designs should be the outcome of own, in-house developments, or, if rights to external design solutions are to be acquired; and (iii) how subcontracted development and production could economically be used. Without doubt, combinations of these alternatives are several and their costs dependable.

The development costs for the new design alternatives outlined in Fig. 14.6 increase with complexity (from A to D). There is an obvious possibility of influencing these by acquiring user rights (IPRs) to such designs. For example, the wearable design has been patent-protected (e.g., Fulkerson and Joseph 2009); the cost for acquiring exclusive user rights could be significantly lower than performing an in-house development of a protected design. Still, there is the cost for verification and regulatory approvals.

Employment of radically novel designs requires substantial expenditures for R&D, regulatory verification and production development, while re-development and refinement of *Dialytica's* present products have a shorter and significantly lower cost profile.

Especially, a wearable system has additional requirements of R&D, production development, new supplies, support, and marketing.

In the estimation given in Table 14.2, three alternatives are included with assumptions based on this reasoning. As in the previous cases (Cases 1–8), the outcome of the evaluation is highly dependent on assessed costs and other assumptions. These should be considered for the actual choices and recommendations.

Costs for subcontracting of new components and supply of raw materials have a decisive effect on the total costs and on the potential market price of *Dialytica's* product.

A potential advantage with subcontracting is that the subcontracted units can be contracted exclusively, thereby hindering competitors using the same designs. Certain supply parts can be included in such contracts. Common supplies (media, connectors, etc.) will, however, not be covered in such exclusivity.

The choice between using subcontracting or in-house production has a profound effect on logistics and production conditions. This concerns especially the production volume (i.e., number of ordered or in-house fabricated units). Table 14.3 indicates the effect on unit costs at varying production volumes.

In Table 14.2, production of single-use units (i.e., optimized hollow-fiber filters, nanofiber filters or zeolite absorptive filters, filters for wearables) is subcontracted at a production volume of 15 million units per year (Wernert et al. 2005; Tsuge et al. 2019; Nareboina et al. 2025). This is applied since the company presently has no production facilities for microdevices, cassettes or novel hollow-fibers. As mentioned, the impact on this cost is sensitive to the production volume. The European market estimate is that 300,000 patients are under permanent hemodialysis treatment. If a market share of 30% of the patients is assumed (target for *Dialytica*), this

Table 14.2 Investment and operational costs for the extracorporeal systems considered

Cost item	An advanced hollow-fiber system (kEUR)I	A new novel separation system (kEUR)	A wearable dialysis system (kEUR)
Investment costs			
Upfront product development			
R&D at external subcontractors	150	500	700
Dialytica's own upfront R&D	150	500	700
Conceiving and filing of patent application	50	100	200
Total upfront R&D cost	*350*	*1100*	*1600*
Equipment and instruments			
Assembling machines at *Dialytica*	150	300	500
Basic production units at subcontractors	50	300	400
Control unit (subcontracted)	50	400	500
Testing equipment at *Dialytica*	100	300	300
Total equipment and instrumentation costs	*350*	*1300*	*1800*
Additional production costs			
Installation of equipment (× 0.5)	175	650	900
Buildings (× 0.30)	105	390	540
Taxation (× 0.1)	35	130	180
Project planning (× 0.3)	105	390	540
Total additional expenditures	*420*	*1500*	*2160*
Total investment costs	**1120**	**3900**	**5560**
Operational costs (annual for 15 million single-use units)			
Consumable costs (15 million single-use units, subcontracted)			
Optimized single-use hollow-fiber units	14,000	–	–
Single-use units with novel separations	–	17,000	–
Single-use units for wearable systems		–	21,000
Auxiliaries (suppliers)	1000	1000	1000
Dialysis machines/ wearables (licensed)	Licensed	Licensed	Licensed
Total consumables for production	*15,000*	*18,000*	*22,000*

(continued)

Table 14.2 (continued)

Cost item	An advanced hollow-fiber system (kEUR)I	A new novel separation system (kEUR)	A wearable dialysis system (kEUR)
Additional annual operational costs			
Labor costs (incl. quality control testing)	2000	1000	1000
External maintenance	50	100	200
Renting of buildings	80	80	80
Taxation	20	20	20
Management	300	300	300
Annual IPR expenditure and licenses	50	100	100
Additional costs for operation	*2500*	*1600*	*1700*
Total operational costs	**17,500**	**19,600**	**23,700**
Yearly payback of investments (5 years)	224	780	1112
Total annual production cost	**17,724**	**20,380**	**24,812**
Production cost per unit (EUR)	1.18	1,36	1,65

Table 14.3 Parameters considered for optimization of the extracorporeal system

Objective for optimization	Expected outcome	Applicable optimization techniques
The key variables of the extracorporeal system	Modelling of the dimensions of the system to optimize its performance regarding rates and purification yield	Mechanistic model, factorial design
Size of extracorporeal unit machine	Minimizing the dimension of the machine to reduce its size and convenience for the patient	Mechanistic modelfactorial design
Properties of the separation/dialytic medium	Selection of filter material properties for efficient dialytic separation	Factorial design (material alternatives to be tested)
Volumetric properties of the treatment	Adaptation of the system to the individual measures of the patient	Mechanistic model
Treatment time	Minimizing the treatment time for the patient	Mechanistic model

will require a production capacity of 15,000,000 dialysis filter units per year (i.e., 100,000 diabetic users) with an average consumption of 3 units per patient per week.

Overall cost estimation for in-house development and production versus subcontracting will significantly influence the total production cost. In the comparison (Table 14.2), it is assumed that the hollow-fiber alternative uses the present

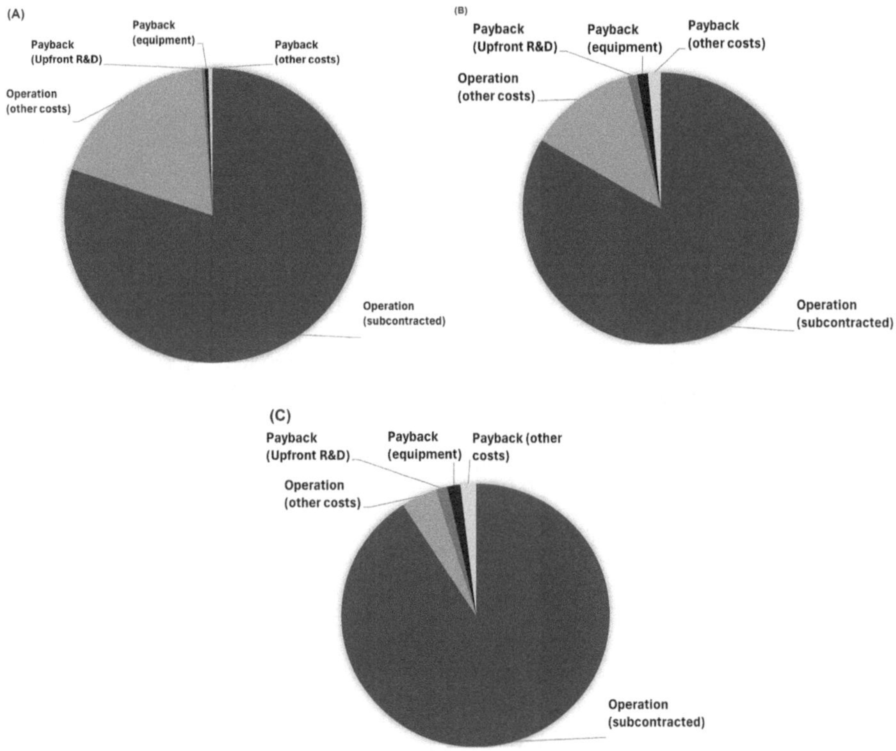

Fig. 14.8 Distribution of costs in the three design alternatives for production of 15 million dialysis filter units

production line where investments are already covered and reimbursed. This trade-off can be changed by implementing in-house production lines for the new products.

The R&D for novel wearable design can be significantly reduced by procuring the user rights to IPR based on external development of these systems. Such costs are partly included in the table. Still, *Dialytica* must spend additional R&D effort to adapt these rights to their own product concept and production and testing, as shown in the table.

Of interest at this stage is the distribution of costs, which indicates where further design efforts could influence the total costs (Fig. 14.8). For example, operational costs seem to dominate and would be worth optimizing further.

To this should be considered the cost for hemodialysis machines at the clinics or wearable devices (the reusable part). The sales price is in the order of 30,000 to 40,000 EUR per machine. The proportion of potential revenues is much favoring the sale of dialysis filter units, and therefore, in this estimation, the machines are considered as a non-profit product where the service and distribution costs are added to the clinic customers, and the production costs are fully reimbursed to the subcontractor.

As the supply of hemodialysis machines to clinics or wearable devices to patients will have considerable effects on the cost structure and the introduction as well as the use of new systems and their practice, these machines/wearables are in this economic estimation licensed. Such a licensing procedure for machines and equipment should cover service agreements, and this would facilitate and enhance marketing. Basically, this will not, at least initially, be a profit-generating business. However, the cost for developing the equipment should be covered by the sales of single-use units, as evident in the evaluation in Table 14.2.

For additional perspectives on estimation of production costs, general literature on production economics is recommended (e.g., Peters et al. 2003; Kristiansen 2007; Ray et al. 2022).

The subcontracting costs in Table 14.2 are based on an annual production volume of 15 million single-use units. This is Dialytica's estimated sales at the current level of requests from the market. If that volume is not reached, a high unit cost needs to be assumed. Here is a preliminary calculation with a reduction factor of 30% at a 5,000,000-unit lower purchase of units from the subcontractor (i.e., at 15,000,000 units, as in the table; at 10,000,000 units/year, 50% high unit cost; at 5,000,000 units/year, 100% high unit cost).

(xxii) *Optimization of the Design Alternatives*

To enhance the overall performance and dialysis capacity of hemodialysis systems, systematic optimization of design parameters across various architectural alternatives presents a critical opportunity (Martins and Ning 2021). This process is a multitask endeavor that spans from microscopic material properties of dialysis membranes to macroscopic system fluidics and separator devices. At the component level, engineers can fine-tune specific parameters, such as fluid flow conditions, membrane porosity, and the precise internal geometry of separation units (Table 14.3). For instance, optimizing the dialysate-to-blood flow ratio or the surface-area-to-volume ratio of the filter can significantly improve solute clearance rates and minimize the risk of clotting or other negative effects on the blood.

However, achieving these gains is resource-demanding. Rigorous optimization requires substantial investments in computational modelling, iterative prototyping, and extensive clinical experimentation to ensure that theoretical improvements translate into safe, real-world efficacy. Given the high costs and lengthy development cycles associated with medical device engineering, a mixed approach is rarely feasible. It is therefore advisable to implement a strategic prioritization framework to identify which specific parameters—such as membrane permeability or sensor-driven control loops—are most likely to provide the highest return on investment in terms of patient satisfaction and system efficiency. By focusing R&D efforts on these high-impact variables, developers can maximize the therapeutic value of the hemodialysis system by a trade-off between the constraints of time and capital.

Optimization of the extracorporeal system design by design of experiment technique Factorial design with design of experiment (DoE) can be applied with several parameters in the design alternatives (Brereton 2003; Mandenius and

Table 14.4 A suggested plan for performing optimization using factorial design according to DoE methodology for the extracorporeal system

Object of optimization	Factors in DoE plan	Response to measure
Dialytic membrane or filter	Different membrane or filter materials, temperature, flow rate, pressure, priming	Filtration yield
Treatment time	Membrane area, blood flow rate	Time for treatment, purity of returning blood
Aspect ratios of dialytic device	Dimensional factors, membrane shape	Filtration yield
Physical variables	Dimensions, flow rates, pressure, temperature	Filtration yield

Brundin 2008; Montgomery 2020) (Table 14.4). A set of design factors can be associated with production. If the units are supplied by subcontractors, it is not an issue for *Dialytica*, but it is still justified when considering costs between alternatives for future in-house production. It may indicate that one of the alternatives has a pronounced advantage. The kind of factors to be included would not differ much from those discussed in previous application cases (Case 1–8).

The choice of plastic materials for filtration can be assumed to influence stability and performance. Again, it is discrete factors to be investigated versus responses that are quantitative.

Finally, conditions for preservation of cuvette consumables are important for distribution of products. This will mostly concern temperature span but also involve packaging materials and conditions. Probably it is of high priority in DoE planning.

Most of the responses are measured by yields of purification. This is the key parameter for assessing the product's filtration capacity. The yield should therefore be very reliable and properly validated. It is recommended to have more than one single measurement to rely on.

There are other potential applications of DoE that could improve the performance of the testing. For example, the geometry of the dialysis unit can be optimized for improving the performance, the surface area available, or the unit volume.

Moreover, the same assays for response measurement can be useful in the mechanistic modelling for generation of data.

Optimization of the design of the extracorporeal system by mechanistic modelling: The separation of glucose or other components in the extracorporeal unit is a dynamic process that can be modelled mechanistically. The transfer rate of the component across the separation zone, whether this is a dialysis ultrafiltering membrane or a forced separation as in a microcentrifugal unit, determines the performance of the hemodialysis system (Nielsen et al. 2011; Doran 2013). A critical parameter is the time needed for the treatment, i.e., to lower the blood plasma concentration of the harmful component to normal and acceptable levels. This parameter is associated with its transferability in the separation zone, governed by the membrane porosity, surface charge of the membrane, and membrane area. Typical values in today's systems are membrane areas of 1.4 to 2.1 m^2 per dialysis

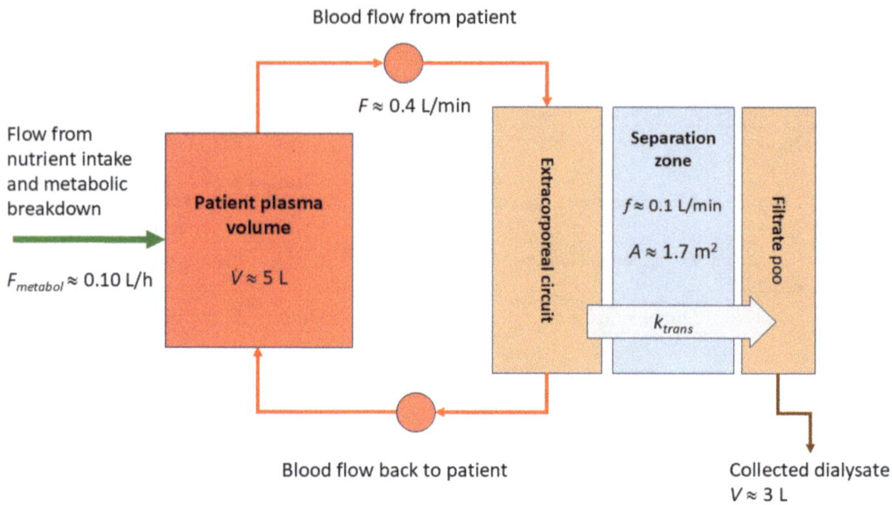

Fig. 14.9 Model structure showing the flows across a dialysis separation unit connected to a patient under treatment

filter unit (with approximately 10,000 capillaries), flow rates 0.3 to 0.5 L/min sampled from the treated patient, and dialysate volume 0.5 to 0.7 L dialysate. Average patient values are a total blood volume of 5.0 L, where 60% of the volume is plasma and 40% is blood cells. To this, there should be an added influx of 2.5 L of liquid from nutrient intake and metabolic liquid per 24 h, with 150 to 200 g of glucose. Normal glucose concentration is 0.7 to 1.1 g/L. Other components than glucose have, of course, other levels.

Figure 14.9 provides a mechanistic structure of the hemodialysis system as a basis for modelling.

The rate of transport across the separation zone, k_{trans}, is the key dependent parameter on (Eq. 14.1):

$$k_{\text{trans}} = f\,(T, p, \text{comp}, \text{membrane}) \tag{14.1}$$

where temperature (T) and pressure (p) increase the rate constant while membrane properties (e.g., *porosity*, *surface charge*, *component size*) will modulate the transport rate.

The variable concentration of the glucose, or other component, can in its most elementary form be expressed as:

$$dc_{\text{component}}/dt = -k_{\text{trans}} \times c_{\text{component}} \times A + F_{\text{internal}} \times c_{\text{nutrient}} \tag{14.2}$$

where the separating cross-section area of the separating zone (A) has a varying shape depending on the design of the separator (e.g., thin bundles of thin capillaries, flat ultrafilter packages, channel size of a microcentrifuge).

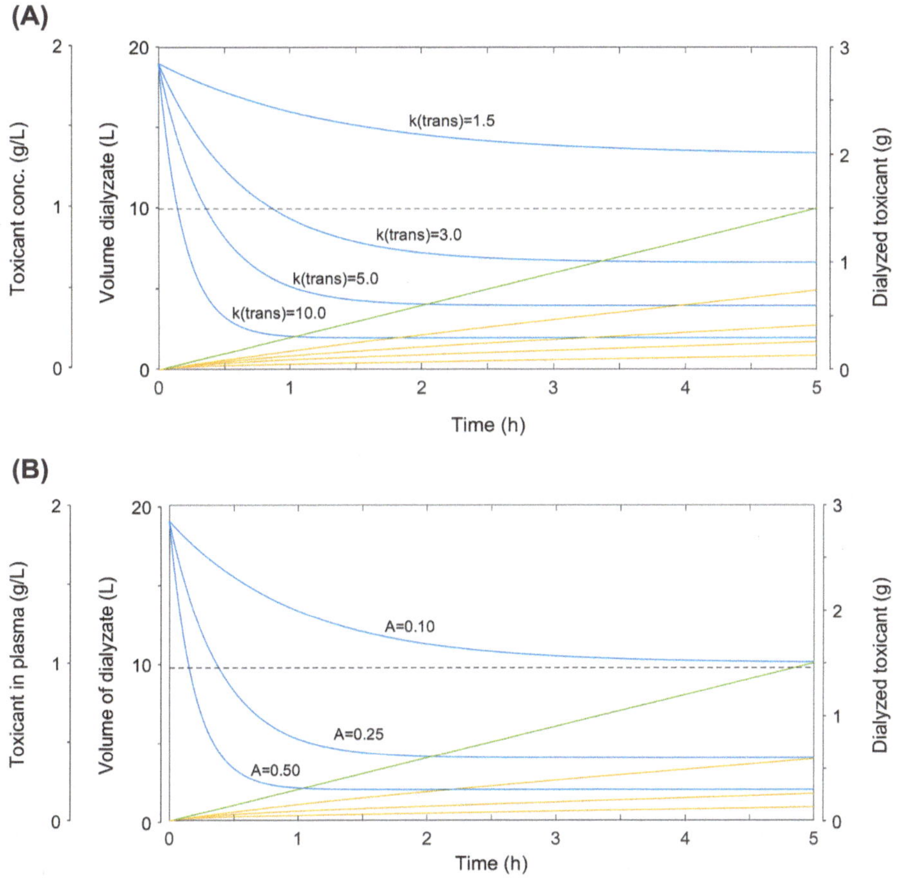

Fig. 14.10 (**a**) Extracorporeal dialysis where the concentration of the toxicant in the blood plasma is reduced (blue lines) at varying transport rates across the dialysis membrane. Yellow lines show dialyzed toxicant, and the green line shows the volume of collected dialyzed liquid. The dashed line indicates a toxicant concentration twice the normal level in plasma. The simulation shows how the toxicant is lowered by transport across the dialysis membrane. (**b**) Alternatively, the area of the dialysis zone, the filtration membrane, or the active separation zone can be varied (0.10–5.0 $m^{2;}$ blue lines). The dotted line indicates normal toxicant level in plasma

Volume of collected dialysate and amount of dialyzed glucose (or other components) can be modelled by Eqs. 14.3 and 14.4. Using these four differential equations, treatment time and dialyzer capacity related to its dimensions can be predicted (Fig. 14.10).

$$dV/dt = F \times f \tag{14.3}$$

and

$$dD_{\text{dialysate}}/dt = c_{\text{component}} \times F \times f \tag{14.4}$$

where V is the volume of the dialysate, F the flow rate from the patient, f the fraction of the flow that passes the separation zone, and $D_{\text{dialysate}}$ the amount of component in the dialysate.

14.4 Conclusive Suggestions for *Dialytica*

Three extracorporeal alternatives are evaluated: (i) conventional hollow-fiber unit with tangential ultrafiltration, (ii) exploitation of novel technologies based on absorptive nanofibers or microcentrifugal microfluidics, and (iii) use of an integrated wearable device.

The following pros and cons of the alternatives should be considered by *Dialytica* in their decision when choosing a commercial product for product development:

- A design based on today's hemodialysis products, such as a hollow-fiber unit, seems to be the least demanding to develop. The same platform technology can be reused for the manufacturing of the platform. The same operative conditions for the user, patient, remain. The clinical practice will follow established experience. The development effort for introducing a new generation of hollow-fiber units should concentrate on optimizing performance, especially the time for operation for each patient. Miniaturization of the unit will require it to shrink in size to allow self-operation.
- However, designs based on novel technology will create a substantial competitive edge for *Dialytica*. Given that the conventional product has been on the market for a long time, it is very likely that a new generation of device is a timely step. Technological advancement in biomaterial properties, use of better digitalized control options, and increasing use expectations motivate new design solutions to remain on the market. The production costs for the alternatives are not radically different. The costs can be reduced, and they can thereby reach a lower unit price for customers. The cost for this may be significant, but as mentioned, microscale fabrication technology has improved, which should be expected to lower production costs very favorably.
- This also strengthens realism in choosing to develop a much more advanced hemodialysis system that allows selectivity toward several toxic components from the patient's blood. The marketing edge for *Dialytica* is favored by their strong position on the market and their strong economy to take on demanding development challenges.
- Thus, both the second and third design alternatives are therefore associated with substantial risk-taking and will need substantial further R&D efforts. This can only be recommended to pursue if a very stark market position is present.

A few risks should also be mentioned:

- Taking the step toward a wearable dialysis system is accompanied by considerable risks. Although the economic evaluation for product development and production seems acceptable, a wearable product is also a paradigm shift from a marketing perspective. This must be very solid to justify continuing development in that direction.
- Due to the diversity of different competencies that are required for novel design alternatives, subcontracting of several of these seems a necessity. Consequently, *Dialytica's* procurement abilities are critical for reaching a competitive manufacturing price that allows a competitive price setting of the product.
- The IPR situation must be secured as well as certification for new inventions.

14.5 Tutorial Perspectives on the Assignment

The assignment is associated with certain challenges and risks that the trainees must gradually understand. The most prominent challenges for the trainees in this assignment are:

- To balance innovation and viability of design alternatives. Identifying and applying state-of-the-art biomedical techniques to create economically feasible products without compromising therapeutic quality.
- To carry out systemic improvements in the designs. Recognizing how novel manufacturing, such as 3D printing, can shift cost structures for mass-produced, single-use devices. Trainees should use modelling tools (e.g., MATLAB kinetic models) to project impacts on performance and manufacturing costs.
- To cage technical Identification and the conceptualization into a realistic frame. Developing the ability to scout and capture emerging technologies. This requires a strong conceptualization phase to bridge the gap between "identifying a solution" and "applying it" to the design.

Certain risks are likely to be associated with the assignment as such:

- The trainees may tend to take too narrow technical focuses. The trainees must adopt a broad perspective early on to understand how constraints influence design alternatives. They should evaluate how small technical adjustments—such as improving analytical precision—reverberate through the entire manufacturing process.
- To deal with subcontracting and external assets. A significant hurdle is understanding the impact of subcontracting costs. Trainees often struggle to allocate these into regular production costs or leverage external development assets effectively.

A few additional pitfalls that are likely to appear:

- Over-precision: Trainees often stall by searching for exact rates and prices. Encourage them to use "rough estimates" for initial evaluations to accelerate the flow of work and focus on comparative analysis.

- Theoretical stagnation: There is a risk of spending too much time in the conceptual stage. Trainees should move quickly toward outlining continuous processing possibilities and then reiterate their concepts based on realistic manufacturing constraints.

The tutorial guidance and actions should focus on monitoring progress in these areas and actively push trainees toward concrete design work by highlighting the following:

- Strategic evaluation: Apply a SWOT-based perspective to guide trainee decision-making.
- Focus on impact: Ensure trainees do not get bogged down in minor details—the "needle in a haystack" and instead remain focused on the most critical design and cost questions.

References

Ashby D, Borman N, Burton J et al (2019) Renal association clinical practice guideline on haemodialysis. BMC Nephrol 20:379. https://doi.org/10.1186/s12882-019-1527-3. ISSN 14 71-2369. PMC 6798406. PMID 31623578

Bieber S, Halldorson JB, Finn E et al. (2013) Extracorporeal delivery of rAAV with metabolic exchange and oxygenation. Sci Rep 3, 1538 doi: 10.1038/srep01538.

Brereton RG (2003) Chemometrics, data analysis for laboratory and chemical plants. Wiley, Chichester

Daugirdas JT, Black PG, Ing TS (2007) Handbook of dialysis, 4th edn. Lippincott Williams & Wilkins, A Wolters Kluwer Business, Philadelphia

Doran PM (2013) Biochemical engineering principles, 2nd edn. Elsevier, Amsterdam. https://doi.org/10.1016/C2009-0-22348-8

Ebara M, Namekawa K, Aoyagi T (2016) Blood purification membrane, method for manufacturing blood purification membrane, and dialysis device. US patent application 2016/0199789 A1

Fissell WH, Dubnisheva A, Eldridge AN et al (2009) High-performance silicon nanopore hemofiltration membranes. J Memb Sci 326(1):58–65. https://doi.org/10.1016/j.memsci.2008.09.039

Fulkerson BN, Joseph RT (2009) Wearable dialysis methods and devices. US patent 2009/0120864 A1

Gauly A, Fleck N, Kircelli F (2022) Advanced hemodialysis equipment for more eco-friendly dialysis. Int Urol Nephrol 54:1059–1065. https://doi.org/10.1007/s11255-021-02981-w

Gura V, Rivara MB, Bieber S et al (2016) A wearable artificial kidney for patients with end-stage renal disease. JCI Insight 1(8):e86397. https://doi.org/10.1172/jci.insight.86397

Hogard ME, Johnson HD, Kelly TD, Long JM, Peterson BA, Preston WG (2001) Method and apparatus for kidney dialysis. US patent 6,284,131 B1 (Baxter)

Hubka V, Eder WE (1988) Theory of technical systems, a total concept theory for engineering design. Springer Verlag, Berlin

Kim EJ, Chen C, Gologorsky R et al (2023) Feasibility of an implantable bioreactor for renal cell therapy using silicon nanopore membranes. Nat Commun 14:4890. https://doi.org/10.1038/s41467-023-39888-2

King JD, Kern MH, Jarr BG (2019) Extracorporeal removal of poisons and toxins (2019). CJASN 14:1408–1415. https://doi.org/10.2215/CJN.02560319

Kristiansen B (2007) Process economics. In: Ratledge C, Kristiansen B (eds) Basic biotechnology, 2nd edn. Cambridge University Press, Cambridge, pp 239–252

Lee GT, Hong YK (2022) Manufacturing and separation characteristics of hemodialysis membranes to improve toxin removal rate. Adv Polymer Technol:2565010. https://doi.org/10.1155/2022/2565010

Mandenius CF, Björkman M (2011) Biomechatronic design in biotechnology: a methodology for development of biotechnology products. John Wiley & Sons, New Jersey. https://doi.org/10.1002/9781118067147

Mandenius CF, Brundin A (2008) Bioprocess optimization using design-of-experiments methodology. Biotechnol Prog 24:1191–1203. https://doi.org/10.1002/btpr.67

Martins JRRA, Ning A (2021) Engineering design optimization. Cambridge University Press, Cambridge. https://doi.org/10.1017/9781108980647

Meidert AS, Saugel B (2018) Techniques for non-invasive monitoring of arterial blood pressure. Front Med 4:231. https://doi.org/10.3389/fmed.2017.00231

Mirakhorli F, Lotfibakalani Z, Ding L et al (2026) Membrane-less microfiltration using microfluidics. Microfluidic Nanofluidic 30:18. https://doi.org/10.1007/s10404-026-02871-6

Montgomery DC (2020) Design and analysis of experiments, 9th edn. John Wiley & Sons, New York, USA. ISBN: 978-1-119-63842-1

Nareboina GSA, Bandaru P, Bekkam U et al (2025) Advanced nanofiber mesh technology for clinical blood detoxification: a new frontier in translational nanomedicine. J Med Clin Case Rep 02(3). https://doi.org/10.61615/JMCCR/2025/AUG027140807

NephCure, Pierce and Associates Inc., P.C. Collegeville, PA 19426, USA.

Nielsen J, Villadsen J, Lidén G (2011) Bioreaction engineering principles, 3rd edn. Springer-Nature, New York

Pahl G, Beitz W, Feldhusen J et al (2007) Engineering design, a systematic approach, 3rd edn. Springer Verlag, Berlin

Park C, Lim W, Song R et al (2024) Efficient separation of large particles and giant cancer cells using an isosceles trapezoidal spiral microchannel. Analyst 149:4496. https://doi.org/10.1039/d4an00750f

Pasitka L, van Noort D, Lim W et al (2018) A microbore tubing based spiral for multistep cell fractionation. Anal Chem 90:12909–12916. https://doi.org/10.1021/acs.analchem.8b03532

Penny JD, Jarosz P, Salerno FR et al (2021) Impact of expanded hemodialysis using medium cut-off dialyzer on quality of life: application of dynamic patient-reported outcome measurement tool. Kidney Med 3(6):992–1002. http://creativecommons.org/licenses/by-nc-nd/4.0

Peters MS, Timmerhaus KD, West RE (2003) Plant design and economics for chemical engineers, 5th edn. McGraw-Hill, New York

Pouchoulin D, Chevallet J (2011) Device and procedure for extracorporeal blood treatment. US patent 2011/0168614 A1

Ray SC, Chambers RG, Kumbhakar SC (2022) Handbook of production economics. Springer Nature, New York

Tsuge M, Takahashi K, Kurimoto R et al (2019) Fabrication of water absorbing nanofiber meshes toward an efficient removal of excess water from kidney failure patients. Fibers 7:39. https://doi.org/10.3390/fib7050039

Ulrich KT, Eppinger SD, Yang MC (2019) Product design and development, 7th edn. McGraw-Hill, New York

Vega-Vega O, Ronco C, Martinez-Rueda J (2023) Pushing the boundaries of hemodialysis, innovations in membranes and sorbents. Rev Investig Clin 75(6):274–288. https://doi.org/10.24875/RIC.23000223

Wernert V, Schäf O, Ghobarker H et al (2005) Adsorption properties of zeolites for artificial kidney applications. Micropor Mesopor Mat 83:101–113. https://doi.org/10.1016/j.micromeso.2005.03.018

Wilt MJ, Demers JA, Grant KL et al (2019) Hemodialysis systems and methods. US patent application 2019/10 449280 B2

Index

A
Aptamer, 264, 270–279, 281–283

B
Bioengineered products, 3–5, 13, 21, 22, 61, 66, 73
Biological systems, 3, 4, 9, 13–16, 18–20, 22, 23, 26, 28–31, 35, 37, 39, 45, 48–52, 55, 74, 85, 97, 98, 101, 103, 104, 113, 141, 158, 169, 170, 191, 209, 234, 259, 295, 305
Biomolecular affinity, 21
Bioprinting, 105, 237, 238, 240, 242, 245, 246, 248, 250, 254–256, 258
Bioproduct, 1–9, 13–16, 18–22, 24–26, 28–31, 35–45, 48, 51–53, 55–63, 71–78, 81, 87, 88, 97, 104, 105, 182, 248, 289
Biosimilar, 27, 103–105, 107–132
Biotherapeutics, 19, 43, 49, 58, 103, 107, 135, 136, 142, 169
Blood glucose testing, 104, 287–306

C
Cardiac cells, 104, 105, 215, 216, 220, 227
Cell expansion, 206, 210, 226, 230
CHO-cells, 139, 143–145, 149, 152, 154–157, 254
Computer-aided design (CAD), 7, 9, 51, 63, 64, 109, 137, 165, 177, 187, 194, 198, 225, 289, 311
Conceptual design, 25, 35, 36, 64, 71, 74, 98, 101, 240
Conceptualization, 43, 45–47, 62, 73, 74, 84–85, 111–114, 139–143, 159, 168–170, 191–194, 221–223, 234, 242–246, 260, 266, 267, 290, 305, 306, 313, 331
Continuous production, 135, 138, 140, 149, 265
Convergence, 17, 18, 38, 44, 86, 93
Conversion rate, 19, 20, 29, 59
Cost assessment, 66, 156, 189
Creativity, 88, 98
Critical filters, 13
Cultured meat, 237–250, 253, 254, 256, 258, 259

D
Design actions, 49, 73, 86, 91
Design alternatives, 39, 49, 52–55, 58, 61, 62, 81, 84–88, 90–94, 96, 108, 110–114, 116, 118, 119, 129, 130, 136, 139, 143, 145, 146, 149, 150, 152, 156, 164, 171, 178, 188, 191, 194, 197–200, 202, 208, 216, 217, 225, 228, 233, 248–259, 263, 266, 269, 273, 275, 279, 282, 284, 293, 295, 297, 298, 303, 305, 316, 321, 322, 325, 326, 330, 331
Design assignment, 74, 75, 78–79, 84–85, 92, 93, 102, 177, 241

C.-F. Mandenius, *Bioengineering Design Methodology*,
https://doi.org/10.1007/978-3-032-33940-9

Design case, 1, 23, 35, 36, 52, 54, 59, 62, 71, 73, 74, 76, 86, 87, 92, 95, 101–105, 167, 177, 312
Design engineering, 16, 24, 94, 194, 208
Design methodology, 5, 7, 9, 13, 14, 25, 35–36, 39, 73, 81, 101, 102, 104, 141
Design mission, 2, 20, 37, 38, 40–44, 47, 56, 73, 78, 81, 91, 102, 103, 110, 111, 180
Design of experiments (DoE), 7, 9, 26, 56–58, 60, 61, 63, 64, 78, 91, 109, 125, 137, 152, 154, 159, 177, 178, 187, 203–206, 212, 228–230, 233, 234, 239, 250, 252, 253, 260, 265, 276–278, 282, 284, 289, 297, 300, 306, 311, 326, 327
Design team, 7–9, 31, 76–78, 89, 102, 204, 264, 288, 311
Design training, 1–9, 71–99, 101–102, 108, 137, 187, 234, 264, 288, 311
Diabetes, 293, 305
Diagnostic antibody, 264
Dialyzer, 310, 318, 329
Digital tools, 35, 37, 54, 63, 64, 66, 67, 196, 221
Divergence, 17
Drug evaluation/drug testing, 103–105, 163, 167, 168, 209

E

Economic evaluation, 38, 53, 54, 62, 64, 85, 88–91, 93, 94, 98, 101, 118, 146–148, 173, 197, 211, 217, 225–228, 246–251, 272, 274, 290, 295, 296, 321, 331

F

Factorial design, 52, 61, 63, 125, 130, 151, 159, 177, 203, 228, 230, 250, 252, 260, 276, 297, 300, 306, 324, 326, 327
Functional food, 104
Functionality, 1, 3, 6–7, 18, 24, 25, 28, 36, 37, 41–45, 47, 48, 51, 54, 84, 98, 105, 121, 140, 143, 166, 169, 179, 182, 191, 211, 220, 222, 240, 268, 269, 290, 313, 319
Fundamental science, 13–16, 74

G

General design engineering, 18
Glucose testing, 104, 287–306
Growth hormone, 104, 105, 107, 123–129

H

Hemodialysis, 104, 105, 309–332
Hollow-fiber capillary, 310
Human growth hormone (hGH), 103, 105, 107–132
Human systems, 51, 243

I

Induced pluripotent cells (iPScs), 85, 187, 193, 196, 199, 202, 204, 210, 216, 219, 221, 223, 225, 231
Industrial experts, 75, 76, 78–81, 88, 89, 97, 98, 109, 131, 182, 212, 240
Information systems, 51, 113
Intellectual property rights (IPR), 25, 43, 50, 63, 73, 85, 87, 90, 92, 108, 109, 111, 113, 120–124, 129, 135–137, 139, 140, 146–148, 159, 164, 165, 169, 171, 173–175, 180, 186, 187, 190, 199–201, 209, 217, 226, 227, 239, 240, 242, 246, 287, 288, 290, 295, 299, 304, 306, 310, 311, 313, 316, 317, 321, 322, 324, 325, 331
Investments, 24, 40, 74, 103, 108, 136, 163, 186, 225, 239, 264, 295, 318

L

Liver tissue, 207

M

Management systems, 51, 113, 167, 193
Manufacturing costs, 9, 37, 54, 200, 235, 242, 248, 250, 288, 303, 305, 311, 331
Mathematical modeling, 9, 36
Mechanistic models, 55, 58–60, 101, 126, 153, 230, 233, 256, 282, 300, 324
Microcarrier, 144, 145, 147, 149, 152, 219, 223, 226, 231, 232, 240, 243–249, 252–258
Microfluidics, 26, 103–105, 185–212, 318, 321, 330
Microphysiological chip, 185, 186, 190, 198, 200, 203–206, 210, 211
Monoclonal antibodies (MAb), 103, 135–159, 270, 271
Myoblasts, 237, 238, 240, 243–248, 250, 252, 257, 259

N

Net income, 24, 25, 54, 89, 110, 116, 119, 131, 165, 175, 179, 188, 200, 219, 225, 226, 228, 248, 250, 259, 274, 288, 297, 302–304

O

Objectives, 1–3, 9, 13, 16, 17, 23, 28, 37, 40, 41, 47, 48, 52–54, 56, 60, 67, 73, 74, 76, 78, 79, 81, 84, 85, 91–93, 97, 98, 107–108, 110, 111, 113, 114, 116, 118, 123, 129, 130, 135–139, 141–143, 146, 152, 157, 164–166, 168, 170, 171, 176, 177, 185–186, 194, 204, 215–217, 219, 222, 225, 228, 234, 237–240, 250, 258, 259, 263–264, 266, 268–270, 272, 282, 283, 287–288, 290, 292, 293, 309–310, 312, 313, 315, 317, 318, 324
Oncogenic drug, 135, 163–165, 167, 182
Operational constraints, 18–22
Operational cost, 25, 53, 54, 59, 74, 81, 86, 89, 90, 119, 120, 130, 136, 137, 142–144, 147–149, 152, 164, 165, 173–177, 181, 198–200, 210, 217, 226–228, 233, 240, 248–250, 265, 273, 274, 289, 295–297, 299, 311, 323–325
Optimization, 1, 22, 36, 73, 118, 139, 165, 190, 222, 248, 266, 297, 318

P

Payback, 24, 25, 27, 54, 89, 90, 95, 131, 158, 164, 181, 198, 228, 229, 239, 242, 248, 249, 251, 259, 274, 296, 299, 324
Perfusion bioreactor, 144, 151, 241, 243, 245, 248
Pluripotent stem cells, 3, 22, 215–235
Point-of-care, 43
Point-of-care diagnostics, 104, 263–284
Production cost, 24, 25, 28, 37, 42, 49, 63, 81, 88, 89, 97, 107–111, 113, 116, 119, 121, 136, 140, 146, 147, 149, 152, 157, 164, 166, 167, 173, 177, 178, 188, 189, 191, 194, 197–200, 209, 210, 216, 219, 220, 226–228, 235, 241, 248, 249, 259, 264, 267, 272, 274, 276–279, 281–283, 295, 296, 299, 303, 304, 317, 321–326, 330, 331
Production economics, 13, 16, 26, 35, 36, 38, 54, 55, 57, 58, 66, 71, 73, 88–91, 102, 118–121, 146–152, 158, 175, 197–200, 211, 225–228, 264, 272, 278, 295, 304, 321, 326
Prototypes, 5, 16–18, 35, 187, 240, 277, 278, 289, 311
Purity, 20, 43, 57, 60, 85, 105, 113, 136, 144, 151, 189, 190, 205, 313, 327

Q

Quality measures, 21, 51

R

Renal replacement therapy, 309
Reporting, 9, 43, 74, 76, 80, 81, 84, 92, 93, 98, 102, 109, 137, 165, 169–171, 173, 174, 177, 181, 187, 217, 240, 265, 289, 312
Reproducibility, 20, 39, 43, 105, 168, 171, 178, 180, 267, 283, 297
Revenue, 24–26, 41, 54, 88, 89, 198, 248, 264, 309, 325
Risk assessment, 13, 51, 103, 181
Robotized testing, 173–176

S

SARS-Covid diagnostic, 104, 105, 263–284
Sensor chips, 282, 283, 297
Service company, 103, 163, 170
Societal expectations, 13, 22–23
Societal needs, 1
Specific antibody, 272
Statistical methods, 63, 71
Subcontracting/subcontractor, 27, 52, 54, 63, 85, 90, 109, 137, 139, 164, 170, 171, 173, 186–188, 195–201, 208, 209, 211, 212, 215, 239, 240, 244–246, 248, 249, 264, 265, 269–274, 281–284, 287–290, 293, 295–297, 299, 304, 306, 311–313, 317, 319, 321–327, 331
SWOT analysis, 38, 62, 63, 91–92, 129–130, 132, 180, 208, 209, 284

T

Technical systems, 20, 27, 37, 45, 51, 78, 85, 112–114, 181, 191, 193, 198, 221, 222
Teeth/Tooth tissue, 185–212
Training case, 98
Training performance, 95–99
Training scenario, 74–76, 79, 80, 92, 108–109, 137, 165, 187, 217, 239–240, 264–265, 288–289, 311–312

Training team, 76, 80, 159
Transformation, 15, 19–21, 39, 44–48, 51, 81, 84, 86, 98, 113, 114, 140, 142, 167–169, 190–192, 218, 221, 222, 243, 254, 268, 269, 290–292, 313–315
Tutor management, 74–76, 78–80, 84, 94, 97

U
Upfront costs, 25, 89, 108, 116, 186, 187, 235, 317
User needs, 37, 41, 42, 74, 84, 96, 98, 99, 102, 104, 139, 141, 219, 265, 266, 269, 270, 284, 293, 317
User requirements, 17, 18, 35, 37, 39–42, 47, 85, 86, 98, 129, 138–139, 165–168, 171, 188–191, 194, 218–221, 234, 240–241, 265, 267, 269, 282, 289, 290, 293, 312, 313

V
Validation, 17, 23, 35–38, 40, 42, 62, 63, 90, 94, 113, 120, 131, 146, 151, 217, 220, 226, 227, 273, 274, 288, 311
Ventricular progenitor cells (VPC), 215, 216, 218, 219, 226
Vocational training, 7, 94–95, 98

W
Wearable device, 319, 325, 326, 330

Z
Zebrafish model, 103–105, 163, 165, 166, 181, 182

FSC
www.fsc.org
MIX
Papier | Fördert
gute Waldnutzung
FSC® C083411

Kolibri 360 GmbH
Ferdinand-Jühlke-Straße 7
99095 Erfurt, Deutschland
produktsicherheit@kolibri360.de